Lecture Notes in Computer Science

Founding Editors

Gerhard Goos
Juris Hartmanis

Editorial Board Members

Elisa Bertino, *Purdue University, West Lafayette, IN, USA*
Wen Gao, *Peking University, Beijing, China*
Bernhard Steffen, *TU Dortmund University, Dortmund, Germany*
Moti Yung, *Columbia University, New York, NY, USA*

The series Lecture Notes in Computer Science (LNCS), including its subseries Lecture Notes in Artificial Intelligence (LNAI) and Lecture Notes in Bioinformatics (LNBI), has established itself as a medium for the publication of new developments in computer science and information technology research, teaching, and education.

LNCS enjoys close cooperation with the computer science R & D community, the series counts many renowned academics among its volume editors and paper authors, and collaborates with prestigious societies. Its mission is to serve this international community by providing an invaluable service, mainly focused on the publication of conference and workshop proceedings and postproceedings. LNCS commenced publication in 1973.

Ujjwal Baid · Reuben Dorent · Sylwia Malec ·
Monika Pytlarz · Ruisheng Su ·
Navodini Wijethilake · Spyridon Bakas ·
Alessandro Crimi
Editors

Brain Tumor Segmentation, and Cross-Modality Domain Adaptation for Medical Image Segmentation

MICCAI Challenges, BraTS 2023 and CrossMoDA 2023
Held in Conjunction with MICCAI 2023
Vancouver, BC, Canada, October 12 and 8, 2024
Proceedings

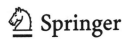

Editors
Ujjwal Baid
Indiana University School of Medicine
Indianapolis, IN, USA

Sylwia Malec
Indiana University School of Medicine
Indianapolis, IN, USA

Ruisheng Su
Eindhoven University of Technology
Eindhoven, The Netherlands

Spyridon Bakas
Indiana University School of Medicine
Indianapolis, IN, USA

Reuben Dorent
Harvard Medical School
Boston, MA, USA

Monika Pytlarz
Sano – Centre for Computational
Personalised Medicine International Research
Foundation
Kraków, Poland

Navodini Wijethilake
King's College London
London, UK

Alessandro Crimi
Sano – Centre for Computational
Personalised Medicine International Research
Foundation
Kraków, Poland

ISSN 0302-9743　　　　　　ISSN 1611-3349 (electronic)
Lecture Notes in Computer Science
ISBN 978-3-031-76162-1　　ISBN 978-3-031-76163-8 (eBook)
https://doi.org/10.1007/978-3-031-76163-8

© The Editor(s) (if applicable) and The Author(s), under exclusive license
to Springer Nature Switzerland AG 2024

This work is subject to copyright. All rights are solely and exclusively licensed by the Publisher, whether the whole or part of the material is concerned, specifically the rights of translation, reprinting, reuse of illustrations, recitation, broadcasting, reproduction on microfilms or in any other physical way, and transmission or information storage and retrieval, electronic adaptation, computer software, or by similar or dissimilar methodology now known or hereafter developed.
The use of general descriptive names, registered names, trademarks, service marks, etc. in this publication does not imply, even in the absence of a specific statement, that such names are exempt from the relevant protective laws and regulations and therefore free for general use.
The publisher, the authors and the editors are safe to assume that the advice and information in this book are believed to be true and accurate at the date of publication. Neither the publisher nor the authors or the editors give a warranty, expressed or implied, with respect to the material contained herein or for any errors or omissions that may have been made. The publisher remains neutral with regard to jurisdictional claims in published maps and institutional affiliations.

This Springer imprint is published by the registered company Springer Nature Switzerland AG
The registered company address is: Gewerbestrasse 11, 6330 Cham, Switzerland

Preface

This volume contains articles from the Brain Tumor Segmentation (BraTS 2023) Challenge, and the Cross-Modality Domain Adaptation (CrossMoDA 2023) Challenge. Both these events were held in conjunction with the Medical Image Computing and Computer Assisted Intervention (MICCAI) conference on the 8th–12th of October 2023 in Vancouver, Canada.

The presented manuscripts describe the research of computational scientists and clinical researchers working on brain lesions, and specifically glioma, multiple sclerosis, cerebral stroke, traumatic brain injuries, vestibular schwannoma, and white matter hyperintensities of presumed vascular origin. This compilation does not claim to provide a comprehensive understanding from all points of view; however, the authors present their latest advances in segmentation, disease prognosis, stroke diagnosis and treatment, and other applications to the clinical context.

The volume is divided into two chapters: The first chapter comprises the accepted paper submissions to the BraTS challenge, and the second chapter covers the CrossMoDA challenge.

The **first chapter** focuses on a selection of papers from the **BraTS 2023** challenge participants. The focus of BraTS 2023 was to identify the current state-of-the-art algorithms for addressing (Task 1) the same adult glioma population as in the RSNA-ASNR-MICCAI BraTS 2021 challenge, as well as (Task 2) the underserved sub-Saharan African brain glioma patient population, (Task 3) patients diagnosed with intracranial meningioma, (Task 4) brain metastasis, (Task 5) as well as pediatric brain tumor patients. Beyond these tumor entities explicit focus was given to address the challenge of (Task 6) global & (Task 7) local missing data. All challenge data were routine clinically acquired, multi-institutional skull-stripped multi-parametric magnetic resonance imaging (mpMRI) scans of brain tumor patients (provided in NIfTI file format).

The **second chapter** contains a selection of papers from the **CrossMoDA 2023** challenge participants. CrossMoDA 2023 was the third edition of the first large and multi-class benchmark for unsupervised cross-modality domain adaptation for medical imagesegmentation. The CrossMoDA challenge, which was held as part of the 9th Brain Lesion workshop (BrainLes 2023), aimed to identify the best-performing methods to build segmentation algorithms that generalize from one image context (contrast-enhanced T1 MR) to another (heterogeneous T2 MR). The segmentation task focuses on key brain structures involved in the follow-up and treatment planning of vestibular schwannoma: the tumor and the cochleas. The 2023 edition extended the segmentation task by including multi-institutional, heterogeneous data acquired for routine surveillance purposes and introduced a sub-segmentation for the tumor (intra- and extra-meatal components), leading to a 3-class problem.

We heartily hope that this volume will promote further exciting computational research on brain-related pathologies.

The organizers,

Ujjwal Baid
Spyridon Bakas
Alessandro Crimi
Reuben Dorent
Sylwia Malec
Monika Pytlarz
Ruisheng Su
Navodini Wijethilake

Organization

Main BrainLes Organizing Committee

Ujjwal Baid	Indiana University, USA
Spyridon Bakas	Indiana University, USA
Alessandro Crimi	Sano Centre for Computational Medicine, Poland
Sylwia Malec	Sano Centre for Computational Medicine, Poland
Monika Pytlarz	Sano Centre for Computational Medicine, Poland

Challenges Organizing Committees

Brain Tumor Segmentation (BraTS) Challenge

Mariam Aboian	Yale University, USA
Sanyukta Adap	Indiana University, USA
Maruf Adewole	Crestview Radiology Ltd., Nigeria
Jake Albrecht	Sage Bionetworks, USA
Udunna Anazodo	Montreal Neurological Institute, McGill University, Canada
Ujjwal Baid	Indiana University, USA
Spyridon Bakas (Lead Organizer)	Indiana University, USA
Hongwei Bran Li	University of Zurich, Switzerland, and Technical University of Munich, Germany
Evan Calabrese	University of California San Francisco, USA
Verena Chung	Sage Bionetworks, USA
Keyvan Farahani	National Institutes of Health, USA
Anahita Fathi Kazerooni	Children's Hospital of Philadelphia, USA
Anastasia Janas	Yale University, USA
Florian Kofler	Helmholtz AI, Germany
Dominic Labella	Duke University Medical Center, USA
Marius George Linguraru	Children's National Hospital, USA
Bjoern Menze	University of Zurich, Switzerland
Ahmed Moawad	Mercy Catholic Medical Center, USA
Jeffrey Rudie	University of California San Francisco, USA
Russell Taki Shinohara	University of Pennsylvania, USA

Cross-Modality Domain Adaptation (CrossMoDA) Challenge

Spyridon Bakas	Indiana University, USA
Stefan Cornelissen	Elisabeth-TweeSteden Hospital, The Netherlands
Reuben Dorent (Lead Organizer)	Harvard University, USA
Marina Ivory	King's College London, UK
Samuel Joutard	King's College London, UK
Aaron Kujawa	King's College London, UK
Patrick Langenhuizen	Elisabeth-TweeSteden Hospital, The Netherlands
Nicola Rieke	NVIDIA, Germany
Jonathan Shapey	King's College London, UK
Tom Vercauteren	King's College London, UK
Navodini Wijethilake	King's College London, UK

Contents

BraTS

Unleash the Power of 2D Pre-trained Model for 3D T1-weighted Brain MRI Inpainting 3
  Jiayu Huo, Yang Liu, Alejandro Granados, Sébastien Ourselin, and Rachel Sparks

The AGU-Net Architecture for Brain Tumor Segmentation: BraTS Challenges 2023 11
  David Bouget, André Pedersen, Ole Solheim, and Ingerid Reinertsen

Ensemble Learning and 3D Pix2Pix for Comprehensive Brain Tumor Analysis in Multimodal MRI 24
  Ramy A. Zeineldin and Franziska Mathis-Ullrich

Denoising Diffusion Models for Inpainting of Healthy Brain Tissue 35
  Alicia Durrer, Philippe C. Cattin, and Julia Wolleb

Brain Tumor Segmentation Based on Self-supervised Pre-training and Adaptive Region-Specific Loss 46
  Yubo Zhou, Lanfeng Zhong, and Guotai Wang

BraSyn 2023 Challenge: Missing MRI Synthesis and the Effect of Different Learning Objectives 58
  Ivo M. Baltruschat, Parvaneh Janbakhshi, and Matthias Lenga

Previous Datasets Performance for Brain Tumor Segmentation of BraTS 2023 Current Dataset 69
  Agus Subhan Akbar, Ahmad Hayam Brilian, Chastine Fatichah, and Nanik Suciati

Enhanced Data Augmentation Using Synthetic Data for Brain Tumour Segmentation 79
  André Ferreira, Naida Solak, Jianning Li, Philipp Dammann, Jens Kleesiek, Victor Alves, and Jan Egger

Attention-Enhanced Hybrid Feature Aggregation Network for 3D Brain Tumor Segmentation 94
  Ziya Ata Yazıcı, İlkay Öksüz, and Hazım Kemal Ekenel

3D ST-Net: A Large Kernel Simple Transformer for Brain Tumor
Segmentation 106
  Jiahao Zheng and Liqin Huang

Multimodal Brain Tumor Segmentation Using Modified 3D UNet3+
Architecture 117
  Xiao Yang and Shaohua Zheng

Enhancing Encoder with Attention Gate for Multimodal Brain Tumor
Segmentation 128
  Yi Li, Zhirui Fang, Di Li, Xin Xie, and Yanqing Guo

Evaluating STU-Net for Brain Tumor Segmentation 140
  Ziyan Huang, Jin Ye, Haoyu Wang, Zhongying Deng, Yanzhou Su,
  Tianbin Li, Junlong Cheng, Jianpin Chen, Sizheng Guo, Yiqing Shen,
  and Junjun He

Automated 3D Tumor Segmentation Using Temporal Cubic PatchGAN
(TCuP-GAN) 152
  Kameswara Bharadwaj Mantha, Ramanakumar Sankar,
  and Lucy Fortson

An Optimization Framework for Processing and Transfer Learning
for the Brain Tumor Segmentation 165
  Tianyi Ren, Ethan Honey, Harshitha Rebala, Abhishek Sharma,
  Agamdeep Chopra, and Mehmet Kurt

All Sizes Matter: Improving Volumetric Brain Segmentation on Small
Lesions 177
  Ayhan Can Erdur, Daniel Scholz, Josef A. Buchner,
  Stephanie E. Combs, Daniel Rueckert, and Jan C. Peeken

3D-TransUNet for Brain Metastases Segmentation in the BraTS2023
Challenge 190
  Siwei Yang, Xianhang Li, Jieru Mei, Jieneng Chen, Cihang Xie,
  and Yuyin Zhou

Towards SAMBA: Segment Anything Model for Brain Tumor
Segmentation in Sub-Saharan African Populations 200
  Mohannad Barakat, Noha Magdy, Jjuuko George William, Ethel Phiri,
  Raymond Confidence, Dong Zhang, and Udunna C. Anazodo

Automated Ensemble Method for Pediatric Brain Tumor Segmentation 211
  Shashidhar Reddy Javaji, Advait Gosai, Sovesh Mohapatra,
  and Gottfried Schlaug

Model Ensemble for Brain Tumor Segmentation in Magnetic Resonance
Imaging 221
    Daniel Capellán-Martín, Zhifan Jiang, Abhijeet Parida, Xinyang Liu,
    Van Lam, Hareem Nisar, Austin Tapp, Sarah Elsharkawi,
    María J. Ledesma-Carbayo, Syed Muhammad Anwar,
    and Marius George Linguraru

Synthesis of Healthy Tissue Within Tumor Area via U-Net 233
    Juexin Zhang, Ke Chen, and Ying Weng

Bridging the Gap: Generalising State-of-the-Art U-Net Models
to Sub-Saharan African Populations 241
    Alyssa R. Amod, Alexandra Smith, Pearly Joubert,
    Confidence Raymond, Dong Zhang, Udunna C. Anazodo,
    Dodzi Motchon, Tinashe E. M. Mutsvangwa, and Sébastien Quetin

nnUNet for Brain Tumor Segmentation in Sub-Saharan Africa Patient
Population 255
    Valeriia Abramova, Uma M. Lal-Trehan Estrada, Cansu Yalçın,
    Rachika E. Hamadache, Albert Clèrigues, Francisco Aarón Tovar Sáez,
    Marc Guirao, Joaquim Salvi, Arnau Oliver, and Xavier Lladó

Advanced Tumor Segmentation in Medical Imaging: An Ensemble
Approach for BraTS 2023 Adult Glioma and Pediatric Tumor Tasks 264
    Fadillah Maani, Anees Ur Rehman Hashmi, Mariam Aljuboory,
    Numan Saeed, Ikboljon Sobirov, and Mohammad Yaqub

Multiscale Encoder and Omni-Dimensional Dynamic Convolution
Enrichment in nnU-Net for Brain Tumor Segmentation 278
    Sahaj K. Mistry, Aayush Gupta, Sourav Saini, Aashray Gupta,
    Sunny Rai, Vinit Jakhetiya, Ujjwal Baid, and Sharath Chandra Guntuku

MenUnet: An End-to-End 3D Neural Network for Meningioma
Segmentation from Multiparametric MRI 291
    Hui Lin, Xi Cheng, and Ziru Chen

Exploring Compound Loss Functions for Brain Tumor Segmentation 300
    Anita Kriz, Raghav Mehta, Brennan Nichyporuk, and Tal Arbel

Local Synthesis of Healthy Brain Tissue Using an Enhanced 3D Pix2Pix
Model for Medical Image Inpainting 312
    M. S. Sadique, M. M. Rahman, W. Farzana, A. Glandon, A. Temtam,
    and K. M. Iftekharuddin

Brain Tumor Segmentation: Glioma Segmentation in Sub-Saharan Africa
Patients Using nnU-Net 322
   M. S. Sadique, M. M. Rahman, W. Farzana, A. Glandon, A. Temtam,
   and K. M. Iftekharuddin

Pediatric Brain Tumor Segmentation Using Multiresolution Fractal Deep
Neural Network 332
   A. Temtam, M. S. Sadique, M. M. Rahman, W. Farzana,
   and K. M. Iftekharuddin

BPML, MLops and 3D-UNet Network Integration in End-to-End
Application Design Applied to the Segmentation of Human Brain Tumors
in Clinic Cases 341
   José Armando Hernández

CrossMoDA

An Efficient Cross-Modal Segmentation Method for Vestibular
Schwannoma and Cochlea on MRI Images 355
   Cancan Chen, Dawei Wang, and Rongguo Zhang

Fine-Grained Unsupervised Cross-Modality Domain Adaptation
for Vestibular Schwannoma Segmentation 364
   Luyi Han, Tao Tan, and Ritse Mann

Learning Site-Specific Styles for Multi-institutional Unsupervised
Cross-Modality Domain Adaptation 372
   Han Liu, Yubo Fan, Zhoubing Xu, Benoit M. Dawant, and Ipek Oguz

MS-MT++: Enhanced Multi-scale Mean Teacher for Cross-Modality
Vestibular Schwannoma and Cochlea Segmentation 386
   Ziyuan Zhao, Ruikai Lin, Kaixin Xu, Xulei Yang, and Cuntai Guan

Author Index 395

BraTS

Unleash the Power of 2D Pre-trained Model for 3D T1-weighted Brain MRI Inpainting

Jiayu Huo[✉], Yang Liu, Alejandro Granados, Sébastien Ourselin, and Rachel Sparks

School of Biomedical Engineering and Imaging Sciences (BMEIS),
King's College London, London, UK
jiayu.huo@kcl.ac.uk

Abstract. The performance of current brain image analysis pipelines can dramatically degrade when handling images with pathologies (*e.g.*, tumors). To address this issue, one solution is using image inpainting to generate synthetic healthy tissues within regions of abnormality. In recent years, image inpainting algorithms have achieved significant improvements due to the rapid development of Convolutional Neural Networks (CNNs). However, brain image inpainting task remains an open challenge because of the insufficient training data and the diversity of brain abnormalities. In this paper, we try to leverage a 2D inpainting model pre-trained on a large dataset of natural images for the 3D brain inpainting task. We effectively fine-tune the 2D inpainting model using brain MRI slices from different views and fuse slice-level predictions to form a volume-level inpainted image. A post-processing strategy is proposed based on the morphological closing operation to refine fused results. Experiments show that the 2D pre-trained inpainting model has a strong generalization ability even without fine-tuning and performance can be further improved with fine-tuning and post-processing applied to the full volume.

Keywords: Brain inpainting · Transfer learning · Fast Fourier convolution

1 Introduction

Image inpainting is a potentially transformative technique in the field of computer vision and image processing to address the task of restoring missing or corrupted portions of an image in a visually coherent manner. This process involves predicting and generating plausible content for the missing regions and then seamlessly blending the generated content into the surrounding original image content. In the context of medical imaging, particularly the domain of neuroradiology, image inpainting could have a pivotal role in enhancing our understanding and analysis of brain images afflicted with tumors. These tumors, while critical to diagnose and treat, can obscure significant portions of the brain, making it challenging for medical professionals to obtain a complete and accurate representation of the patient's brain anatomy. By employing image inpainting methods, it becomes possible to fill in the tumor areas with healthy brain tissue, facilitating a comprehensive assessment of the cerebral structures and aiding in more precise diagnosis and treatment planning. This fusion of image inpainting with medical imaging holds the potential to revolutionize how clinicians interpret brain images, leading to more informed decisions and improving patient care.

To this end, methods for brain MRI inpainting have been presented in the literature. For instance, Manjon et al. [9] designed a U-shaped model for brain lesion inpainting. This model takes T1 brain images with a random region removed as input and uses the original image as the ground truth. Such a design can lead to over-fitting when the dataset is small. Additionally, a masked image can have multiple plausible inpainted solutions, thus directly learning the mapping between the masked image and the ground truth will make the generated contents less diverse. Kang et al. [3] developed a dense convolutional model for brain inpainting using small image patches as input. A patch-based model performs poorly on the full-size brain image and using sliding window inference can lead to unnatural transitions between patches. Liu et al. [7] proposed a symmetric constraint for brain inpainting, to use the contra-lateral side of the image to help guide inpainting. This method requires the midline of the brain to be aligned correctly, and may not be effective for regions of the brain with distinct differences in the hemispheres. Overall, these frameworks have limitations when applied to the full-size T1-weighted brain MRI inpainting task.

In this paper, we unleash the power of a 2D pre-trained inpainting model for the 3D T1-weighted brain MRI inpainting task. Concretely, we freeze the trainable parameters in the encoder and bottleneck and fine-tune only the parameters in the decoder with a small learning rate. Once the training process is finished, we fuse the predictions from three different views and apply the morphological closing operation for prediction refinement. Experimental results on the BraTS 2023 Inpainting Challenge dataset demonstrate that our framework can achieve plausible and realistic brain inpainting MRI.

2 Methodology

We try to predict the plausible content given a gray image x and a binary mask m (1 for the mask area and 0 for the background). Specifically, we create the input by concatenating the image to be inpainted, $x' = x \odot m$, and the mask area m, for inpainting network $f_\theta(\cdot)$. The final inpainted image $\hat{x} = f_\theta(x', m)$ output from the model should be realistic, and the boundary of the inpainted area should be seamless with the surrounding image region.

2.1 Inpainting with Fast Fourier Convolution (FFC)

Figure 1 represents our inpainting framework. Our model is based on Big LaMa [11] which contains a down-scaling, bottleneck, and up-scaling part. We use convolutions and transpose convolutions for the down-scaling part and the up-scaling part, respectively. For the bottleneck, we use the Fast Fourier Convolution (FFC) [1] to capture global semantic feature information. FFC is based on Fast Fourier Transform (FFT), thus it naturally has a receptive field that covers the entire image. For FFC, we first apply the $FFT2d$ decomposition to get the real and imaginary parts of the FFT and then we concatenate each component in the channel dimension and apply a convolution kernel on both components of the frequency domain. We reshape the components and use the inverse transform ($iFFT2d$) to remap the output to the original feature space.

For the model inputs, we randomly select slices from the axial, coronal, and sagittal views of the image. Each extracted slice is considered independent in the inpainting network to make the network robust to view variation. We add random brightness adjustments to make the inpainting model more robust to different intensity distributions in the image. After the training process is finished, we perform inference using all three view images and obtain three independent volume-level predictions for each scan. We then calculate the average value across the three predictions. Since the model is trained on the slice level, fusing three predictions on different views results in an intensity discontinuity, so as a post-processing step, we apply a morphological closing operation to reduce the image artifacts and make the appearance more plausible.

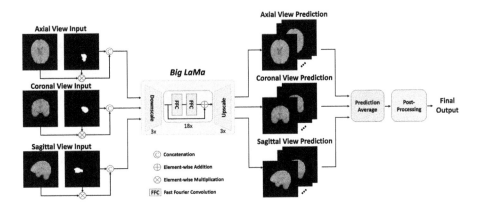

Fig. 1. Our pipeline for T1-weighted brain MRI inpainting.

2.2 Fine-Tuning Based on Pre-trained Weights

Big LaMa is trained on natural images, yet it shows strong generalization ability on the brain MRI inpainting task (see Table 1). However, the performance of this model can be further boosted since natural images only contain the image intensity pattern but do not contain the shape and structure knowledge of T1-weighted brain scans. Based on this assumption, we decided to fine-tune the pre-trained Big LaMa model weights. We only fine-tune the up-scaling part of the network because the down-scaling and the FFC residual blocks have the ability to extract general feature maps and we do not want to cause a catastrophic forgetting problem during model training [12].

2.3 Loss Functions

The inpainting problem tries to predict the plausible intensity values for a masked area of an image, which means one image may have multiple feasible inpainting predictions. To this end, we introduce a joint loss function to optimize our inpainting model. First, we utilize the L_1 loss to constrain predictions from the spatial domain. It can be formulated as:

$$\mathcal{L}_{hole} = \|x - \hat{x}\|_1 \odot m, \quad (1)$$
$$\mathcal{L}_{valid} = \|x - \hat{x}\|_1 \odot (1 - m), \quad (2)$$
$$\mathcal{L}_{rec} = \lambda_{hole}\mathcal{L}_{hole} + \lambda_{valid}\mathcal{L}_{valid}. \quad (3)$$

Here x is the ground-truth image, $\hat{x}$ is the prediction, m is a binary mask, and $\odot$ denotes the element-wise multiplication. λ_{hole} and λ_{valid} are set to 3 and 10, determined empirically, to prevent over-fitting to a specific content. Furthermore, we add the high receptive field perceptual loss $\mathcal{L}_{PL}$ formulated as:

$$\mathcal{L}_{PL} = \|\phi_{PL}(x) - \phi_{PL}(\hat{x})\|_1, \quad (4)$$

where ϕ is a pre-trained segmentation ResNet50 model with dilated convolutions. However, only using $\mathcal{L}_{rec}$ and $\mathcal{L}_{PL}$ may lead to fuzzy predictions. To sharpen the model outputs, we add an adversarial loss term formulated as:

$$\mathcal{L}_D = -\mathbb{E}_x\left[\log D(x)\right] - \mathbb{E}_{x,m}\left[\log D(\hat{x}) \odot m\right] \\ -\mathbb{E}_{x,m}\left[\log\left(1 - D(\hat{x})\right) \odot (1-m)\right], \quad (5)$$
$$\mathcal{L}_G = -\mathbb{E}_{x,m}\left[\log D(\hat{x})\right], \quad (6)$$
$$\mathcal{L}_{r1} = \mathbb{E}_x\|\nabla_x D(x)\|^2, \quad (7)$$
$$\mathcal{L}_{adv} = \mathcal{L}_D + \mathcal{L}_G + 0.001\mathcal{L}_{r1}. \quad (8)$$

Here, the discriminator D forces the generator (a.k.a. the inpainting network) to give realistic predictions that are similar to the real T1 images according to $\mathcal{L}_D$. Also, we add $\mathcal{L}_{r1}$ to penalize large gradients to make the training process more stable. Additionally, we add a feature match loss term $\mathcal{L}_{fm}$ (L_1 loss computed between discriminator features of true and fake images) to stabilize training and slightly boost model performance.

Overall, the final loss function for model training is defined as:

$$\mathcal{L}_{total} = \lambda_{rec}\mathcal{L}_{rec} + \lambda_{PL}\mathcal{L}_{PL} + \lambda_{fm}\mathcal{L}_{fm} + \lambda_{adv}\mathcal{L}_{adv}, \quad (9)$$

where $\lambda_{rec} = 1$, $\lambda_{PL} = 100$, $\lambda_{fm} = 30$, and $\lambda_{adv} = 10$.

3 Experiments

3.1 Experiment Settings

Dataset. We use the BraTS 2023 Inpainting Challenge dataset [5] to evaluate the performance of our inpainting model. This dataset was developed based on T1 scans from the multi-modal BraTS 2022 segmentation challenge, which contains 1251 brain MRIs. All images were registered to the SRI24 template [10] and resampled to a uniform isotropic resolution ($1mm^3$). Two types of masks (unhealthy and healthy masks) were provided. The unhealthy mask is the ensemble of tumor core, enhanced tumor, and edema area, and the healthy mask is generated through a standard pipeline (refer to [5] for more details). We randomly select 150 cases as the local validation set, and let the remaining (1101 cases) be the training set. For each training case, we extract slices from three views. Then all slices are padded and resized to 256×256. The inpainting mask is generated on the fly but does not overlap with the unhealthy part. For each validation case, we utilize the healthy mask for the performance evaluation. The final results are evaluated through the MedPerf platform [4].

Implementation Details. The network structure stays the same with Big LaMa [11], which contains 3 downsampling blocks, 18 residual blocks, and 3 upsampling blocks. We use AdamW optimizer [8] and set the initial learning rates to 1e-5 for inpainting and discriminator networks. The model is fine-tuned for 20 epochs with a batch size of 8 on a Nvidia Quadro RTX 5000 (16GB) GPU. Three metrics are utilized to evaluate the inpainting performance, *i.e.*, mean square error (MSE), peak signal-to-noise ratio (PSNR), and structural similarity index (SSIM). For each metric, the mean value and the standard deviation are both reported.

3.2 Experimental Results

Quantitative Validation Results. We quantitatively compare the image inpainting results with Big LaMa, one of the SOTA image inpainting model, results are shown in Table 1. Notably, the training set of Big LaMa does not contain any brain MRI data, but it shows great generalization ability on the BraTS 2023 Inpainting Challenge dataset. This is because the large inpainting model trained on millions of natural images has already learned to complete intrinsic image patterns, therefore the fake inpainted content predicted by Big LaMa seems to be reasonable. However, if we use the challenge data to fine-tune the decoder part of Big LaMa, we can find remarkable improvement in all three metrics. We believe the fine-tuning process teaches the model some shape and structure information about the brain so that the model can do better on the validation set. In addition, we can obtain the best performance when we use the morphological closing operation to refine the fused prediction. The morphological closing operation helps eliminate some subtle artifacts (*e.g.*, black stripes caused by inter-slice inconsistency) so that the evaluation metrics could be higher compared to the fine-tuning results.

Table 1. Quantitative results on the BraTS 2023 Inpainting Challenge validation set. The best results are highlighted in bold. The results of Auto-Encoder, Pix2Pix [2] and PConv [6] do not show in this table since we do not submit the predictions for evaluation. Ours-pp means we add the post-processing to the fused prediction. The standard deviation is computed over the samples.

Method	MSE↓	PSNR↑	SSIM↑
Big LaMa [11]	0.0081 ± 0.0052	21.96 ± 3.37	0.7934 ± 0.1245
Ours	0.0079 ± 0.0052	22.14 ± 3.56	0.7950 ± 0.1241
Ours-pp	**0.0077 ± 0.0049**	**22.18 ± 3.50**	**0.7956 ± 0.1243**

Quantitative Test Results. Table 2 presents the quantitative performance of our model evaluated on the hidden test set. The hidden test set contains 568 T1-weighted images. The mask generation pipeline is described in [5]. As shown in Table 2, different samples exhibit large performance disparities. For example, the best MAE is 0.0002 while the worst is 0.5455. This might be caused by different mask sizes and tissue varieties.

Table 2. Quantitative results on the BraTS 2023 Inpainting Challenge hidden test set. The hidden test set contains 568 T1-weighted images. The standard deviation is computed over the samples

	MSE↓	PSNR↑	SSIM↑
Best	0.0002	36.91	0.9992
75th Percentile	0.0080	20.68	0.9357
Median	0.0134	18.39	0.8645
25th Percentile	0.0203	16.34	0.7552
Worst	0.5455	2.63	0.1981
Average	0.0173 ± 0.0258	18.79 ± 3.82	0.8342 ± 0.1267

Inpainting Results Visualization. We also visualize the outputs of different models in Fig. 2. Here we show the inpainting results of three views from two subjects. Voided T1 images contain both healthy and unhealthy mask areas with zero value. The AE and Pix2Pix models were realized by the organizer, it can be found that the inpainted content of these two models is over-smoothing and lacks realistic textures. Also, the boundary of the inpainted area is quite abrupt. Besides, we re-implement a 3D version of the partial convolution inpainting network [6]. The texture information of results generated by PConv is more abundant and diverse compared to the previous two models. However, some weirdly highlighted areas within the generated result make it not realistic. The last two columns are our results. Our proposed model can give seamless transitions from the background area to the inpainted area, which means our model can capture the global appearance information over the whole image and predict reasonable contents with the same style. In addition, the texture of the generated images is more realistic compared to other results. By applying the post-processing strategy, the stripe artifacts are alleviated.

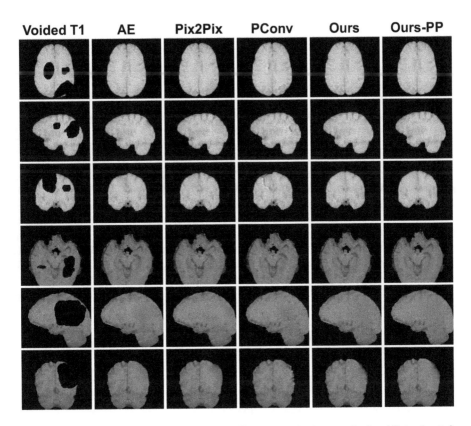

Fig. 2. Qualitative comparison between different inpainting methods. AE is short for auto-encoder, PConv stands for partial convolution [6]

4 Conclusion and Discussion

In this paper, we apply the 2D inpainting model for the 3D brain inpainting task. It is surprising to find that the publicly available 2D pre-trained weights can achieve relatively good performance on brain MRI data, but some results still look weird which may be caused by a lack of prior knowledge of the brain structure. By only fine-tuning the decoder part of the model with a small learning rate, we achieve better results compared to the pre-trained model. Moreover, the post-processing strategy based on the morphological closing operation can further improve the model performance. However, the inter-slice consistency cannot be guaranteed since we train the model in a 2D manner, and no supervision on inter-slice consistency is introduced during the model training. In the future, we aim to refine current predictions, and some strategies on video inpainting and video generation may be applied.

References

1. Chi, L., Jiang, B., Mu, Y.: Fast Fourier convolution. Adv. Neural. Inf. Process. Syst. **33**, 4479–4488 (2020)
2. Isola, P., Zhu, J.Y., Zhou, T., Efros, A.A.: Image-to-image translation with conditional adversarial networks. In: Proceedings of the IEEE Conference on Computer Vision and Pattern Recognition, pp. 1125–1134 (2017)
3. Kang, S.K., et al.: Deep learning-based 3D inpainting of brain MR images. Sci. Rep. **11**(1), 1673 (2021)
4. Karargyris, A., et al.: Federated benchmarking of medical artificial intelligence with MedPerf. Nat. Mach. Intell. **5**(7), 799–810 (2023)
5. Kofler, F., et al.: The brain tumor segmentation (brats) challenge 2023: local synthesis of healthy brain tissue via inpainting. arXiv preprint arXiv:2305.08992 (2023)
6. Liu, G., Reda, F.A., Shih, K.J., Wang, T.-C., Tao, A., Catanzaro, B.: Image inpainting for irregular holes using partial convolutions. In: Ferrari, V., Hebert, M., Sminchisescu, C., Weiss, Y. (eds.) ECCV 2018. LNCS, vol. 11215, pp. 89–105. Springer, Cham (2018). https://doi.org/10.1007/978-3-030-01252-6_6
7. Liu, X., Xing, F., Yang, C., Kuo, C.-C.J., El Fakhri, G., Woo, J.: Symmetric-constrained irregular structure inpainting for brain MRI registration with tumor pathology. In: Crimi, A., Bakas, S. (eds.) BrainLes 2020. LNCS, vol. 12658, pp. 80–91. Springer, Cham (2021). https://doi.org/10.1007/978-3-030-72084-1_8
8. Loshchilov, I., Hutter, F.: Decoupled weight decay regularization. arXiv preprint arXiv:1711.05101 (2017)
9. Manjón, J.V., et al.: Blind MRI brain lesion inpainting using deep learning. In: Burgos, N., Svoboda, D., Wolterink, J.M., Zhao, C. (eds.) SASHIMI 2020. LNCS, vol. 12417, pp. 41–49. Springer, Cham (2020). https://doi.org/10.1007/978-3-030-59520-3_5
10. Rohlfing, T., Zahr, N.M., Sullivan, E.V., Pfefferbaum, A.: The SRI24 multichannel atlas of normal adult human brain structure. Hum. Brain Mapp. **31**(5), 798–819 (2010)
11. Suvorov, R., et al.: Resolution-robust large mask inpainting with Fourier convolutions. In: Proceedings of the IEEE/CVF Winter Conference on Applications of Computer Vision, pp. 2149–2159 (2022)
12. Zhao, Y., Zhang, Y., Sun, Z.: Unsupervised transfer learning for generative image inpainting with adversarial edge learning. In: Proceedings of the 2022 5th International Conference on Sensors, Signal and Image Processing, pp. 17–22 (2022)

The AGU-Net Architecture for Brain Tumor Segmentation: BraTS Challenges 2023

David Bouget[1(✉)], André Pedersen[1], Ole Solheim[3,4], and Ingerid Reinertsen[1,2]

[1] Department of Health Research, SINTEF Digital, 7465 Trondheim, Norway
{david.bouget,andre.pedersen,ingerid.reinertsen}@sintef.no
[2] Department of Circulation and Medical Imaging, Norwegian University of Science and Technology (NTNU), 7491 Trondheim, Norway
[3] Department of Neurosurgery, Trondheim University Hospital, St. Olavs hospital, 7491 Trondheim, Norway
[4] Department of Neuromedicine and Movement Science, Norwegian University of Science and Technology (NTNU), 7491 Trondheim, Norway
ole.solheim@ntnu.no

Abstract. For patients suffering from brain tumors, prognosis estimation and treatment decisions are made by a multidisciplinary team of medical doctors based on a set of MR scans. Currently, the lack of automatic, standardized, and robust methods for tumor characterization represents a major hurdle for use in clinical practice. This paper describes our contribution to the BraTS 2023 Continuous Evaluation challenge for the segmentation of all tumor types, using our single-stage AGU-Net architecture and various training strategies. Performance over the training sets were reported using our custom pixel-wise, patient-wise, and lesion-wise metrics. For the tumor core, an average lesion-wise Dice score of 85% was obtained over the glioma challenges, 80% for the meningioma challenge, and 73% for the metastasis challenge. Performance reported over the validation and test sets were officially computed by the challenge team. Over the test sets, an average lesion-wise Dice score of 75% to 80% was achieved for the tumor core over the glioma and meningioma challenges, while a lower score of 43% was reached for the metastasis challenge. The proposed method performed well and showed an ability to generalize on challenges with sufficient data.

Keywords: Glioma · Meningioma · Metastasis · MRI · Deep learning · Segmentation

1 Introduction

All possible tumors originating from the brain or spinal cord are collectively assembled under the central nervous system (CNS) tumors nomenclature. From iterative editions of the World Health Organization [23], CNS tumors have been further classified into more than 100 subtypes. The heterogeneity in a tumor expression (e.g., location, size, invasiveness, or growth rate) leads to varying survival expectancy ranging from weeks to several decades depending on the tumor type and grade. Many patients experience neurological and cognitive deficits over time [10]. The vast majority of CNS tumors are primary tumors, emanating from the brain itself or its supporting tissues. Conversely, cancer can originate elsewhere in the body and find its way to the brain in form of metastases, which are considered secondary tumors. For primary tumors, the glioma subtype represents those arising from the brain's glial tissue while the meningioma subtype covers those emanating from the meninges. A further categorization of gliomas can be made whereby the most aggressive ones are entitled glioblastomas, whereas the less aggressive entities are labelled diffuse lower-grade gliomas. Glioblastomas remain among the most difficult cancers to treat with an extremely short overall survival [19]. Upon initial tumor discovery, treatment decisions and preoperative prognosis assessment are made from the analysis of a set of magnetic resonance (MR) scans. The multidisciplinary team of surgeons, radiologists, and oncologists must uphold the utmost accuracy during the diagnostics phase in order to optimize patient outcome. The radicality of surgery and the risks of postoperative complications hinge on the tumor characteristics gleaned from the MR scans (e.g., volume, location, or cortical profile) [16]. While reliable and standardized measurements of tumor characteristics are instrumental in patient care, the current lack of automatic and robust methods represents a major hurdle. In clinical practice, manual tumor delineation or assessment by radiologists is time-consuming and subject to intra- and inter-rater variability [4].

The task of automatic brain tumor segmentation from preoperative MR scans is an active research topic [13,31,32]. Generic segmentation models, not considering the different CNS tumor types, have been investigated with concurrent tasks such as classification or survival estimation [26,29,30]. A large majority of studies related to brain tumor segmentation have focused on the glioma subtype, leveraging the public dataset from the BraTS challenges [24]. The current state-of-the-art baseline is the nnU-Net framework [14], a typical encoder-decoder architecture, coupled to a smart parameters optimization scheme for preprocessing and training catering to any input dataset. Overall, average Dice scores about 90% have been reached over combinations of contrast-enhancing tumor, necrosis, and edema regions [33]. The task of meningioma segmentation has been considerably less studied over the last decade [27], probably due to the lack of open-access annotated datasets. Using well-know neural network architectures, such as DeepLabV3 [9] or DeepMedic [15], Dice scores around 80% were reached over limited patient cohorts of up to 200 patients [20,21]. Using the AGU-Net architecture [6], cross-validation studies over a dataset of up to 600 patients reported an average Dice score of 88% for the tumor core segmentation over contrast-enhanced T1-weighted MRI volumes [6]. Finally, the body of work regarding brain metastasis segmentation is equally scarce. Grovik et al. used a multicentric and multi-sequence dataset of 165 metastatic patients to train a segmentation model with the DeepLabV3 architecture [11,12]. Other prior studies, using contrast-enhanced T1-weighted MRI volumes as input, obtained average

Table 1. Overview of the different BraTS challenge training datasets. ET stands for the Gd-enhancing tumor, NCR stands for the necrotic tumor core, and ED stands for the peritumoral edematous/invaded tissue.

Challenge	Nb patients	Class volume (ml)			Nb patients per class combination					
		ET	NCR	ED	ET-NCR-ED	ET-ED	ET-NCR	NCR-ED	ED	ET
Glioma	1251	21.44 ± 18.05	14.30 ± 20.64	60.21 ± 42.24	1180	37	1	27	6	0
Glioma SSA	43	31.66 ± 29.29	28.06 ± 38.58	100.7 ± 63.22	40	3	0	0	0	0
Meningioma	1000	21.35 ± 29.42	01.09 ± 05.40	20.59 ± 39.21	404	257	35	1	0	303
Metastasis	165	09.99 ± 11.70	03.01 ± 06.75	46.79 ± 55.16	110	51	0	0	0	4

Dice scores over the contrast-enhancing tumor approximating 75%, with almost 8 false positive detections per patient [8,22]. Over a dataset of 400 patients, cross-validation studies reported an average Dice of 87% using the AGU-Net architecture in a patch-wise fashion, with a patch dimension of 160^3 voxels [5].

In this study, we propose to test the AGU-Net architecture for which documented segmentation performances between 85–90% Dice scores were obtained for gliomas, meningiomas, and metastases [5,7]. The initial architecture was used over single input (i.e., contrast-enhanced T1-weighted MRI scan) and for a single class (i.e., combination of contrast-enhancing tumor and necrosis regions), which was slightly adapted for the multi-inputs and multi-classes use-case featured in the challenge.

2 Data

The datasets used in this study were made available for the BraTS challenge edition 2023, namely a glioma dataset [2,3,24], a meningioma dataset [18], a metastasis dataset [25], and a glioma dataset with Sub-Sahara-Africa patients [1] denoted glioma SSA. For all patients, four input MR scans are available: contrast-enhanced T1-weighted (T1w-CE), T1-weighted (T1w), T2-weighted (T2), and T2 Fluid Attenuated Inversion Recovery (FLAIR). All datasets have been annotated manually, by one to four raters, following the same annotation protocol, and their annotations were approved by experienced neuro-radiologists. Annotations comprise the Gd-enhancing tumor (ET), the peritumoral edematous/invaded tissue (ED), and the necrotic tumor core (NCR). In addition, all input MR scans have undergone the following preprocessing steps: co-registration to the same anatomical template, resampling to an isotropic space of $1\,mm^3$, and skull-stripping. All preprocessed MRI scans have the following dimensions: $240 \times 240 \times 155$ voxels. An overall overview of the classes distribution for the different training datasets is reported in Table 1.

3 Methods

Architecture. All CNS tumor segmentation models have been trained with the AGU-Net architecture [6] using five levels with $\{16, 32, 128, 256, 512\}$ as filter sizes, deep supervision, multiscale input, and single attention modules. Unlike the originally published architecture leveraging downsampled full head MRI volumes, a patch-wise approach for training and inference was followed, with 160^3 voxels as patch dimension, and non-overlapping patches.

Preprocessing. Since the BraTS data already underwent some extent of preprocessing, the additionally implemented steps were limited to intensity clipping to remove the 0.05% highest values, followed by intensity normalization and scaling to $[0, 1]$.

Training Strategy. Training has been performed using mixed precision, with batch size four, the Adam optimizer with an initial learning rate of $5 \cdot 10^{-4}$, and using the focal Dice loss with a gamma of 2. In addition, a gradient accumulation of 8 steps was performed, resulting in a virtual batch size of 32 samples, using the open TensorFlow model wrapper implementation [28]. An early stopping scheme was setup to stop training after 25 consecutive epochs without validation loss improvement. Given the varying magnitude of the datasets' size across the different challenges, the number of steps per epoch has been set to 512 for the glioma and meningioma challenges, reduced to 256 for the metastasis challenge, and further limited to 64 for the glioma SSA challenge.

For the data augmentation during training, the following transforms were applied to each input sample with a probability of 50%: horizontal and vertical flipping, random rotation in the range $[-20°, 20°]$, translation up to 10% along the axial axis, zoom in the range $[0.5, 1.5]$. No test-time data augmentation was considered in this study.

Training Protocol. For the glioma segmentation task, the model has been trained from scratch. For the other three segmentation tasks (i.e., glioma SSA, meningioma, and metastasis), the models were trained by fine-tuning the best glioma segmentation model. The glioma subset contains the largest amount of patients, almost all featuring the three classes of interest. As such, leveraging weights pre-trained on such dataset should help other models to converge faster and possibly generalize better. The glioma and meningioma models were trained under a 10-fold cross-validation paradigm, while a 5-fold cross-validation was used for the metastasis and glioma SSA models given their limited dataset magnitude. In turns, one fold was used as validation set, one fold as test set, and all remaining folds constituted the training set. For the glioma segmentation task, all patients featured in the training subset were used and randomly split to populate the ten folds. Similarly for the glioma SSA and metastasis segmentation tasks, all patients featured in the training subset were used, but randomly split to populate five folds only. Finally for the meningioma, a selection was performed to exclude patients inside class combination categories with less than 50 cases (cf. Table 1), leaving a total of 964 patients for training. In addition, the remaining patients from each class combination category were randomly and evenly split to populate the ten folds.

4 Results

Experiments were carried out on multiple machines with the following specifications: Intel Xeon W-2135 CPU @3.70 GHz x 12, 64 GB of RAM, NVIDIA Tesla V100S (32 GB), and a regular hard-drive. The implementation was done in Python 3.7, TensorFlow v2.8 for training the segmentation models, and ONNX Runtime v1.12.1 for running model inference.

Pooled estimates [17] are reported for each measurement as mean and standard deviation (indicated by ±) in the tables. Results reported over the training datasets only include performances from the model trained on the first fold given time and resource constraints, and have been computed using our own metrics implementation [7]. The pixel-wise (PiW) metrics consider each pixel independently, the patient-wise metrics asses the disease screening performance, and finally the lesion-wise metrics assess the performance in identifying each components (i.e. focus) of a tumor. For the results reported over the validation datasets, performances were computed officially by the BraTS challenge team. Additional segmentation classes were virtually put together for reporting segmentation performances. As such, the tumor core (TC) consists of both the contrast-enhancing tumor and necrotic tumor core, while the whole tumor (WT) comprises the tumor core and the peritumoral edematous/invaded tissue. Lastly, some classes are not featured in all patients across all challenges, and as such the segmentation performances are furthermore reported solely for the true positive cases of the class, denoted by (TP) in the tables. Performance comparison of AGU-Net with other baselines such as nnU-Net has already been reported previously [6] and as such not included in the tables.

4.1 Challenge 1: Glioma Segmentation Performance

Segmentation performances obtained over the training dataset, for the first fold only, are reported in Table 2. The tumor core and whole tumor are consistently correctly segmented with an average Dice score of 89% and HD95 of 5 mm, without any tumor being missed. However, when looking more carefully at the enhancing tumor and necrotic tumor core classes, only 83% and 77% average Dice are reached respectively. The model has a tendency to get slightly confused between the two classes composing the tumor core. The Dice score and HD95

Table 2. Segmentation performances over the training dataset for the glioma segmentation challenge, for each class (first fold only).

Class	Pixel-wise			Patient-wise			Lesion-wise			HD95
	Dice	Recall	Precision	F1-score	Recall	Precision	Dice	Recall	Precision	
ET	83.86 ± 20.20	85.41 ± 20.41	84.90 ± 20.42	99.18	99.99	98.38	77.07 ± 24.60	91.01 ± 22.48	93.56 ± 19.61	3.23 ± 05.35
NCR	73.03 ± 29.96	74.52 ± 31.38	78.07 ± 27.31	97.07	98.30	95.86	66.63 ± 29.98	78.37 ± 30.32	83.49 ± 25.97	6.47 ± 10.74
NCR (TP)	76.97 ± 25.65	77.93 ± 27.93	82.47 ± 20.93	99.14	98.30	99.99	66.33 ± 29.07	78.60 ± 29.22	84.49 ± 24.09	6.39 ± 10.82
ED	80.24 ± 15.45	81.16 ± 17.36	82.48 ± 15.53	99.99	99.99	99.99	58.54 ± 28.50	81.44 ± 25.36	85.50 ± 22.84	5.79 ± 08.99
TC	88.23 ± 17.18	89.02 ± 19.60	90.08 ± 13.79	99.99	99.99	99.99	83.70 ± 21.29	94.49 ± 17.01	95.96 ± 15.34	4.84 ± 10.11
WT	90.51 ± 07.05	91.59 ± 10.87	90.46 ± 06.01	99.99	99.99	99.99	81.34 ± 21.51	88.84 ± 21.93	90.50 ± 20.24	5.49 ± 10.47

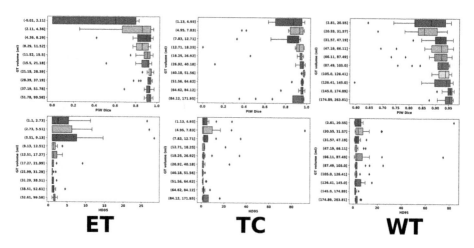

Fig. 1. Boxplots showing pixel-wise Dice (top row) and HD95 (bottom row) performances against tumor volume for the glioma type and the following classes: Gd-enhancing tumor (ET), tumor core (TC), and whole tumor (WT).

Table 3. Segmentation performances over the whole training dataset for the Sub-Sahara-Africa glioma segmentation challenge, for each class, using the best glioma segmentation model.

Class	Pixel-wise			Patient-wise			Lesion-wise			HD95
	Dice	Recall	Precision	F1-score	Recall	Precision	Dice	Recall	Precision	
ET	69.03 ± 23.08	72.64 ± 24.42	74.91 ± 24.02	98.82	97.67	99.99	59.85 ± 29.20	74.40 ± 30.48	86.43 ± 22.52	13.86 ± 21.52
NCR	53.60 ± 36.03	61.05 ± 34.12	58.35 ± 41.30	92.49	92.49	92.49	46.26 ± 34.42	72.57 ± 40.33	75.11 ± 37.34	12.33 ± 13.72
ED	73.07 ± 17.43	78.45 ± 20.94	71.48 ± 18.20	99.99	99.99	99.99	58.65 ± 26.04	86.64 ± 22.21	77.46 ± 29.62	11.52 ± 16.00
TC	69.56 ± 29.63	84.83 ± 15.57	67.69 ± 32.83	99.99	99.99	99.99	64.38 ± 32.17	85.11 ± 23.49	83.72 ± 24.50	14.19 ± 18.47
WT	87.70 ± 08.14	93.45 ± 05.65	83.72 ± 11.73	99.99	99.99	99.99	83.07 ± 15.19	91.47 ± 19.48	83.33 ± 27.31	11.49 ± 15.80

performances, relative to the tumor size, have been included in Fig. 1 using boxplots with equally populated bins. Unsurprisingly, the model performs on average better the larger a tumor is, whether considering the Dice score or HD95 distance. Some outliers are visible in almost every bin, indicating difficult cases for reasons such as different tumor contrast uptake or unusual location in the brain. Visual performances for five selected patients are reported in Fig. 2, with varying segmentation quality. While the whole tumor is generally well segmented, a larger extent of erroneous labelling between the ET, NCR, and ED classes is visible in the bottom three patients. Overall, tumor core false positives tend to appear over contrast-enhancing blood vessels either around the ventricles or at the base of the brain.

4.2 Challenge 2: Sub-Sahara-Africa Glioma Segmentation Performance

For the patients comprising the Sub-Sahara-Africa glioma dataset, the best glioma segmentation model trained from the Challenge 1 dataset was used as-is,

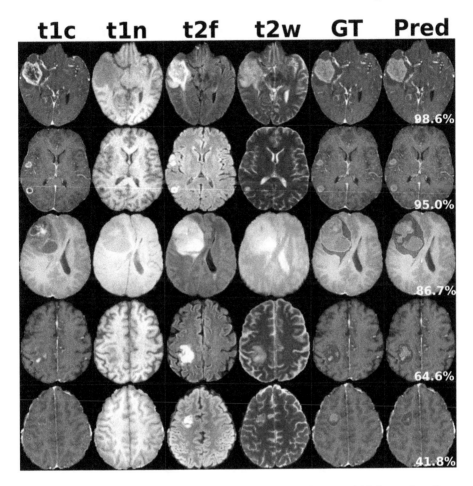

Fig. 2. Examples of segmentation performances over the test fold from the glioma challenge training dataset, one patient featured per row. The NCR, ET, and ED classes are shown in green, red, and blue respectively. The Dice score for the TC category is shown in white for each patient. (Color figure online)

Table 4. Segmentation performances over the training dataset for the Sub-Sahara-Africa glioma segmentation challenge after fine-tuning, for each class (first fold only).

Class	Pixel-wise			Patient-wise			Lesion-wise			HD95
	Dice	Recall	Precision	F1-score	Recall	Precision	Dice	Recall	Precision	
ET	84.02 ± 05.78	83.74 ± 10.23	85.78 ± 08.59	99.99	99.99	99.99	82.36 ± 07.38	96.29 ± 10.47	72.96 ± 25.01	4.75 ± 02.92
NCR	67.91 ± 34.94	72.00 ± 37.97	75.19 ± 28.95	94.11	88.88	99.99	62.63 ± 36.69	72.22 ± 41.57	88.88 ± 22.22	6.08 ± 04.51
ED	83.71 ± 15.60	84.10 ± 20.21	85.90 ± 07.26	99.99	99.99	99.99	81.25 ± 22.70	94.44 ± 15.71	85.18 ± 26.28	6.90 ± 08.89
TC	89.06 ± 05.26	89.41 ± 07.77	89.76 ± 08.80	99.99	99.99	99.99	86.61 ± 07.38	100.0 ± 00.00	79.62 ± 23.27	4.04 ± 02.76
WT	92.06 ± 03.51	93.18 ± 06.79	91.48 ± 04.74	99.99	99.99	99.99	92.39 ± 02.96	92.59 ± 20.95	91.11 ± 25.14	7.57 ± 10.08

and the performances are reported in Table 3. In addition, the best glioma segmentation was fine-tuned for the first fold of the glioma SSA dataset, and results are shown in Table 4. The major visible difference is the improved overall performances when fine-tuning an already competitive glioma segmentation model over the SSA dataset, even if the number of patients featured in the test set decreased from 43 to 9 due to the 5-fold cross-validation split. The TC average Dice went up from 70% to 89%, for a significant reduction in HD95 from 14 mm to 4 mm. After fine-tuning, segmentation performances over the SSA dataset are similar to the ones obtained over the initial glioma dataset. However, the direct use of the best glioma segmentation model over the SSA patients shows a struggle in the ability to generalize and seamlessly perform on differently acquired MR scans or a different population.

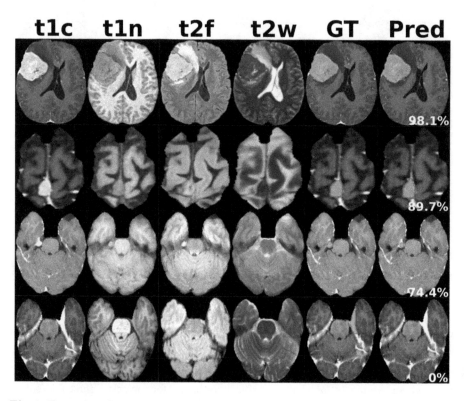

Fig. 3. Examples of segmentation performances over the test fold from the meningioma challenge training dataset, one patient featured per row. The NCR, ET, and ED classes are shown in green, red, and blue respectively. The Dice score for the TC category is shown in white for each patient. (Color figure online)

4.3 Challenge 3: Meningioma Segmentation Performance

Segmentation performances obtained over the training dataset, for the first fold only, are reported in Table 5. For the ET and TC categories, an average Dice score of 80% and HD95 of 6 mm is reached while the WT category only attain 77%

Table 5. Segmentation performances over the training dataset for the meningioma segmentation, for each class (first fold only).

Class	Pixel-wise			Patient-wise			Lesion-wise			HD95
	Dice	Recall	Precision	F1-score	Recall	Precision	Dice	Recall	Precision	
ET	80.52 ± 30.62	80.13 ± 32.42	84.04 ± 28.75	95.13	90.72	99.99	80.45 ± 30.66	87.75 ± 31.99	96.25 ± 13.57	05.94 ± 17.01
NCR	16.95 ± 29.67	17.18 ± 31.38	21.20 ± 35.02	78.68	92.30	68.57	76.11 ± 37.00	78.11 ± 36.58	88.04 ± 28.36	16.96 ± 15.55
NCR (TP)	53.48 ± 30.63	54.14 ± 34.59	66.44 ± 28.49	95.99	92.30	99.99	51.48 ± 31.74	57.88 ± 33.67	78.03 ± 27.95	16.67 ± 12.82
ED	38.30 ± 42.29	40.44 ± 43.91	38.98 ± 42.80	84.48	90.74	79.03	66.94 ± 40.02	69.29 ± 40.41	77.48 ± 37.66	11.27 ± 15.59
ED (TP)	69.51 ± 32.80	72.15 ± 34.34	70.74 ± 32.84	95.14	90.74	99.99	62.23 ± 35.23	66.49 ± 36.48	79.50 ± 32.20	08.32 ± 12.07
TC	80.57 ± 30.28	80.86 ± 32.22	83.12 ± 28.46	95.13	90.72	99.99	80.06 ± 30.53	84.52 ± 33.26	95.06 ± 17.20	05.91 ± 16.53
WT	77.65 ± 30.98	79.79 ± 31.47	80.49 ± 29.52	95.18	91.75	98.88	79.19 ± 29.51	87.75 ± 31.18	91.49 ± 21.98	09.23 ± 21.09

Dice score and 9 mm HD95. Segmenting the edema region appears to be more challenging in patients suffering from meningiomas. In many instances, either the NCR or ED classes are not featured which is visible from the gap in average Dice scores when considering the true positive cases only. Visual performances for five selected patients are reported in Fig. 3. The bottom row patient features a meningioma in a peculiar location, with a very challenging appearance that could locally resemble a blood vessel, which explains the model's struggle.

4.4 Challenge 4: Metastasis Segmentation

Segmentation performances obtained over the training dataset, for the first fold only, are reported in Table 6. For the TC and WT categories, an average Dice score of 70% and HD95 of 21 mm are reached, indicating a more difficult nature for this tumor type to be segmented. The metastases are the smallest of all tumors featured in the four BraTS challenges considered, with an average ET volume of 10 ml and often with a multifocal aspect. As such, oversegmentation, undersegmentation, or false positive segmentation will have a greater impact on the reported metrics.

4.5 Overall Performances on Validation and Test Subsets

Segmentation performances obtained over the validation and test subsets for each challenge are reported in Table 7 and Table 8 respectively, using the metrics computed by the BraTS challenge team.

Table 6. Segmentation performances over the training dataset for the metastasis segmentation, for each class (first fold only).

Class	Pixel-wise			Patient-wise			Lesion-wise			HD95
	Dice	Recall	Precision	F1-score	Recall	Precision	Dice	Recall	Precision	
ET	65.01 ± 28.45	68.42 ± 29.63	66.15 ± 28.95	91.80	93.33	90.32	67.67 ± 26.10	67.15 ± 33.62	87.85 ± 24.08	18.68 ± 27.70
NCR	38.70 ± 38.06	38.29 ± 40.04	44.32 ± 38.70	83.72	89.99	78.26	62.50 ± 37.76	70.17 ± 42.14	84.59 ± 33.21	08.73 ± 16.86
NCR (TP)	63.86 ± 28.00	63.17 ± 32.75	73.13 ± 26.60	94.73	89.99	99.99	63.12 ± 28.52	75.78 ± 36.22	94.58 ± 13.50	08.73 ± 16.86
ED	61.14 ± 34.28	63.88 ± 35.34	61.45 ± 32.92	96.66	93.54	99.99	53.67 ± 30.85	72.27 ± 35.36	85.77 ± 26.32	15.39 ± 25.88
ED (TP)	65.09 ± 31.53	68.00 ± 32.39	65.42 ± 29.91	96.66	93.54	99.99	53.91 ± 29.17	73.70 ± 33.70	84.85 ± 26.90	15.39 ± 25.88
TC	71.04 ± 30.77	75.80 ± 30.75	70.99 ± 30.44	91.80	93.33	90.32	72.86 ± 27.04	68.46 ± 32.87	84.29 ± 24.61	21.69 ± 27.58
WT	68.55 ± 31.49	74.15 ± 32.11	66.67 ± 29.68	95.23	90.90	99.99	68.94 ± 27.17	71.81 ± 34.24	80.66 ± 28.76	21.02 ± 29.17

Table 7. Segmentation performances over the validation subset for challenges 1–4, reporting the official lesion-wise metrics and custom pixel-wise metrics.

Challenge	# cases	Lesion-wise						Pixel-wise					
		Dice			HD95			Dice			HD95		
		ET	TC	WT	ET	TC	WT	ET	TC	WT	ET	TC	WT
1 (GLI)	219	75.98	78.06	82.60	44.97	40.30	28.18	77.08	80.29	85.67	26.69	18.76	08.25
2 (GLI SSA)	15	69.94	76.54	69.11	72.28	53.68	75.29	80.83	83.35	78.71	28.26	29.28	36.38
3 (MEN)	141	73.01	73.37	70.86	74.67	74.80	80.92	78.78	79.19	77.26	54.57	53.48	47.34
4 (MET)	31	44.33	47.74	48.32	164.03	163.78	152.65	65.33	71.30	67.93	51.82	52.08	39.15

Table 8. Segmentation performances over the test subset for challenges 1–4, reporting the official lesion-wise metrics, sensitivity, and specificity.

Challenge	Lesion-wise											
	Dice			HD95			Sensitivity			Specificity		
	ET	TC	WT	ET	TC	WT	ET	TC	WT	ET	TC	WT
1 (GLI)	79.83 ± 24.2	80.41 ± 28.7	81.61 ± 22.3	34.60 ± 89.5	39.69 ± 97.3	38.40 ± 81.8	85.52 ± 22.7	85.26 ± 26.2	88.75 ± 15.5	99.96 ± 0.04	99.96 ± 0.07	99.88 ± 0.42
2 (GLI SSA)	70.23 ± 30.0	74.32 ± 32.9	79.37 ± 25.0	59.17 ± 122	63.45 ± 126	46.79 ± 101	66.15 ± 28.2	71.84 ± 31.0	84.33 ± 22.6	99.97 ± 0.05	99.97 ± 0.04	99.83 ± 0.17
3 (MEN)	77.54 ± 30.5	77.28 ± 30.7	75.02 ± 30.6	61.41 ± 117	61.61 ± 118	64.17 ± 119	83.16 ± 29.1	82.19 ± 29.8	81.18 ± 29.6	99.98 ± 0.02	99.98 ± 0.02	99.94 ± 0.08
4 (MET)	39.35 ± 28.6	43.21 ± 31.4	42.54 ± 32.3	174.5 ± 136	172.1 ± 137	171.1 ± 137	61.63 ± 35.0	64.86 ± 36.5	68.90 ± 36.8	99.92 ± 0.39	99.84 ± 0.82	99.59 ± 1.87

5 Discussion

In this study, we have investigated the segmentation performances of models trained using the AGU-Net architecture over four different datasets from the BraTS challenge 2023: glioma, Sub-Sahara-Africa glioma, meningioma, and metastasis. Overall, the best segmentation performances across all metrics were obtained on the glioma challenge, including the largest number of patients. In addition, almost all patients are concurrently featuring the three classes (i.e., ET, NCR, and ED), with average volumes for each class above 15 ml, being favourable conditions for training a robust segmentation model. Surprisingly, a direct use of the best glioma segmentation model over African patients did not yield comparable performances, which could only be reached after performing a round of fine-tuning. Such variations could be explained by differences in data acquisition (e.g., scanner type or protocol), in patients' characteristics, or in the selection bias for such a limited sample size. Similarly, fine-tuning the best glioma segmentation model for the segmentation of meningioma and metastasis types generated competitive results, reduced training time, and bypassed potential issues due to the higher class imbalance and smaller volumes in those two challenges' datasets. The remaining challenges to address are: improving the segmentation of smaller tumors, better handling of the outliers and hard-cases, and finally reducing the inter-class confusion.

Acknowledgements. Data were processed in digital labs at HUNT Cloud, Norwegian University of Science and Technology, Trondheim, Norway.

D.B., I.R., and O.S. are partly funded by the Norwegian National Research Center for Minimally Invasive and Image-Guided Diagnostics and Therapy.

References

1. Adewole, M., et al.: The brain tumor segmentation (brats) challenge 2023: glioma segmentation in Sub-Saharan Africa patient population (brats-Africa). arXiv preprint arXiv:2305.19369 (2023). https://doi.org/10.48550/arXiv.2305.19369
2. Baid, U., et al.: The RSNA-ASNR-MICCAI BraTS 2021 benchmark on brain tumor segmentation and radiogenomic classification. arXiv preprint arXiv:2107.02314 (2021)
3. Bakas, S., et al.: Advancing the cancer genome atlas glioma MRI collections with expert segmentation labels and radiomic features. Sci. Data **4**(1), 1–13 (2017)
4. Binaghi, E., Pedoia, V., Balbi, S.: Collection and fuzzy estimation of truth labels in glial tumour segmentation studies. Comput. Methods Biomech. Biomed. Eng. Imaging Visual. **4**(3–4), 214–228 (2016). https://doi.org/10.1080/21681163.2014.947006
5. Bouget, D., et al.: Raidionics: an open software for pre-and postoperative central nervous system tumor segmentation and standardized reporting. arXiv preprint arXiv:2305.14351 (2023)
6. Bouget, D., Pedersen, A., Hosainey, S.A.M., Solheim, O., Reinertsen, I.: Meningioma segmentation in T1-weighted MRI leveraging global context and attention mechanisms. Front. Radiol. **1**, 711514 (2021). https://doi.org/10.3389/fradi.2021.711514
7. Bouget, D., et al.: Preoperative brain tumor imaging: models and software for segmentation and standardized reporting. Front. Neurol. 1500 (2022). https://doi.org/10.3389/fneur.2022.932219
8. Charron, O., Lallement, A., Jarnet, D., Noblet, V., Clavier, J.B., Meyer, P.: Automatic detection and segmentation of brain metastases on multimodal MR images with a deep convolutional neural network. Comput. Biol. Med. **95**, 43–54 (2018). https://doi.org/10.1016/j.compbiomed.2018.02.004
9. Chen, L.C., Papandreou, G., Schroff, F., Adam, H.: Rethinking atrous convolution for semantic image segmentation. arXiv preprint (2017). https://doi.org/10.48550/arXiv.1706.05587
10. Day, J., et al.: Neurocognitive deficits and neurocognitive rehabilitation in adult brain tumors. Curr. Treat. Options. Neurol. **18**(5), 1–16 (2016). https://doi.org/10.1007/s11940-016-0406-5
11. Grøvik, E., et al.: Handling missing MRI sequences in deep learning segmentation of brain metastases: a multicenter study. NPJ Digit. Med. **4**(1), 33 (2021). https://doi.org/10.1038/s41746-021-00398-4
12. Grøvik, E., Yi, D., Iv, M., Tong, E., Rubin, D., Zaharchuk, G.: Deep learning enables automatic detection and segmentation of brain metastases on multisequence MRI. J. Magn. Reson. Imaging **51**(1), 175–182 (2020). https://doi.org/10.1002/jmri.26766
13. Havaei, M., et al.: Brain tumor segmentation with deep neural networks. Med. Image Anal. **35**, 18–31 (2017). https://doi.org/10.1016/j.media.2016.05.004
14. Isensee, F., Jaeger, P.F., Kohl, S.A., Petersen, J., Maier-Hein, K.H.: nnU-Net: a self-configuring method for deep learning-based biomedical image segmentation. Nat. Methods **18**(2), 203–211 (2021). https://doi.org/10.1038/s41592-020-01008-z
15. Kamnitsas, K., et al.: DeepMedic for brain tumor segmentation. In: Crimi, A., Menze, B., Maier, O., Reyes, M., Winzeck, S., Handels, H. (eds.) BrainLes 2016. LNCS, vol. 10154, pp. 138–149. Springer, Cham (2016). https://doi.org/10.1007/978-3-319-55524-9_14

16. Kickingereder, P., et al.: Radiomic profiling of glioblastoma: identifying an imaging predictor of patient survival with improved performance over established clinical and radiologic risk models. Radiology **280**(3), 880–889 (2016). https://doi.org/10.1148/radiol.2016160845
17. Killeen, P.R.: An alternative to null-hypothesis significance tests. Psychol. Sci. **16**(5), 345–353 (2005). https://doi.org/10.1111/j.0956-7976.2005.01538.x
18. LaBella, D., et al.: The ASNR-MICCAI brain tumor segmentation (BraTs) challenge 2023: intracranial meningioma. arXiv preprint arXiv:2305.07642 (2023). https://doi.org/10.48550/arXiv.2305.07642
19. Lapointe, S., Perry, A., Butowski, N.A.: Primary brain tumours in adults. The Lancet **392**(10145), 432–446 (2018). https://doi.org/10.1016/S0140-6736(18)30990-5
20. Laukamp, K.R., et al.: Automated meningioma segmentation in multiparametric MRI: comparable effectiveness of a deep learning model and manual segmentation. Clin. Neuroradiol. **31**, 357–366 (2021). https://doi.org/10.1007/s00062-020-00884-4
21. Laukamp, K.R., et al.: Fully automated detection and segmentation of meningiomas using deep learning on routine multiparametric MRI. Eur. Radiol. **29**, 124–132 (2019). https://doi.org/10.1007/s00330-018-5595-8
22. Liu, Y., et al.: A deep convolutional neural network-based automatic delineation strategy for multiple brain metastases stereotactic radiosurgery. PLoS ONE **12**(10), e0185844 (2017). https://doi.org/10.1371/journal.pone.0185844
23. Louis, D.N., et al.: The 2021 WHO classification of tumors of the central nervous system: a summary. Neuro Oncol. **23**(8), 1231–1251 (2021). https://doi.org/10.1093/neuonc/noab106
24. Menze, B.H., et al.: The multimodal brain tumor image segmentation benchmark (BRATS). IEEE Trans. Med. Imaging **34**(10), 1993–2024 (2014). https://doi.org/10.1109/TMI.2014.2377694
25. Moawad, A.W., et al.: The brain tumor segmentation (BraTS-METS) challenge 2023: Brain metastasis segmentation on pre-treatment MRI. arXiv preprint arXiv:2306.00838 (2023). https://doi.org/10.48550/arXiv.2306.00838
26. Naser, M.A., Deen, M.J.: Brain tumor segmentation and grading of lower-grade glioma using deep learning in MRI images. Comput. Biol. Med. **121**, 103758 (2020). https://doi.org/10.1016/j.compbiomed.2020.103758
27. Neromyliotis, E., et al.: Machine learning in meningioma MRI: past to present. A narrative review. J. Magn. Reson. Imaging **55**(1), 48–60 (2022). https://doi.org/10.1002/jmri.27378
28. Pedersen, A., de Frutos, J.P., Bouget, D.: andreped/GradientAccumulator: v0.4.0 (2023). https://doi.org/10.5281/zenodo.7831244
29. Pereira, S., Pinto, A., Alves, V., Silva, C.A.: Brain tumor segmentation using convolutional neural networks in MRI images. IEEE Trans. Med. Imaging **35**(5), 1240–1251 (2016). https://doi.org/10.1007/s10916-019-1416-0
30. Ranjbarzadeh, R., Bagherian Kasgari, A., Jafarzadeh Ghoushchi, S., Anari, S., Naseri, M., Bendechache, M.: Brain tumor segmentation based on deep learning and an attention mechanism using MRI multi-modalities brain images. Sci. Rep. **11**(1), 1–17 (2021). https://doi.org/10.1038/s41598-021-90428-8
31. Tiwari, A., Srivastava, S., Pant, M.: Brain tumor segmentation and classification from magnetic resonance images: review of selected methods from 2014 to 2019. Pattern Recogn. Lett. **131**, 244–260 (2020). https://doi.org/10.1016/j.patrec.2019.11.020

32. Wadhwa, A., Bhardwaj, A., Verma, V.S.: A review on brain tumor segmentation of MRI images. Magn. Reson. Imaging **61**, 247–259 (2019). https://doi.org/10.1016/j.mri.2019.05.043
33. Zeineldin, R.A., Karar, M.E., Burgert, O., Mathis-Ullrich, F.: Multimodal CNN networks for brain tumor segmentation in MRI: a brats 2022 challenge solution. arXiv preprint arXiv:2212.09310 (2022)

Ensemble Learning and 3D Pix2Pix for Comprehensive Brain Tumor Analysis in Multimodal MRI

Ramy A. Zeineldin(✉) and Franziska Mathis-Ullrich

Department of Artificial Intelligence in Biomedical Engineering (AIBE),
Friedrich-Alexander-University Erlangen-Nürnberg (FAU), Erlangen, Germany
`ramy.zeineldin@fau.de`

Abstract. Motivated by the need for advanced solutions in the segmentation and inpainting of glioma-affected brain regions in multi-modal magnetic resonance imaging (MRI), this study presents an integrated approach leveraging the strengths of ensemble learning with hybrid transformer models and convolutional neural networks (CNNs), alongside the innovative application of 3D Pix2Pix Generative Adversarial Network (GAN). Our methodology combines robust tumor segmentation capabilities, utilizing axial attention and transformer encoders for enhanced spatial relationship modeling, with the ability to synthesize biologically plausible brain tissue through 3D Pix2Pix GAN. This integrated approach addresses the BraTS 2023 cluster challenges by offering precise segmentation and realistic inpainting, tailored for diverse tumor types and sub-regions. The results demonstrate outstanding performance, evidenced by quantitative evaluations such as the Dice Similarity Coefficient (DSC), Hausdorff Distance (HD95) for segmentation, and Structural Similarity Index Measure (SSIM), Peak Signal-to-Noise Ratio (PSNR), and Mean-Square Error (MSE) for inpainting. Qualitative assessments further validate the high-quality, clinically relevant outputs. In conclusion, this study underscores the potential of combining advanced machine learning techniques for comprehensive brain tumor analysis, promising significant advancements in clinical decision-making and patient care within the realm of medical imaging.

Keywords: BraTS · Ensemble Learning · GAN · MRI · Tumor Inpainting

1 Introduction

Brain tumors, particularly malignant gliomas, represent a formidable challenge in neuro-oncology, given their complex biological behavior and impact on patient survival [1]. The heterogeneity of gliomas in terms of appearance, growth patterns, and response to therapy complicates the task of accurately diagnosing and delineating tumor boundaries within the intricate brain anatomy [2]. Magnetic resonance imaging (MRI) serves as the gold standard in the non-invasive assessment of these tumors, offering detailed insights into their characteristics and progression [3]. However, the interpretation of MRI data demands precise segmentation of tumor regions, a task that remains labor-intensive and subject to variability when performed manually [4]. This necessity underscores the motivation for developing automated segmentation tools capable of reliably identifying tumor extents, thus facilitating targeted treatment planning, monitoring of disease evolution, and evaluation of therapeutic efficacy.

The Brain Tumor Segmentation (BraTS) Challenge, initiated by the Medical Image Computing and Computer-Assisted Intervention Society (MICCAI), represents a concerted effort to address these challenges [4–6]. By providing a platform for the development and benchmarking of advanced segmentation algorithms, BraTS encourages innovation in the field of medical image analysis [2, 5–8]. The main BraTS Glioma (GLI) challenge focuses on the segmentation of gliomas from multi-parametric MRI scans, offering a diverse dataset that includes high-grade and low-grade gliomas across various age groups and populations. The inclusion of a broad spectrum of data aims to ensure that developed algorithms are robust, versatile, and applicable in real-world clinical settings, contributing to the improvement of patient outcomes.

Moreover, the BraTS Sub-Saharan Africa (SSA) [9] and BraTS Pediatric (PED) [10] challenges have markedly advanced the field of medical imaging by fostering an environment of collaboration among researchers, clinicians, and technologists focused on the distinct challenges presented by the diverse patient populations in sub-Saharan Africa and the complexities of pediatric brain tumors, respectively. Through the establishment of a rigorous benchmarking environment tailored to these specific demographics, these challenges have catalyzed the rapid development of technology, leading to more accurate, efficient, and contextually relevant automated tumor segmentation and analysis. These efforts underscore the transformative potential of machine learning and artificial intelligence in enhancing healthcare delivery and patient outcomes, particularly in underserved regions and vulnerable age groups within the sphere of brain tumor management.

Most recently, the BraTS challenge has expanded to include the Local Synthesis of Healthy Brain Tissue via Inpainting (Inpaint) [11]. This novel component addresses the critical need for processing algorithms capable of 'normalizing' brain images affected by tumors, facilitating the application of standard analysis tools designed for healthy brains. The goal is to synthesize 3D healthy brain tissue within areas impacted by tumors, enabling the seamless integration of tumor patients' scans into existing frameworks for brain image analysis. This initiative not only enhances the practicality of automatic processing tools but also paves the way for innovations in the understanding of tumor biology and the development of targeted therapies.

Our research introduces a novel approach that synergizes ensemble learning with hybrid transformer models and convolutional neural networks (CNNs) for precise brain tumor segmentation and employs 3D Pix2Pix Generative Adversarial Network (GAN) for the realistic inpainting of glioma-affected brain areas within multi-modal MRI scans. The ensemble learning methodology capitalizes on the strengths of transformers and CNNs to capture the essential spatial relationships and contextual information, which are pivotal for the accurate demarcation of tumor boundaries. This is particularly relevant in heterogenous gliomas, enabling the algorithm to adapt to the diverse presentations of tumors in MRI imaging effectively.

The integration of 3D Pix2Pix GAN for inpainting proposes an innovative use of GAN technology in medical imaging, focusing on the synthesis of healthy brain tissue in regions impacted by gliomas. This aspect of our research is aimed at facilitating the application of standard brain image segmentation algorithms to tumor cases without the need to be altered. By effectively "removing" the tumor from images, our method allows for improved accuracy in segmentation and offers new insights into the relationship between tumor presence and brain structure, potentially enhancing surgical planning and treatment outcomes.

This work aligns with the objectives set forth by the MICCAI and the BraTS 2023 challenge, which seeks to push the boundaries of what is currently achievable in automated brain tumor segmentation. By addressing the diverse aspects of the challenge, including the segmentation of various tumor entities, consideration of pediatric cases, and the inclusion of data from low- and middle-income countries, our approach demonstrates a commitment to inclusivity and broad applicability.

Automated deep learning methods are at the forefront of transforming brain tumor segmentation, markedly enhancing precision, efficiency, and clinical applicability. CNNs have demonstrated significant efficacy in medical image analysis, including the segmentation of brain tumors, by adeptly learning complex features from data [12, 13]. This capability positions them as essential tools for identifying the intricate and varied characteristics of brain tumors visible in multi-parametric MRI scans. Through training on extensively annotated datasets, CNNs adeptly distinguish between tumor sub-regions, such as enhancing tumors, peritumoral edema, and necrotic components, enabling accurate and consistent segmentation. Furthermore, the application of Transformers [14], initially designed for natural language processing and now adapted for image analysis, presents new avenues for brain tumor segmentation. The self-attention mechanisms of Transformers are adept at recognizing long-range dependencies, crucial for understanding spatial relationships and contextual nuances vital for precise tumor segmentation. Their ability to holistically process images is invaluable in identifying complex tumor boundaries that cross multiple sub-regions.

By integrating CNNs with Transformers, this approach significantly enhances the capability of automated brain tumor segmentation [15]. This combination allows for a comprehensive analysis of multi-parametric MRI data, extracting detailed spatial and contextual information while ensuring accuracy down to the finest details. Employing these advanced methodologies on diverse datasets streamlines the segmentation process, minimizes manual intervention, reduces subjectivity, and accelerates the path from diagnosis to treatment planning for brain tumors. As deep learning evolves, it promises to make substantial contributions to improving patient care and outcomes in brain tumor management.

The main contributions of our study are manifold. Firstly, we introduce a novel ensemble learning model that combines the robust feature-extraction capabilities of CNNs with the long-range contextual understanding of transformers, optimizing segmentation accuracy. Secondly, we adopt an enhanced 3D Pix2Pix GAN for the inpainting of glioma-affected regions, presenting a new avenue for enhancing the utility of MRI scans in clinical practice. Thirdly, our methodology demonstrates significant improvements in segmentation precision and inpainting across a variety of tumor types and sub-regions, as validated by comprehensive evaluations and qualitative analyses.

2 Methodology

2.1 Ensemble Learning for Segmentation

Our ensemble learning approach for brain tumor segmentation capitalizes on the synergy between the baseline 3D U-Net architecture [16, 17] and a transformer encoder [18], complemented by an innovative axial attention decoder. The baseline network architecture, based on the renowned 3D U-Net encoder-decoder structure, has proven effective for various medical image segmentation tasks, as detailed in our previous paper [12]. It combines an encoder that extracts high-level features from input data with a decoder that upsamples these features to produce the final segmentation map.

Transformer. To accommodate the computational demands of processing 3D volumetric data with Transformers, our method draws inspiration from the Vision Transformer (ViT) [15, 18], implementing a strategy that segments the image into fixed-size patches and converts each into a token. This preprocessing reduces the sequence length, making the computational load manageable. However, to preserve the local context across spatial and depth dimensions critical for volumetric segmentation, we applied $3 \times 3 \times 3$ convolution blocks with downsampling. This strategy encodes the input into a low-resolution yet richly featured representation, which is then fed into the Transformer encoder. This process enables the model to discern both local and global contexts, significantly enhancing segmentation performance [21].

The integration of an axial attention decoder marks a pivotal advancement in the U-Net architecture. Axial attention, borrowing from advancements in natural language processing [13] and adapted for the vision domain [20], addresses the computational complexity of applying self-attention to 3D data. By applying self-attention sequentially across each axis, the model achieves linear computational complexity relative to the image size, facilitating the inclusion of this mechanism with volumetric data [19].

BraTS-specific Modifications. Our approach incorporates several BraTS-specific modifications to enhance the model's performance on the challenge dataset. These optimizations draw inspiration from the winning solutions of previous editions of the BraTS challenge, aiming to tailor the model more effectively to the unique characteristics of the data. First, given the memory-intensive demands of 3D CNNs, particularly with 3D data, we replace batch normalization with group normalization [19]. Group normalization has proven effective in scenarios with low batch sizes, as demonstrated by previous challenge winners [12, 20]. We use a default value of 32 groups unless stated otherwise, enabling better utilization of limited GPU memory during training. Second, to align with the BraTS evaluation metrics focusing on tumor subregions, we modify our network architecture's loss function and activation function. We replace the softmax nonlinearity with a sigmoid activation, and we optimize the three tumor subregions independently using binary cross-entropy (CE), inspired by [16].

Post-processing. We adopted a post-processing technique meticulously designed to enhance the segmentation accuracy. Specifically, we implemented measures to adjust enhancing tumor predictions based on predefined thresholds and thus optimizing the performance metrics while minimizing false positives. In addition, complemented by connected component analysis was utilized to refine predictions of small enhancing tumor regions, ensuring that only the most probable regions were classified as such.

2.2 GAN for Inpainting

In addressing the BraTS inpainting challenge, our methodology employs the capabilities of 3D Pix2Pix GAN, inspired by the transformative techniques detailed in a recent denoising diffusion-based study [21, 22]. This section outlines our approach, integrating advanced image translation with our DeepSeg model [13], which has been specifically fine-tuned for the BraTS dataset to optimize brain tumor segmentation and inpainting tasks. This task was intricately linked to the dataset from the BraTS 2022 segmentation challenge, consisting of T1-weighted MRI scans marked for inpainting.

Our GAN-based inpainting methodology was designed to address the challenge of filling inpainting targets with convincingly synthesized healthy tissue. The dataset, a retrospective collection from multiple institutions, presented a unique set of challenges due to the variation in clinical conditions, equipment, and imaging protocols. To navigate these complexities, we employed a strategy that amalgamated multi-class tumor delineations into a singular area of interest, subsequently dilated to encompass mass effects. Furthermore, the training, validation, and testing phases were meticulously structured to leverage surrogate inpainting masks generated within the healthy portions of the tumor-bearing brain images. These masks were pivotal in training our supervised infill algorithms, enabling the precise synthesis of healthy tissue in areas previously occupied by tumors.

These methods were assessed for their effectiveness in generating high-quality images, with peak signal-to-noise ratio (PSNR) serving as the primary quality metric. Subsequent segmentation of the synthesized images leveraged our DeepSeg framework, a novel adaptation that supersedes traditional UNet models, demonstrating superior performance in brain tumor segmentation within MRI scans. Further, to adapt our 3D image translation strategy to the complexities of volumetric data, several key modifications were implemented. These included the removal of attention layers to conserve GPU resources, the substitution of concatenation skip connections with additive operations for efficiency, and the incorporation of position embeddings to augment spatial accuracy. Training procedures utilized 3D patches within a fully convolutional framework, ensuring the applicability to images of variable dimensions during inference—a pioneering step in the realm of 3D medical image translation.

3 Results

3.1 Evaluation Metrics

Our submissions to the BraTS challenge were evaluated based on lesion-wise Dice Similarity Coefficients (DSC) scores and the 95th percentile Hausdorff Distance (HD95), applied to whole, core, and active tumor regions. The DSC score measures the accuracy of our predicted segmentations against the ground truth, while the HD95 assesses the maximum deviation between predicted and actual segmentations. Lesion-wise calculations penalize false positives and negatives by assigning a 0 Dice score and 374 for HD95, before averaging these scores for each case ID, ensuring a detailed assessment of segmentation precision.

For the inpainting task, statistical validation via paired t-tests compared PSNR and DSC across models to verify our improvements. This analysis confirmed our methodological enhancements significantly increased the quality and accuracy of brain tumor inpainting. Further, performance was measured using Structural Similarity Index Measure (SSIM), PSNR, and Mean Square Error (MSE), focusing on the realism of synthesized versus actual healthy tissue regions. An equally weighted rank-sum across these metrics determined the final MICCAI challenge rankings, with participants ranked per case for each metric. This evaluation framework rigorously quantifies the success of our inpainting efforts, underscoring our models' ability to generate realistic, accurate brain tissue infills.

3.2 Quantitative Results

In the rigorous evaluation of our models for the BraTS 2023 challenge, performance metrics were obtained using the validation datasets for GLI, PED, and SSA. The results of this evaluation are presented in Table 1 and Table 2. Using Synapse, the online platform provided by Sage Bionetworks, we reported the lesion-wise DSC and the lesion-wise HD95 to quantify the segmentation accuracy and the spatial consistency between the predicted and ground truth tumor sub-regions. These metrics provide a lesion-specific assessment, revealing how effectively each model detects and segments abnormalities, ensuring that models adept at identifying smaller lesions are not overlooked in favor of those that capture only larger lesions. Additionally, Table 2 lists the legacy DSC and HD95 as calculated in the previous BraTS Challenges.

Table 1. Comparative performance of segmentation models on BraTS 2023 GLI, PED, and SSA validation datasets: "WT" Denotes Whole Tumor, "ET" Refers to Enhancing Tumor, and "TC" Indicates Tumor Core components.

Dataset	Model	Lesion-wise DSC ↑				Lesion-wise HD95 ↓			
		ET	TC	WT	Avg	ET	TC	WT	Avg
GLI	TransBTS	0.77	0.81	0.75	0.78	46.97	36.68	72.15	51.93
	nnU-Net	0.81	0.85	0.86	0.84	**30.09**	**18.14**	30.25	27.35
	DeepSCAN	0.80	0.83	**0.90**	0.84	34.81	28.08	**14.11**	**26.16**
	SPARC	**0.82**	**0.86**	0.85	0.84	31.82	19.08	35.84	28.91
SSA	SPARC	0.75	0.76	0.75	0.76	56.04	57.41	77.12	63.52
PED	SPARC	0.74	0.61	0.84	0.73	61.36	16.34	26.00	34.57

- Bold values correspond to higher scores for the BraTS-GLI dataset.

Table 2. Comparative performance of SPARC model on BraTS 2023 GLI, PED, and SSA validation datasets using the legacy DSC and HD95 scores. All reported values were computed by the online evaluation platform Synapse.

Dataset	Model	DSC (%) ↑				HD95 ↓			
		ET	TC	WT	Avg	ET	TC	WT	Avg
GLI	SPARC	84.49	87.86	92.91	88.42	16.19	7.88	4.21	9.43
SSA	SPARC	83.56	85.08	91.37	86.67	17.75	11.56	4.15	11.15
PED	SPARC	84.23	87.62	92.70	88.19	17.50	7.53	3.60	9.54

In our experiments, the ensemble model, namely SPARC, utilized five distinct models, each generated with different cross-validation training configurations on the BraTS GLA dataset. The individual lesion-wise scores for the enhancing tumor (ET), tumor core (TC), and the whole tumor (WT) regions were then averaged to provide an overall performance metric for each model, as indicated in the "Avg" column of Table 1.

Statistical evaluation on the PED and SSA datasets was to gauge the transfer learning capabilities of the proposed SPARC model. In the BraTS-GLI dataset, SPARC showed a robust ability to segment brain tumors, with an average lesion-wise DSC of 0.84 and lesion-wise HD95 of 28.91. In the PED and SSA datasets, SPARC achieved lesion-wise DSCs of 0.73 and 0.76, respectively, reflecting its reliable performance and adaptability to diverse clinical settings. The ensemble approach ensures a comprehensive assessment, effectively capturing various tumor sub-regions and maintaining consistent performance across different datasets. These quantitative results validate the effectiveness of our models in addressing the challenges posed by BraTS 2023, with transfer learning efficacy highlighted in datasets beyond its initial training scope.

3.3 Segmentation Output

Figure 1 presents a comparative display of tumor segmentation using the SPARC ensemble model on tumor scans within the BraTS GLA, SSA, and PED validation datasets. The figure highlights the precision of the ensemble model in identifying tumor regions, delineating boundaries distinctly aligned with ground truth annotations. When examining the third row of Figure 1, which represents results from the BraTS PED dataset, SPARC efficiently segments the enhancing tumor (ET), depicted in green. However, a classification challenge is noted where Edema is erroneously identified as a non-enhancing tumor (NC), indicated in red. This specific error aligns with common automated segmentation challenges detailed in [10], particularly prevalent in pediatric tumor analysis due to their distinct morphological characteristics.

Such misclassification affects SPARC's performance metrics in the tumor core (TC) category within the PED dataset, as reflected in Table 1. The TC comprises both the ET and NC, and inaccuracies in classification can lead to decreased performance scores, elucidating the need for refined algorithmic precision tailored to pediatric oncological imaging.

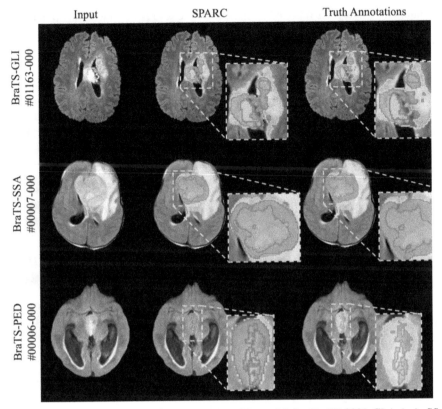

Fig. 1. Visual segmentation outputs by our ensemble model for BraTS 2023 GLA (*up*), SSA (*middle*), and PED (*down*) sets. Tumor labels are Edema in *yellow* (ED), Enhancing Tumor in *green* (ET), and Non-enhancing Component (NC) in *red*. (Color figure online)

3.4 Inpainting Output

Our enhanced 3D Pix2Pix GAN model was evaluated in the BraTS 2023 Inpainting Challenge, where it achieved good results. Table 3 details the performance metrics, including MSE, PSNR, and SSIM. Specifically, the model achieved an MSE of 0.0533, PSNR of 16.4413, and SSIM of 0.6956 for the validation set, while it showed improved performance on the test set, with an MSE of 0.0665, PSNR of 17.2619, and SSIM of 0.7242. These findings affirm the robustness and generalizability of the proposed inpainting model.

Visual representations provided in Fig. 2 augment the quantitative data, where various stages of the inpainting process are shown. Each row presents a phase in the inpainting process: the top row features voided T1 scans, the middle row shows the regions masked for inpainting, and the bottom row displays the predictions generated by our model. The enhanced GAN model demonstrates particularly effective inpainting for smaller tumor regions, where the predictions closely align with the expected healthy tissue patterns. The high-resolution generated samples depict a high degree of structural accuracy while showing seamless reconstruction of complex brain tissues, reaffirming the quantitative outcomes reported in Table 3. These results underscore the potential of our approach for clinical applications, providing a valuable tool for medical professionals in the assessment and planning of brain tumor treatments.

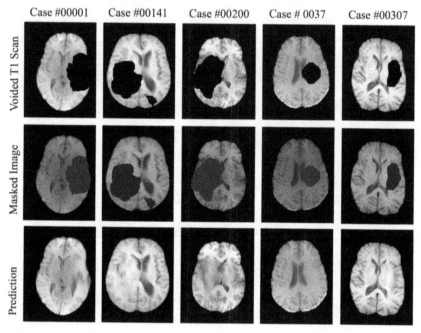

Fig. 2. Enhanced Pix2Pix GAN model predictions on 2D transversal T1 MRI slices.

Table 3. Results of the enhanced 3D Pix2Pix model on the BraTS 2023 Inpainting Challenge.

Dataset	MSE	PSNR	SSIM
Valid	0.0533	16.4413	0.6956
Test	0.0665	17.2619	0.7242

4 Discussion

The extensive evaluations of our models within the BraTS 2023 challenges have unveiled the strengths and potential limitations of our proposed methodologies. Through these analyses, we have elucidated the capabilities of our ensemble learning model, SPARC, and the enhanced 3D Pix2Pix GAN, across the diverse datasets of GLA, SSA, and PED.

The results, as presented in Table 1, outline the performance metrics across the different models: TransBTS, nnU-Net, DeepSCAN, and SPARC model. The nnU-Net model exhibits robust performance in terms of lesion-wise DSC scores, outperforming

TransBTS and DeepSCAN in most metrics. Notably, our SPARC model, leveraging post-processing strategies, shows promising results, particularly in the enhancing tumor sub-region. This underscores the efficacy of ensemble learning in enhancing the robustness and generalization capabilities of our segmentation models.

Furthermore, the scores of SPARC on the PED and SSA tasks are presented in Table 3. These results demonstrate competitive DSC values, indicating that our model can achieve accurate segmentations across varying clinical and imaging environments. However, as the PED dataset analysis suggests, segmentation challenges remain, particularly in pediatric cases where distinguishing between tumor types can be difficult due to their varied morphology. This is evidenced by the misclassification of ED as NC, an issue that resonates with common errors in automated pediatric brain tumor segmentations, as outlined in the literature [10].

Additionally, this methodology, set within the context of the BraTS inpainting challenge, signifies a notable advancement in the field of medical image analysis. By integrating cutting-edge 3D Pix2Pix GAN with our bespoke DeepSeg model—optimized for the specific nuances of the BraTS dataset—we have established a comprehensive framework for the effective inpainting, and segmentation of glioma-affected brain regions as listed in Table 3. For an in-depth exploration of the techniques and their implications, we direct readers to the detailed publications [13, 21].

Despite the promising results, challenges remain, such as optimizing post-processing strategies to balance the trade-off between false positives and true positives. Additionally, addressing the domain gap between training and test datasets, particularly evident in the BraTS challenge, remains an essential area for improvement. Further exploration of advanced data augmentation techniques and normalization strategies, as well as investigation of more complex architectures and domain adaptation methods, could be beneficial for enhancing our model's performance in the future.

In conclusion, our methodology for the BraTS challenges of 2021 and 2023 represents a comprehensive effort to advance the field of medical imaging for brain tumor analysis. By integrating ensemble learning for segmentation with GAN-based techniques for inpainting, we have outlined a robust framework capable of addressing some of the most pressing challenges in neuro-oncology imaging. Our approach demonstrates the potential of combining multiple AI techniques for medical image analysis and also sets a new benchmark for future research in the domain.

References

1. Patel, A.P., et al.: Global, regional, and national burden of brain and other CNS cancer, 1990–2016: a systematic analysis for the Global Burden of Disease Study 2016. Lancet Neurol. **18**, 376–393 (2019)
2. Baid, U., et al.: The RSNA-ASNR-MICCAI BraTS 2021 benchmark on brain tumor segmentation and radiogenomic classification. arXiv:2107.02314 (2021)
3. Gritsch, S., Batchelor, T.T., Gonzalez Castro, L.N.: Diagnostic, therapeutic, and prognostic implications of the 2021 World Health Organization classification of tumors of the central nervous system. Cancer **128**, 47–58 (2021)
4. Menze, B.H., et al.: The multimodal brain tumor image segmentation benchmark (BRATS). IEEE Trans. Med. Imaging **34**, 1993–2024 (2015)

5. Bakas, S., et al.: Advancing the cancer genome atlas glioma MRI collections with expert segmentation labels and radiomic features. Sci. Data **4** (2017)
6. Karargyris, A., et al.: Federated benchmarking of medical artificial intelligence with MedPerf. Nat. Mach. Intell. **5**, 799–810 (2023)
7. Bakas, S., Akbari, H., Sotiras, A.: Segmentation labels for the pre-operative scans of the TCGA-GBM collection. The Cancer Imaging Archive (2017)
8. Bakas, S., et al.: Segmentation labels and radiomic features for the pre-operative scans of the TCGA-LGG collection. Cancer Imaging Archive **286** (2017)
9. Adewole, M., et al.: The brain tumor segmentation (BraTS) challenge 2023: glioma segmentation in Sub-Saharan Africa patient population (BraTS-Africa). arXiv:2305.19369 (2023)
10. Fathi Kazerooni, A., et al.: The brain tumor segmentation (BraTS) challenge 2023: focus on pediatrics (CBTN-CONNECT-DIPGR-ASNR-MICCAI BraTS-PEDs). arXiv:2305.17033 (2023)
11. Kofler, F., et al.: The brain tumor segmentation (BraTS) challenge 2023: local synthesis of healthy brain tissue via inpainting. arXiv:2305.08992 (2023)
12. Zeineldin, R.A., Karar, M.E., Burgert, O., Mathis-Ullrich, F.: Multimodal CNN Networks for Brain Tumor Segmentation in MRI: A BraTS 2022 Challenge Solution. Brainlesion: Glioma, Multiple Sclerosis, Stroke and Traumatic Brain Injuries, pp. 127-137 (2023)
13. Zeineldin, R.A., Karar, M.E., Coburger, J., Wirtz, C.R., Burgert, O.: DeepSeg: deep neural network framework for automatic brain tumor segmentation using magnetic resonance FLAIR images. Int. J. Comput. Assist. Radiol. Surg. **15**, 909–920 (2020). https://doi.org/10.1007/s11548-020-02186-z
14. Vaswani, A., et al.: Attention is all you need. In: Advances in Neural Information Processing Systems, vol. 30 (2017)
15. Zeineldin, R.A., et al.: Explainable hybrid vision transformers and convolutional network for multimodal glioma segmentation in brain MRI. Sci. Rep. **14**, 3713 (2024)
16. Isensee, F., Jaeger, P.F., Kohl, S.A.A., Petersen, J., Maier-Hein, K.H.: NnU-Net: a self-configuring method for deep learning-based biomedical image segmentation. Nat. Methods **18**, 203–211 (2020)
17. Ronneberger, O., Fischer, P., Brox, T.: U-net: Convolutional networks for biomedical image segmentation. In: Navab, N., Hornegger, J., Wells, W., Frangi, A. (eds.) Medical Image Computing and Computer-Assisted Intervention. Lecture Notes in Computer Science, vol. 9351, pp. 234–241. Springer, Cham (2015). https://doi.org/10.1007/978-3-319-24574-4_28
18. Dosovitskiy, A., et al.: An image is worth 16x16 words: transformers for image recognition at scale. arXiv preprint arXiv:2010.11929 (2020)
19. Yuxin, W., He, K.: Group normalization. In: Ferrari, V., Hebert, M., Sminchisescu, C., Weiss, Y. (eds.) Computer Vision – ECCV 2018: 15th European Conference, Munich, Germany, September 8-14, 2018, Proceedings, Part XIII, pp. 3–19. Springer, Cham (2018). https://doi.org/10.1007/978-3-030-01261-8_1
20. Luu, H.M., Park, S.H.: Extending nn-UNet for brain tumor segmentation. In: Crimi, A., Bakas, S. (eds.) Brainlesion: Glioma, Multiple Sclerosis, Stroke and Traumatic Brain Injuries. Lecture Notes in Computer Science, vol. 12963, pp. 173–186. Springer, Cham (2022). https://doi.org/10.1007/978-3-031-09002-8_16
21. Graf, R., et al.: Denoising diffusion-based MRI to CT image translation enables automated spinal segmentation. Eur. Radiol. Exp. **7**, 70 (2023). https://doi.org/10.1186/s41747-023-00385-2
22. Isola, P., Zhu, J.-Y., Zhou, T., Efros, A.A.: Image-to-image translation with conditional adversarial networks. In: Proceedings of the IEEE Conference on Computer Vision and Pattern Recognition, pp. 1125–1134 (2017)

Denoising Diffusion Models for Inpainting of Healthy Brain Tissue

Alicia Durrer(✉), Philippe C. Cattin, and Julia Wolleb

Center for Medical Image Analysis and Navigation, Department of Biomedical Engineering, University of Basel, Allschwil, Switzerland
`alicia.durrer@unibas.ch`

Abstract. This paper is a contribution to the "BraTS 2023 Local Synthesis of Healthy Brain Tissue via Inpainting Challenge". The task of this challenge is to transform tumor tissue into healthy tissue in brain magnetic resonance (MR) images. This idea originates from the problem that MR images can be evaluated using automatic processing tools, however, many of these tools are optimized for the analysis of healthy tissue. By solving the given inpainting task, we enable the automatic analysis of images featuring lesions, and further downstream tasks.

Our approach builds on denoising diffusion probabilistic models. We use a 2D model that is trained using slices in which healthy tissue was cropped out and is learned to be inpainted again. This allows us to use the ground truth healthy tissue during training. In the sampling stage, we replace the slices containing diseased tissue in the original 3D volume with the slices containing the healthy tissue inpainting. With our approach, we achieve the second place in the challenge. On the test set our model achieves a mean SSIM of 0.8271, a PSNR of 20.4949 and a MSE of 0.0115. In future we plan to extend our 2D model to a 3D model, allowing to inpaint the region of interest as a whole without losing context information of neighboring slices.

Keywords: BraTS challenge · Inpainting · Diffusion Models

1 Introduction

Magnetic Resonance (MR) images of the brain and the subsequent automatic processing of these images are essential for monitoring pathologies. However, many automatic processing tools are built to e.g., register or segment only healthy tissue and are not as reliable for processing diseased brain regions [1–3]. As illustrated in Fig. 1, it is therefore required to transform diseased tissue into healthy tissue to benefit from these automatic processing tools. This paper is a contribution to the "BraTS [4–7] 2023 Local Synthesis of Healthy Brain Tissue via Inpainting Challenge" [8] that focuses on synthesizing healthy brain tissue in brains affected by tumors by transforming tumor tissue into healthy tissue. The challenge organizers provide T1-scans from the multi-modal BraTS 2022 segmentation challenge [4–6,9]. In these scans, the areas affected by glioma, tumors originating from glial cells in the brain or spinal cord [10], need to be inpainted in three dimensions with healthy brain tissue. For this task, we propose a method based on denoising diffusion probabilistic models (DDPMs) [11–13]. We build on a method we previously applied to the task of contrast harmonization between different MR scanners [14].

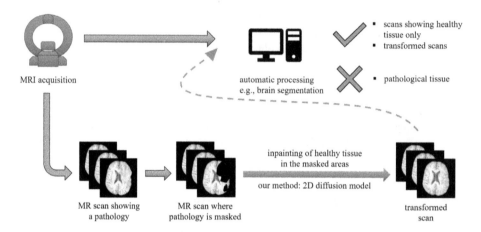

Fig. 1. Illustration of the problem. MR scans not showing pathologies can be fed directly into automatic processing tools. Often, scans containing pathologies need to be modified first. The task of this challenge is to replace pathological brain tissue with healthy brain tissue. The suggested inpainting requires a masked scan, whereby the masked region will be filled by an inpainting process, for which we suggest a DDPM-based model, visualized by the bold blue arrow. The output, denoted as the transformed scan, then shows a healthy scan. The transformed scan can then be fed into automatic processing tools for further analysis, denoted by the dashed blue arrow. (Color figure online)

1.1 BraTS Challenge

BraTS [4–7], short for "International Brain Tumor Segmentation", provides challenges within the International Conference for Medical Image Computing and Computer-Assisted Intervention (MICCAI). The here discussed challenge "Local Synthesis of Healthy Brain Tissue via Inpainting" [8], is one of several challenges offered in the BraTS 2023 cluster of challenges.

1.2 Contribution

Based on our existing image-to-image translation method [14], we train a slice-wise 2D DDPM to solve this inpainting task.

2 Method

2.1 Denoising Diffusion Probabilistic Models

DDPMs are generative models consisting of an iterative noising process q and a learned denoising process p_θ. Gaussian noise is added to an image x for T time steps t during the noising process q. Each resulting image $x_0, x_1, ..., x_T$ contains a higher amount of noise than the previous image, as the noise level increases with each time step t until it reaches a maximum at $t = T$. The equation

$$q(x_t|x_{t-1}) := \mathcal{N}(x_t; \sqrt{1-\beta_t}x_{t-1}, \beta_t \mathbf{I}), \tag{1}$$

describes the forward noising process q, whereby $\mathbf{I}$ is the identity matrix and $\beta_1, ..., \beta_T$ are the forward process variances. Defining $\alpha_t := 1 - \beta_t$, $\overline{\alpha}_t := \prod_{s=1}^{t} \alpha_s$ and applying the reparameterization trick, x_t can be written as

$$x_t = \sqrt{\overline{\alpha}_t} x_0 + \sqrt{1-\overline{\alpha}_t} \epsilon, \quad \text{with } \epsilon \sim \mathcal{N}(0, \mathbf{I}). \tag{2}$$

During the denoising process p_θ, the goal is to reverse the forward process. Therefore, we want to predict x_{t-1} from x_t for $t \in \{T, ..., 1\}$, whereby p_θ is defined as a normal distribution with mean μ_θ and variance Σ_θ. The aim is to determine μ_θ and Σ_θ such that p_θ and q match. The denoising process p_θ can be written as

$$p_\theta(x_{t-1}|x_t) := \mathcal{N}\big(x_{t-1}; \mu_\theta(x_t, t), \Sigma_\theta(x_t, t)\big). \tag{3}$$

By learning μ_θ, a model ϵ_θ can be trained to denoise an image step by step. In [11] it was shown that Σ_θ can be fixed to $\sigma_t^2 \mathbf{I}$ and does not need to be learned. The model ϵ_θ is a U-Net [15] that predicts the noise pattern $\epsilon_\theta(x_t, t)$ at time step t to generate a slightly denoised image x_{t-1}. In their original form, DDPMs are generative models that can sample images starting from random noise. This sampling process is given through:

$$x_{t-1} = \frac{1}{\sqrt{\alpha_t}} \left(x_t - \frac{1-\alpha_t}{\sqrt{1-\overline{\alpha}_t}} \epsilon_\theta(x_t, t) \right) + \sigma_t \mathbf{z}, \quad \text{with } \mathbf{z} \sim \mathcal{N}(0, \mathbf{I}), \tag{4}$$

whereby we start from $x_T \sim \mathcal{N}(0, \mathbf{I})$ and apply Eq. 4 for all time steps $t \in \{T, ..., 1\}$. The final prediction is x_0. Section 2.2 describes how this well-known method is modified for inpainting.

2.2 Inpainting of Masked Region

The goal of this challenge is to replace tumor tissue with healthy tissue. We use the great performance of DDPMs in image synthesis to inpaint healthy tissue in masked regions of the brain. Figure 2 gives an overview.

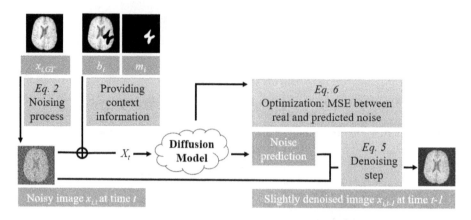

Fig. 2. Overview of the training process. Context information is provided through the concatenation of input b_i and mask m_i with the noisy image $x_{i,t}$, which originated from the ground truth $x_0 = x_{i,GT}$ using Eq. 2. The concatenated image X_t is used by the diffusion model to predict a slightly denoised image $x_{i,t-1}$ from $x_{i,t}$ using Eq. 5. The diffusion model is trained using an MSE loss between the real and the predicted noise, summarized in Eq. 6.

Training. For the training process of the proposed approach, we need the ground truth image x_{GT}, a predefined mask m that masks out some healthy tissue of the ground truth image, as well as the masked ground truth image denoted as b. Due to the high computation costs of 3D volumes, we propose a 2D approach on slices of the respective volumes. Therefore, we slice all 3D volumes into 2D slices, and consider only the slices i with a non-zero mask for training. We take a random time step $t \in \{1, ..., T\}$ and compute a noisy image $x_{i,t}$ from the ground truth slice $x_{i,GT}$ by applying Eq. 2 with $x_0 = x_{i,GT}$. The goal is to predict the slightly denoised $x_{i,t-1}$. We add the slice context information of our baseline image b_i and the mask m_i through channel-wise concatenation. The concatenated image $X_t := x_{i,t} \oplus b_i \oplus m_i$ serves as input for our diffusion model. The computation of $x_{i,t-1}$ can be done via a denoising step with

$$x_{i,t-1} = \frac{1}{\sqrt{\alpha_t}}\left(x_{i,t} - \frac{1-\alpha_t}{\sqrt{1-\bar{\alpha}_t}}\epsilon_\theta(X_t,t)\right) + \sigma_t \mathbf{z}, \quad \text{with } \mathbf{z} \sim \mathcal{N}(0,\mathbf{I}), \quad (5)$$

where $\epsilon_\theta(X_t, t)$ is the diffusion model output at time step t, σ_t is the variance scheme and $\mathbf{z}$ covers the stochastic component of the process. As shown in [14], to train the diffusion model ϵ_θ the following loss term with $\epsilon \sim \mathcal{N}(0,\mathbf{I})$ is used:

$$||\epsilon - \epsilon_\theta(X_t,t)||^2 = ||\epsilon - \epsilon_\theta((\sqrt{\bar{\alpha}_t}x_{i,0} + \sqrt{(1-\bar{\alpha}_t)}\epsilon) \oplus b_i \oplus m_i), t)||^2. \quad (6)$$

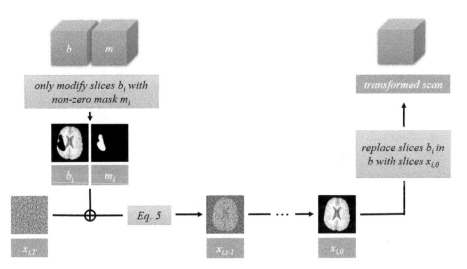

Fig. 3. Sampling method. During sampling, we apply the denoising described by Eq. 5 for each of the T denoising steps for each slice b_i with a non-zero mask m_i. We then replace the slices b_i in b with the samples $x_{i,0}$, containing the inpainting, to obtain our transformed 3D scan.

Sampling. During sampling, shown in Fig. 3, we loop through the slices of the masked 3D volume and only modify the slices with a non-zero mask. For each of these slices, the starting point $x_{i,T}$ is set to random Gaussian noise $\sim \mathcal{N}(0, \mathbf{I})$. We use the masked T1 slice b_i and the corresponding mask m_i to guide the denoising process for each time step t for each of the slices. This means, we start from $x_{i,1000} \sim \mathcal{N}(0, \mathbf{I})$ and apply Eq. 5 until we get the prediction $x_{i,0}$ for each slice affected by a lesion. We replace the masked slices b_i in the 3D scan b with the predicted slices $x_{i,0}$ to get the transformed scan. This transformed scan can be used for further downstream tasks, as illustrated in Fig. 1.

3 Data Set and Training Details

3.1 Data Preprocessing

The data set consists of T1 scans from the multi-modal BraTS 2022 glioma segmentation challenge [4–6,9]. The data is a retrospective collection of brain tumor MR scans originating from multiple different institutions using different equipment and imaging protocols but all working under standard clinical conditions. For each patient, the challenge organizers provide T1 scans of brains affected by tumors, masks of the tumor regions, masks of healthy tissue regions, combined masks of the tumor and healthy regions as well as "T1-voided" scans, in which the combined masks are cropped out from the original T1 image. For our approach, we use the T1 images and the healthy region masks during training. As our final goal is to learn to replace healthy tissue, for training, we crop out the healthy masks from the T1 images to obtain a masked T1 image in which only a healthy region is missing. We remove the top and bottom 0.1 percentile of voxel intensities and normalize the scans to voxel values between 0 and 1. As our model is constructed for 2D data, we slice each 3D scan into axial slices that are then cropped to a size of [224, 224]. Only background pixels are affected by the cropping. For training, we only use slices showing a non-zero mask. The provided training set consists of 1251 subjects which were used for a two-fold cross-validation, each using 1241 subjects for training and 10 for validation.

3.2 Training Details

We trained our model on an NVIDIA A100-SXM4-40GB with batch size 8 for 2'850'000 iterations, taking about two and a half weeks. The number of channels in the first layer of the model is 128, as proposed in [13]. Furthermore, one attention head is used at resolution 16, resulting in 113'672'066 model parameters. The learning rate is set to 10^{-4} for the used Adam optimizer. T is defined as 1000. For the evaluation of the validation and test set, we use the model saved with an exponential moving average (EMA) over model parameters with a rate of 0.9999. Further details on hyperparameters and architecture can be found in [16].

3.3 Postprocessing and Evaluation

After sampling, we apply a Gaussian filter with a standard deviation $sigma = 1.075$ for the Gaussian kernel to smooth borders between the slices. In addition to the training data, the challenge organizers provided a validation set of 219 subjects that could be evaluated using our model and submitted to the Synapse [17] platform to obtain structural similarity index measure (SSIM), peak signal-to-noise ratio (PSNR) and mean squared error (MSE). For submission to the Synapse platform, each model output is normalized to the intensity range of the corresponding input image from which the first and last 0.5 percentile were clipped. After submission of the final model as a MLCube [18], it was evaluated by the challenge organizers on a non-public test set of 568 cases.

4 Results

4.1 Cross-Validation Using Train-Validation Splits from Training Data Set

We evaluated both models we trained for the cross-validation on our validation splits using the evaluation script provided by the organizers. The calculated metrics are SSIM, PSNR and MSE for the inpainted region only. Table 1 provides the results of our cross-validation.

Table 1. Results of the two-fold cross validation.

	SSIM	PSNR	MSE
Model 1	0.8003 [±0.1081]	18.7572 [±1.8850]	0.0146 [±0.0063]
Model 2	0.7764 [±0.1292]	18.7310 [±1.5019]	0.0142 [±0.0049]
Average	**0.7884** [±0.1187]	**18.7441** [±1.6935]	**0.0144** [±0.0056]

Figure 4 provides examples of a given 2D masked slice, the corresponding mask, the generated sample and the ground truth. In 2D, our approach manages to generate consistent results. However, if we look at the whole 3D volume, stripe artifacts appear in the sagittal and coronal plane if multiple sequential axial slices are replaced within the volume. This is shown in Fig. 5. One possibility to reduce the visibility of these artifacts is the application of a Gaussian filter, also demonstrated in Fig. 5.

4.2 Validation on Synapse Server

We evaluated both models that we trained for the cross-validation on the validation set provided by the organizers. The evaluation was performed on the Synapse server. Again, SSIM, PSNR and MSE are only evaluated for the inpainted region. Table 2 provides the results for our cross-validation. Regarding all metrics, we achieve comparable results as the other challenge participants.

Table 2. Results of the evaluation of our model's performance on the validation set, evaluated on the Synapse server.

	SSIM	PSNR	MSE
Model 1	0.7802 [±0.1273]	20.3220 [±2.8306]	0.0113 [±0.0076]
Model 2	0.7805 [±0.1255]	20.3830 [±2.7619]	0.0112 [±0.0074]
Average	**0.7804** [±0.1264]	**20.3525** [±2.7963]	**0.0113** [±0.0075]

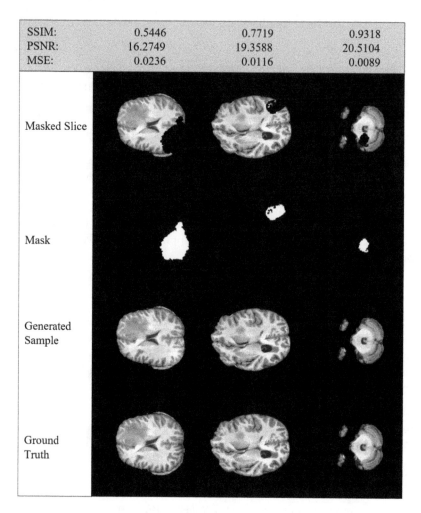

Fig. 4. Axial slices of images from our validation set. The masked slice, the mask, the generated sample, and the ground truth are provided. In general, the 2D generated samples are of good quality. Moreover, they show a high similarity to the corresponding ground truth. The SSIM, MSE and PSNR that are reported refer to the comparison of the whole generated volume (obtained by stacking of the generated slices) and the corresponding ground truth volume.

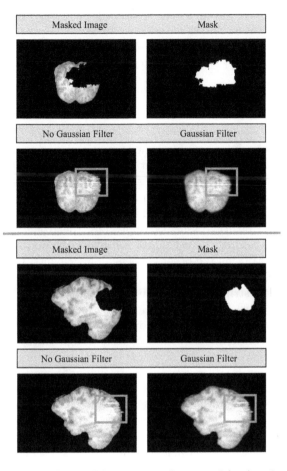

Fig. 5. Exemplary image of our validation set in the coronal (top) and sagittal (bottom) view. We observe stripe artifacts (blue boxes) due to the stacking of multiple axial slices. These artifacts can be reduced by applying a Gaussian filter (standard deviation $sigma = 1.075$ for Gaussian kernel). (Color figure online)

4.3 Test Set Scores

Model 2 was submitted as a MLCube for the evaluation on the non-public test set. The evaluation was performed by the challenge organizers. Table 3 provides the obtained results. Again, SSIM, PSNR and MSE are only evaluated for the inpainted region. Using this model, we achieve the second place in the inpainting challenge.

Table 3. Results of the evaluation of our model on the non-public test set.

	SSIM	PSNR	MSE
Model 2	0.8271 [±0.1308]	20.4949 [±3.1141]	0.0115 [±0.0096]

5 Discussion

We present an approach for healthy tissue inpainting based on 2D DDPMs. Taking advantage of the excellent image synthesis performance of DDPMs, we apply these models to masked brain MR images. Image context of the masked image is provided by concatenating the masked image to the input of the diffusion model in every time step t. These concatenated images are created to guide the denoising process. As only healthy tissue is cropped out, the ground truth is available during training. Regarding the validation, we achieve similar results in terms of SSIM, PSNR and MSE as the other challenge participants. Our model creates good results in 2D, but a drawback of our method is that the stacking of the 2D slices can lead to stripe artifacts, which we tried to reduce using a Gaussian filter. As an alternative, we tried to avoid the stripe artifacts using a sequential approach, where we included the previous ground truth slice as an additional channel that was concatenated with the noisy image during training. During sampling, the previously sampled slice was concatenated with the noisy image. However, this approach still needs modifications, as it seemed as if the errors accumulated over the sequence of slices. An advantage of the model we used for this challenge is that due to the two-dimensionality, it needs less computational resources than 3D models and shows a stable training progression. Nevertheless, in future, we aim to expand our approach to a 3D model, e.g., similar to [19]. So far we experimented with a 3D model using the same framework as presented in this paper, but it was limited regarding memory consumption, which led to limitations in network architecture tuning. A drawback of diffusion models in general is the slow sampling speed compared to other generative models. We aim to improve this using e.g., Heun sampling schemes [20] or consistency models [21]. We conclude that our method provides a baseline that shows a good performance for the task, resulting in the second place in the competition, and has potential to be fine-tuned using different architectural and sampling changes.

References

1. Jenkinson, M., Beckmann, C.F., Behrens, T.E., Woolrich, M.W., Smith, S.M.: FSL. Neuroimage **62**(2), 182–790 (2012)
2. Farazi, M. R., Faisal, F., Zaman, Z., Farhan, S.: Inpainting multiple sclerosis lesions for improving registration performance with brain atlas. In: International Conference on Medical Engineering, Health Informatics and Technology (2016)
3. Almansour, M., Ghanem, N. M., Bassiouny, S.: High-Resolution MRI Brain Inpainting. In: IEEE EMBS International Conference on Biomedical and Health Informatics (2021)

4. Menze, B.H., et al.: The multimodal brain tumor image segmentation benchmark (BRATS). IEEE Trans. Med. Imaging **34**(10), 1993–2024 (2014)
5. Bakas, S., et al.: Advancing the cancer genome atlas glioma MRI collections with expert segmentation labels and radiomic features. Sci. Data **4**(1), 1–13 (2017)
6. Bakas, S., et al.: Identifying the best machine learning algorithms for brain tumor segmentation, progression assessment, and overall survival prediction in the brats challenge. arXiv preprint arXiv:1811.02629 (2018)
7. Baid, U., et al.: The RSNA-ASNR-MICCAI BraTS 2021 benchmark on brain tumor segmentation and radiogenomic classification. arXiv preprint arXiv:2107.02314 (2021)
8. Kofler, F., et al.: The brain tumor segmentation (BraTS) challenge 2023: local synthesis of healthy brain tissue via inpainting. arXiv preprint arXiv:2305.08992 (2023)
9. Karargyris, A., et al.: Federated benchmarking of medical artificial intelligence with MedPerf. Nat. Mach. Intell. **5**, 799–810 (2023)
10. Mamelak, A.N., Jacoby, D.B.: Targeted delivery of antitumoral therapy to glioma and other malignancies with synthetic chlorotoxin (TM-601). Expert Opin. Drug Deliv. **4**(2), 175–182 (2007)
11. Ho, J., Jain, A., Abbeel, P.: Denoising diffusion probabilistic models. Adv. Neural. Inf. Process. Syst. **33**, 6840–6851 (2020)
12. Saharia, C., et al.: Palette: Image-to-image diffusion models. In: ACM SIGGRAPH 2022 Conference Proceedings, pp. 1–10 (2022)
13. Wolleb, J., Sandkühler, R., Bieder, F., Valmaggia, P., Cattin, P.C: Diffusion models for implicit image segmentation ensembles. In: Medical Imaging with Deep Learning, pp. 1336–1358. PMLR (2022)
14. Durrer, A., et al.: Diffusion models for contrast harmonization of magnetic resonance images. arXiv preprint arXiv:2303.08189 (2023)
15. Ronneberger, O., Fischer, P., Brox, T.: Convolutional networks for biomedical image segmentation. In: International Conference on Medical Image Computing and Computer-Assisted Intervention, pp. 234–241. Springer (2021)
16. Nichol, A. Q., Dhariwal, P.: Improved denoising diffusion probabilistic models. In: International Conference on Machine Learning, pp. 8162–8171. PMLR (2021)
17. Synapse Homepage. https://www.synapse.org/. Accessed 11 Aug 2023
18. MLCube. https://mlcommons.github.io/mlcube/. Accessed 11 Aug 2023
19. Bieder, F., Wolleb, J., Durrer, A., Sandkuehler, R., Cattin, P.C.: Memory-efficient 3D denoising diffusion models for medical image processing. In: Medical Imaging with Deep Learning (2023)
20. Karras, T., Aittala, M., Aila, T., Laine, S.: Elucidating the design space of diffusion-based generative models. Adv. Neural. Inf. Process. Syst. **35**, 26565–26577 (2022)
21. Song, Y., Dhariwal, P., Chen, M., Sutskever, I.: Consistency models. arXiv preprint arXiv:2303.01469 (2023)

Brain Tumor Segmentation Based on Self-supervised Pre-training and Adaptive Region-Specific Loss

Yubo Zhou, Lanfeng Zhong, and Guotai Wang[✉]

School of Mechanical and Electrical Engineering, University of Electronic Science and Technology of China, Chengdu, China
guotai.wang@uestc.edu.cn

Abstract. Automatic segmentation of pediatric brain tumors has garnered increasing attention due to its crucial role in diagnosis and treatment planning, which is challenging due to tumors' rarity and heterogeneity. This work presents a high-performance segmentation method based on nnU-Net for the pediatric brain tumor segmentation (BraTS-PEDs) challenge 2023. Firstly, we leverage the BraTS-PEDs 2023 dataset to pre-train our network with self-supervised learning strategies that encourage the network to grasp both global and local features inherent to pediatric brain tumors. Secondly, we leverage an adaptive region-specific training loss to tackle the challenges posed by the heterogeneity of magnetic resonance imaging (MRI) and the imbalance between different tissue categories during training, which effectively enhances the network's ability to learn from difficult regions. Our approach achieves lesion-wise Dice scores of 82.68%, 74.06%, and 59.63% with corresponding lesion-wise HD95 (mm) values of 22.85, 29.22, and 121.02 for the whole tumor (WT), non-enhancing component (NC), and enhancing tumor (ET) respectively, as determined by the online evaluation platform. We also validate our method on the BraTS meningioma challenge 2023 at the online evaluation platform and get lesion-wise Dice scores of 79.69%, 80.61%, and 79.97% with corresponding lesion-wise HD95 (mm) values of 49.37, 47.18, and 47.38 for the non-enhancing tumor core (NT), edema (ED), and ET.

Keywords: Brain tumor · Segmentation · Adaptive loss · Self-supervised learning

1 Introduction

Pediatric brain tumors have unfortunately led to a significant number of disease-related deaths among children. The median overall survival (OS) of diffuse intrinsic pontine glioma (DIPG), one type of pediatric brain tumor, is 9 months, and less than 10% of patients are alive at 2 years after diagnosis [1,2]. An effective and automated tumor segmentation process is crucial for accurate diagnosis and treatment planning, ultimately leading to a reduction in death rates. While numerous automatic tumor segmentation tools have been developed for adult brain tumors [3–7], disparities in imaging characteristics and clinical presentations between pediatric and adult brain tumors constrain the applicability of these tools to the pediatric context. Compounding this challenge is the pronounced heterogeneity exhibited by pediatric brain tumors, a factor that contributes to their elusive nature and makes accurate segmentation even more difficult. Adding to the complexity, these tumors can manifest randomly within the brain [8]. Given these unique attributes, it becomes imperative to develop a specialized automatic segmentation tool tailored explicitly to pediatric brain tumors.

By leveraging neural networks to learn from medical images and make predictions, deep learning has greatly solved the problems of burdensome workload and substantial inter-operator variability in manual segmentation [9]. In the context of the BraTS competition, a huge effort has been made to find suitable segmentation methods for glioma, and winners of the recent competitions had employed deep learning. For example, the winners from 2020 to 2022 all applied nnU-Net, a self-configuring deep learning framework that automatically adapts U-Net to a particular dataset, for glioma segmentation [10–13]. To be specific, Isensee et al. utilized nnU-Net with region-based training [11], Luu et al. extended the U-Net architecture with a larger encoder and added axial attention [12], Zeineldin et al. ensembled nnU-Net and other two CNN networks for more accurate segmentation of glioma [13], Wu et al. proposed the TISS-Net that obtains the synthesized target modality and segmentation of brain tumors end-to-end with high performance [14]. However, for pediatric brain tumors, there are only a handful of dedicated automatic segmentation tools, some of them are developed based on 2D images which ignore the volumetric information of MRI, and others only focus on one modality (e.g. T2 fluid attenuated inversion recovery (FLAIR)) [15–17]. In this work, we aim to extend nnUNet with 3D configuration for pediatric brain tumor segmentation.

Self-supervised learning is a type of machine learning strategy that has gained more and more popularity in recent years. Pretraining a model based on such self-supervision can get useful weights to initialize the subsequent model for downstream tasks based on data with limited labels [18]. Given sparse labeled medical data, diverse self-supervised pre-training strategies [18–20] enhance global and local medical image feature understanding, yielding favorable outcomes. Inspired by this, we adopted self-supervised pre-training to bolster our network's grasp of global and local tumor features.

Furthermore, medical image segmentation commonly employs Dice loss for network optimization [21]. Yet, the heterogeneity and size imbalance across tissue regions hinder Dice loss from effectively leveraging region-specific information. In response, Chen et al. introduced adaptive region-specific loss [22] for medical image segmentation. Given the heterogeneity of pediatric brain tumors, this loss could augment network predictions. Considering that pediatric brain tumors are also heterogeneous, adaptive region-specific loss might assist the prediction of the network.

For our entry to the challenge, we extended the nnUNet in two aspects. Firstly, we employed and improved self-supervised training strategies of the Model Genesis [19] to pre-train the network with given BraTS-PEDs 2023 data (no additional public and/or private data). Secondly, we integrated the adaptive region-specific loss [22] during the training of the segmentation task. Experiment results with validation data from the online evaluation platform showed that our method has a positive impact on the network performance.

2 Materials and Methods

2.1 Dataset

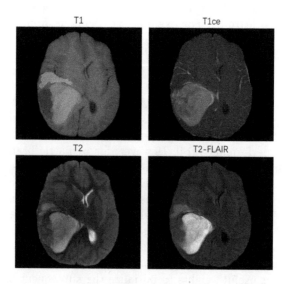

Fig. 1. Axial slices from one subject (BraTS-PED-00004) representing the four different sequences with segmentation labels for the 3 tumor sub-regions on the T1 image. Blue: enhancing tumor (ET), red: non-enhancing Component (NC), green: edema (ED). (Color figure online)

A retrospective multi-institutional cohort of multi-parametric MRI scans from 228 patients with pediatric high-grade glioma was chosen for the BraTS-PEDs 2023 competition, and they were divided into three datasets: 99 cases for training, 45 cases for validation at the online evaluation platform, and 84 cases for the private leaderboard and final ranking of the participants. The dataset included four MRI sequences: pre- and post-gadolinium T1-weighted (T1 and T1ce), T2-weighted (T2), and T2-weighted fluid-attenuated inversion recovery (T2-FLAIR) images. To generate the definitive labels of the data, two automated deep learning segmentation models [23,24] were employed initially to produce original segmentations, and three attending board-certified neuroradiologists reviewed the segmentations. This process was followed iteratively until the approvers found the refined tumor subregion segmentations acceptable for public release and the challenge conduction. The final labels for the segmentation tasks included enhancing tumor (ET), non-enhancing component (NC), and edema (ED). All the MRI scans were preprocessed with a conversion of the DICOM files to the NIfTI file format, co-registration to the same anatomical template (SRI24), resampling to an isotropic resolution (1 mm^3), and skull-stripping. Slices representing the four sequences of a patient's MRI scans are depicted in Fig. 1.

For the BraTS meningioma challenge 2023, there are 1000 cases for training and 141 cases for online evaluation, respectively. The dataset included the same four MRI sequences as the BraTS-PEDs dataset, and the labels of data included enhancing tumor (ET), non-enhancing tumor core (NT), and edema (ED). All the MRI scans were preprocessed with the same procedure as BraTS-PEDs.

2.2 Methods

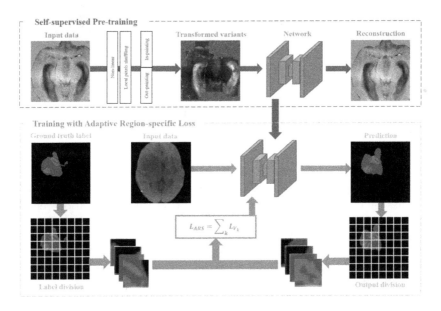

Fig. 2. The workflow of our work. The blue dashed box illustrated the self-supervised pre-training of the network, and the orange dashed box illustrated segmentation task training with adaptive region-specific loss. (Color figure online)

This section will describe the details of our methods, including two modifications we made to nnU-Net for better performance on pediatric brain tumors and meningioma. We utilize self-supervised pre-training strategies to enrich the network's comprehension of both local and global features and leverage adaptive region-specific loss to bolster the network's ability to learn from critical regions (Fig. 2).

Self-supervised Pre-training. Model Genesis learns from scratch on unlabeled images, with an objective to yield a common visual representation that is generalizable and transferable across diseases, organs, and modalities [19]. In our method, we use similar self-supervised training strategies as the Model Genesis to pre-train the model with the provided BraTS PEDs 2023 dataset. Throughout pre-training, the model reconstructs original patches from their transformed variants, thereby imbibing the appearance, texture, and context of 3D pediatric brain tumor images. The transformed variants can be generated following the transformations in Fig. 3.

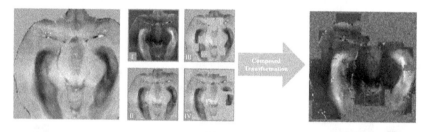

Fig. 3. The transformations made to the original patch during the pre-training. I:Non-linear transformation, II:local pixels shuffling, III: in-painting, IV: out-painting. By randomly composing those transformations to get the transformed variants of the original patch.

Learning Appearance via Non-linear Transformation. Absolute or relative intensity values of pixels in medical images contain crucial information reflecting structures and organs. We integrate the Bézier Curve - a smooth, monotonous transformation function, which assigns every pixel a unique value, ensuring a one-to-one mapping. This approach encourages self-supervised pre-training to focus on acquiring knowledge about organ appearance, encompassing shape and intensity distribution. Figure 3-I shows an example of non-linear transformation.

Learning Texture via Local Pixel Shuffling. Local pixel shuffling entails sampling a window from a patch and rearranging pixels, creating a transformed patch. Window size is smaller than the model's receptive field, preserving global content. Unlike PatchShuffling, local pixels shuffling can prompt the model to remember local textures and boundaries. Figure 3-II shows a local shuffling example.

Learning Context via Out-Painting and in-Painting. For self-supervised learning, out-painting involves layering windows of varied sizes to create a complex shape. Pixels outside the window get random values, while inner pixels retain the original intensities. In in-painting, outer intensities remain, and inner ones are set to random values. Those two strategies encourage the model to grasp global geometry (out-painting) and local continuity (in-painting). See Fig. 3-III and Fig. 3-IV for in-painting and out-painting examples.

Those four kinds of transformations will be randomly composed to generate transformed variants, and the pre-training model will learn the features of the dataset by reconstructing the image. The mean squared error (MSE) loss is used for the optimization of the pre-training model, for a given volume V it can be calculated as follow:

$$L_{MSE} = \frac{1}{n} \sum_{i \in V} (g_i - p_i)^2 \quad (1)$$

where i is the voxel index, n is the number of the voxels, g_i is the untransfromed image and p_i is the prediction of the model.

Training with Adaptive Region-Specific Loss. Our work builds upon nnU-Net [10], the core of which is a 3D-Uet that has an encoder-decoder structure with skip connections linking the two pathways. The number of convolutional filters was initialized at 32, 64, 128, 256, and 320 for every reduction of resolution. The weights of the pre-trained model's encoder and decoder will be loaded into the segmentation model, facilitating further training for tumor segmentation. Leveraging the pre-trained model, the network will gain enhanced insight into both local and global characteristics intrinsic to pediatric brain tumors. It is worth noting that nnU-Net facilitates region-based training, this entails the network utilizing region labels (e.g., WT comprising ET, NC, and ED) during training, in contrast to the traditional approach involving mutually exclusive tumor sub-region labels (ET, NC, and ED).

The nnU-Net employs the conventional Dice loss function for segmentation loss computation, yet this approach presents two primary drawbacks. Firstly, it assigns equal weight to all input volume regions, disregarding MRI heterogeneity, where only a part of regions will significantly impact network performance. Secondly, it treats FP and FN errors with equal emphasis. In medical image segmentation, FN errors tend to outweigh FP errors due to the limited segmentation target size, causing an imbalance in error types. To enhance nnU-Net performance, our work introduces an adaptive region-specific loss. This approach acknowledges the unique characteristics of different regions and addresses the FN error prevalence in medical image segmentation [22].

The computation of the adaptive region-specific loss involves three sequential steps. Firstly, the network output and corresponding segmentation label are partitioned into several sub-regions (e.g., $8 \times 8 \times 8$ in our study). Subsequently, for a given sub-region V_k, there are two main coefficients based on the fraction of FP and FN errors will be calculated as follows:

$$\alpha = A + B \cdot \frac{FP}{FP + FN}$$
$$= A + B \cdot \frac{\sum_{i \in V_k} p_i(1-g_i) + \varepsilon}{\sum_{i \in V_k} p_i(1-g_i) + \sum_{i \in V_k}(1-p_i)g_i + \varepsilon} \quad (2)$$

$$\beta = A + B \cdot \frac{FN}{FP + FN}$$
$$= A + B \cdot \frac{\sum_{i \in V_k}(1-p_i)g_i + \varepsilon}{\sum_{i \in V_k} p_i(1-g_i) + \sum_{i \in V_k}(1-p_i)g_i + \varepsilon} \quad (3)$$

A and B are two constant scalers. The adaptive coefficients α and β will be used to control the magnitude of the penalty for FP and FN, respectively. Lastly, these adaptive coefficients are employed to compute the adaptive loss for each individual sub-region. The cumulative loss across all sub-regions yields the adaptive region-specific loss, serving as a foundational element for subsequent training enhancements

$$L_{ARS} = \sum_k (1 - \frac{\sum_{i \in V_k} p_i g_i + \varepsilon}{\sum_{i \in V_k} p_i g_i + \alpha \sum_{i \in V_k} p_i(1-g_i) + \beta \sum_{i \in V_k}(1-p_i)g_i + \varepsilon}) \quad (4)$$

Cross-entropy loss is one of the most representative loss functions for the segmentation task, it can measure the pixel-wise difference between the two inputs, for a volume V, its L_{CE} can be calculated as:

$$L_{CE} = -\sum_{i \in V} g_i \log p_i \quad (5)$$

For the training, a combination of cross-entropy loss and adaptive region-specific loss will be used for the model optimization:

$$L = \lambda L_{ARS} + L_{CE} \quad (6)$$

where λ correspond to the weights of the L_{ARS}.

3 Experiments and Results

3.1 Implementation Details

For the pre-training of the model, all the BraTS PEDsa 2023 training datasets were used for self-supervised training, and the validation was done on the training dataset as well. No additional data augmentations were employed, aside from the resize and crop transformations facilitated by the nnUNet framework and the transformations outlined in Model Genesis [19]. This procedure last 500 epochs, with each epoch consisting of 250 minibatches. The validation loss was used to monitor the training progress, model with the lowest validation loss was used as the pre-trained model for the segmentation task training.

There are two notable improvements we have made to the original Model Genesis self-supervised training strategies. (1) We perform sub-volume extraction and transformations during training, in contrast to completing these steps prior to training as Model Genesis did. This modification expands the diversity of transformed sub-volumes, enriching the learning process. (2) We fine-tune transformation parameters to optimize pre-training performance on the BraTS PEDs 2023 dataset. *e.g.*, shrinking the size and increasing the number of out-painting blocks to ensure the preservation of tumors instead of complete erasure. These refinements collectively bolster the efficacy of our approach.

For the segmentation task training, we followed the training framework of nnUNet with 5-fold cross-validation. To bolster generalization, on-the-fly data augmentation was implemented during training, encompassing random rotation, scaling, Gaussian noise, Gaussian blur, contrast adjustments, additive brightness variation, and gamma scaling. Inspired by the winner of BraTS 2021, the batch adaptive region-specific loss was used instead of the sample adaptive region-specific loss [12]. For the internal 5-fold cross-validation and online valuation, each training run lasted 300 epochs, and for the testing on unseen data, each training run lasted 1000 epochs, with each epoch consisting of 250 minibatches. The Dice score on the validation set of each fold was used to monitor the training progress. We set the constant coefficients A and B at 0.3 and 0.4 for the calculation of adaptive region-specific loss.

For both pre-training and segmentation task training, the batch size was set to 2, the patch size was set to 128 × 128 × 128, the networks were optimized with stochastic gradient descent with a Nesterov momentum of 0.99, The initial learning rate was 0.01 and was decayed following a polynomial schedule:

$$lr = 0.01 \times (1 - \frac{epoch\_id}{epoch\_num})^{0.9} \qquad (7)$$

The training setting of the BraTS meningioma challenge [25] is mostly the same as the BraTS-PEDs challenge, except that we set the patch size to 128 × 160 × 112, and we train the model for 1000 epochs and only validate it on the online evaluation platform.

All experiments were conducted with Pytorch 2.0.1 on NVIDIA RTX 2080 Ti GPU with 11 GB VRAM and NVIDIA RTX 3090 GPU with 24GB VRAM. The final model will be wrapped in MLCube and submitted to MedPerf [26] for testing.

3.2 Quantitative Results

The following models were developed to enable comprehensive evaluation and comparison, considering different configurations and strategies: (1) BL: baseline nnUNet, without pre-trained weights. (2) BL + L_{ARS}: baseline nnUNet with adaptive region-specific loss, no pre-trained weights. (3) BL + L_{ARS} + pre-train: baseline nnUNet with adaptive region-specific loss and pre-trained weights.

Table 1 and Table 2 showed the Dice and HD95 computed by the online evaluation platform and displayed in the public leaderboard. All predicted segmentation labels were ensembled from 5 folds. Evidently, our approach has demonstrated a large improvement in performance, particularly noteworthy for the ET region, a challenging segment to accurately delineate in pediatric brain tumor segmentation. The results underscore the remarkable strides achieved through our method, as reflected in the improved metrics showcased on the public leaderboard.

Table 1. Dice (%) metrics of the networks on online evaluation platform for BraTS-PEDs challenge. ET: enhancing tumor, NC: non-enhancing component, WT: whole tumor

Model	Lesion-wise Dice (%) ↑		
	ET	NC	WT
BL	51.10 ± 41.77	75.04 ± 22.51	82.26 ± 19.25
BL+L_{ARS}	53.79 ± 42.22	**75.05 ± 21.21**	**83.27 ± 18.30**
BL+L_{ARS}+pre-train	**59.63 ± 42.02**	74.06 ± 23.54	82.68 ± 19.39

Table 2. HD95 (mm) metrics of the networks on online evaluation platform for BraTS-PEDs challenge. ET: enhancing tumor, NC: non-enhancing component, WT: whole tumor

Model	Lesion-wise HD95 (mm) ↓		
	ET	NC	WT
BL	145.58 ± 170.16	34.37 ± 77.96	26.45 ± 70.91
BL+L_{ARS}	135.94 ± 171.67	**25.49 ± 65.91**	**22.35 ± 66.45**
BL+L_{ARS}+pre-train	**121.02 ± 163.24**	29.22 ± 70.34	22.85 ± 66.47

We also validate our method on the BraTS meningioma challenge and the Table 3 has shown that our method can achieve satisfactory results on this dataset.

3.3 Qualitative Results

Figure 4 shows the different models' predictions on BraTS-PED-00003. It's obvious that all the methods failed to predict the edema, that's mainly because the edema is not the label of the final prediction, instead, edema is included in WT. By adding adaptive region-specific loss and self-supervised pre-training subsequently, the prediction of the whole region was improved. Besides, the BL + L_{ARS} + pre-train can achieve the best performance on the ET, which showed the superiority of our method.

Table 3. Dice (%) and HD95 (mm) metrics of the networks on online evaluation platform for BraTS meningioma challenge with BL+L_{ARS}+pre-train. NT: the non-enhancing tumor core, ED: edema, ET: enhancing tumor

Metric	NT	ED	ET
Lesion-wise Dice (%)	79.69 ± 29.56	80.61 ± 28.92	79.97 ± 28.73
Lesion-wise HD95 (mm)	49.37 ± 109.35	47.18 ± 107.25	47.38 ± 106.13

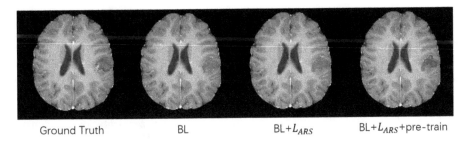

Ground Truth   BL   BL+L_{ARS} BL+L_{ARS}+pre-train

Fig. 4. Different models' predictions of the BraTS-PED-00003 on the T1ce sequence. Blue: enhancing tumor (ET), red: non-enhancing Component (NC), green: edema (ED). (Color figure online)

4 Discussion

Our approach incorporates self-supervised techniques inspired by Model Genesis [19] for model pre-training. Yet, a plethora of alternative self-supervised strategies remains unexplored, potentially offering superior pre-training solutions for pediatric brain tumor and meningioma segmentation. Furthermore, acknowledging the presence of noisy labels in the provided datasets, we recognize the potential for performance enhancement through denoising methods such as label smoothing or knowledge distillation. These avenues warrant further exploration to amplify network performance and label quality.

5 Conclusion

In this paper, we proposed a nnU-Net based method for the BraTS-PEDs 2023 challenge. Drawing inspiration from recent BraTS winners' methodologies and an assessment of pediatric brain tumor MRI quality, we extended the nnU-Net framework in two aspects. Self-supervised training strategies from Model Genesis are applied and improved by us to pre-train the network with BraTS PEDs 2023 training dataset. Pre-training can help the network to gain more local and global features of the images, which will assist in further segmentation task training. Besides, the adaptive region-specific loss is added into the nnU-Net to replace the conventional Dice loss, helping the network to focus on the regions that contribute more to the performance. The experiment results on the online evaluation platform have affirmed the efficacy of our approach. The presented methods significantly enhance the nnU-Net's ability to deliver more satisfactory outcomes in pediatric brain tumor segmentation.

Acknowledgements. This work was supported in part by the National Natural Science Foundation of China under Grant 62271115, and in part by the Fundamental Research Funds for the Central Universities under Grant ZYGX2022YGRH019.

References

1. Hargrave, D., Bartels, U., Bouffet, E.: Diffuse brainstem glioma in children: critical review of clinical trials. Lancet Oncol. **7**(3), 241–248 (2006)
2. Jansen, M.H.A., Van Vuurden, D.G., Vandertop, W.P., Kaspers, G.J.L.: Diffuse intrinsic pontine gliomas: a systematic update on clinical trials and biology. Cancer Treat. Rev. **38**(1), 27–35 (2012)
3. Menze, B.H., et al.: The multimodal brain tumor image segmentation benchmark (BRATS). IEEE Trans. Med. Imaging **34**(10), 1993–2024 (2014)
4. Yang, S., Guo, D., Wang, L., Wang, G.: Cascaded coarse-to-fine neural network for brain tumor segmentation. In: Brainlesion: Glioma, Multiple Sclerosis, Stroke and Traumatic Brain Injuries, pp. 458–469. Springer (2021)
5. Wang, G., Li, W., Ourselin, S., Vercauteren, T.: Automatic brain tumor segmentation based on cascaded convolutional neural networks with uncertainty estimation. Front. Comput. Neurosci. **13**, 56 (2019)
6. Bakas, S., et al. Identifying the best machine learning algorithms for brain tumor segmentation, progression assessment, and overall survival prediction in the BRATS challenge. arXiv:1811.02629 (2018)
7. Baid, U., et al. The RSNA-ASNR-MICCAI BRATS 2021 benchmark on brain tumor segmentation and radiogenomic classification. arXiv:2107.02314 (2021)
8. Kazerooni, A.F., et al.: The brain tumor segmentation (BraTS) challenge 2023: Focus on pediatrics (CBTN-CONNECT-DIPGR-ASNR-MICCAI BraTS-PEDs). arXiv:2305.17033 (2023)
9. Bakas, S., et al.: GLISTRboost: combining multimodal MRI segmentation, registration, and biophysical tumor growth modeling with gradient boosting machines for glioma segmentation. In: Brainlesion: Glioma, Multiple Sclerosis, Stroke and Traumatic Brain Injuries, pp. 144–155. Springer (2016)
10. Isensee, F., Jaeger, P.F., Kohl, S.A.A., Petersen, J., Maier-Hein, K.H.: nnU-net: a self-configuring method for deep learning-based biomedical image segmentation. Nat. Methods **18**(2), 203–211 (2021)
11. Isensee, F., Jäger, P.F., Full, P.M., Vollmuth, P.: nnU-net for brain tumor segmentation, pp. 118–132. Springer (2021)
12. Luu, H.M., Park, S.-H.: Extending nn-UNet for brain tumor segmentation. In: International MICCAI Brainlesion Workshop, pp. 173–186. Springer (2021)
13. Zeineldin, R.A., Karar, M.E., Burgert, O., Mathis-Ullrich, F.: Multimodal CNN networks for brain tumor segmentation in MRI: a BraTS 2022 challenge solution. arXiv:2212.09310 (2022)
14. Jianghao, W., et al.: TISS-net: brain tumor image synthesis and segmentation using cascaded dual-task networks and error-prediction consistency. Neurocomputing **544**, 126295 (2023)

15. Nalepa, J., et al.: Segmenting pediatric optic pathway gliomas from MRI using deep learning. Comput. Biol. Med. **142**, 105237 (2022)
16. Jansen, M.H., et al.: Survival prediction model of children with diffuse intrinsic pontine glioma based on clinical and radiological criteria. Neuro-Oncol. **17**(1), 160–166 (2015)
17. Peng, J., et al.: Deep learning-based automatic tumor burden assessment of pediatric high-grade gliomas, medulloblastomas, and other leptomeningeal seeding tumors. Neuro-Oncol. **24**(2), 289–299 (2022)
18. Chen, L., Bentley, P., Mori, K., Misawa, K., Fujiwara, M., Rueckert, D.: Self-supervised learning for medical image analysis using image context restoration. Med. Image Anal. **58**, 101539 (2019)
19. Zhou, Z., et al.: Models genesis: generic autodidactic models for 3D medical image analysis. In: Medical Image Computing and Computer Assisted Intervention–MICCAI 2019, pp. 384–393. Springer (2019)
20. Gao, Y., Wang, H., Liu, X., Huang, N., Wang, G., Zhang, S.: A denoising self-supervised approach for COVID-19 pneumonia lesion segmentation with limited annotated CT images. In: 2021 43rd Annual International Conference of the IEEE Engineering in Medicine & Biology Society (EMBC), pp. 3705–3708. IEEE (2021)
21. Ma, J., et al.: Loss odyssey in medical image segmentation. Med. Image Anal. **71**, 102035 (2021)
22. Chen, Y., et al.: Adaptive region-specific loss for improved medical image segmentation. IEEE Trans. Pattern Anal. Mach. Intell. (2023)
23. Kazerooni, A.F., et al.: Automated tumor segmentation and brain tissue extraction from multiparametric MRI of pediatric brain tumors: a multi-institutional study. Neuro-Oncol. Adv. **5**(1), vdad027 (2023)
24. Liu, X., et al.: From adult to pediatric: deep learning-based automatic segmentation of rare pediatric brain tumors. In: Society of Photo-Optical Instrumentation Engineers (SPIE) Conference Series, vol. 12465, p. 1246505 (2023)
25. LaBella, D., et al.: The ASNR-MICCAI brain tumor segmentation (BraTS) challenge 2023: Intracranial meningioma. arXiv:2305.07642 (2023)
26. Karargyris, A., et al.: Federated benchmarking of medical artificial intelligence with MedPerf. Nat. Mach. Intell. 1–12 (2023)

BraSyn 2023 Challenge: Missing MRI Synthesis and the Effect of Different Learning Objectives

Ivo M. Baltruschat[✉], Parvaneh Janbakhshi, and Matthias Lenga

Bayer AG, Müllerstr. 178, 13353 Berlin, Germany
{ivo.baltruschat,parvaneh.janbakhshi,matthias.lenga}@bayer.com

Abstract. This work addresses the Brain Magnetic Resonance Image Synthesis for Tumor Segmentation (BraSyn) challenge, which was hosted as part of the Brain Tumor Segmentation (BraTS) challenge in 2023. In this challenge, researchers are invited to synthesize a missing magnetic resonance image sequence, given other available sequences, to facilitate tumor segmentation pipelines trained on complete sets of image sequences. This problem can be tackled using deep learning within the framework of paired image-to-image translation. In this study, we propose investigating the effectiveness of a commonly used deep learning framework, such as Pix2Pix, trained under the supervision of different image-quality loss functions. Our results indicate that the use of different loss functions significantly affects the synthesis quality. We systematically study the impact of various loss functions in the multi-sequence MR image synthesis setting of the BraSyn challenge. Furthermore, we demonstrate how image synthesis performance can be optimized by combining different learning objectives beneficially.

1 Introduction

Automatic localization and segmentation of brain tumors in magnetic resonance imaging (MRI) has been an emerging research area that aims to provide clinicians with efficient and objective aid in diagnosing and monitoring patients. Tumor biological properties can be captured differently depending on the MRI sequence. Therefore, many of the recent deep learning-based segmentation algorithms require multiple input MRI sequences during the inference stage, e.g., typically T1-weighted images with and without contrast enhancement (T1-N and T1-C, respectively), T2-Weighted (T2-W) images, and T2-FLAIR (T2-F) images. However, the challenge in such multi-modal approaches arises when an MR sequence is missing due to time constraints and/or motion artifacts.

The *Brain MR Image Synthesis for Tumor Segmentation* (BraSyn) challenge as part of the Brain Tumor Segmentation (BraTS) challenge 2023 provides an opportunity for researchers to address the problem of missing MRI sequence by synthesizing it given multiple available MRI sequences [5]. Therefore, researchers are invited to work on MRI synthesis or MRI image-to-image translation algorithms, the solution of which can later facilitate automatic brain tumor segmentation pipelines where the missing sequence can be substituted by its synthesized counterpart [5]. This work focuses on the BraSyn challenge, where the specific goal is to synthesize one missing MRI sequence given the other three available sequences. The synthesized MRI scans should be perceptually as similar as possible to the missing sequences and provide the necessary information (as in the real missing scans) for a downstream task such as tumor segmentation.

The problem lies in the scope of paired image-to-image translation for either converting MRI sequences to one another or producing a Gadolinium-based contrast agent enhanced post-contrast T1 image from pre-contrast MRI scans. Most recent image synthesis approaches exploit Pix2Pix [4], i.e., U-Net style encoder-decoder architecture trained using different penalties, i.e., loss functions, to encourage appropriate similarities between real and synthesized images. In [12], a Pix2Pix model is used to synthesize T2-F and T2-W images from T1-w images by incorporating edge information into the typical loss functions used in Pix2Pix (i.e., adversarial and L1 norm) to enforce the synthesized image to have a similar edge map as the real image. In [6], the missing data imputation is formulated as a sequence-to-sequence prediction problem, where a sequence of (available) input sequences of variable length can be converted to the sequence of (missing) output sequences using transformer models trained based on a combination of L1 norm and adversarial loss functions.

In the literature, image-to-image translation approaches based on the Pix2Pix model, despite their simplicity, have shown promising performance in many applications. However, depending on the synthesis task, the networks have been trained under the supervision of a wide range of image-quality loss functions, which makes it difficult to interpret the contributions of each proposed architecture variant decoupled from the effects of the different training objectives.

Addressing the BraSyn challenge, in this work, we proposed to investigate the effectiveness of a commonly used deep learning image-to-image translation approach, such as Pix2Pix trained under the supervision of different image-quality loss functions. The right choice of loss function dictates the quality of synthetic images and can be crucial for the convergence of the network, in particular in scenarios with limited availability of training data. We aim to establish a baseline framework for the task at hand while providing a comprehensive comparison and benchmarking of different training procedures for brain MRI sequence synthesis (which is lacking in the literature) and validating the effectiveness of each against the evaluation scenarios considered by the challenge organizers.

We aim to investigate the contributions of various loss functions to the synthesis of realistic brain MRI images. Specifically, we consider loss functions based on pixel-to-pixel similarities (e.g., $\mathcal{L}_1$ norm and its variants), adversarial training, Structural Similarity Index (SSIM), frequency domain consistency, and latent feature (VGG-based perceptual) consistency. Experimentally, we will verify which loss function guides the network to produce more realistic images.

Furthermore, we aim to investigate whether there are any differences among the synthesized sequences with respect to the loss functions used. By combining different loss functions, we demonstrate the possibility of achieving more optimal image synthesis performance.

2 Method

This section describes the dataset, the synthesis framework, i.e., the network architecture, its training procedure based on different loss functions, and the inference procedure. Our general synthesis framework, i.e., training and inference stages, are depicted in Fig. 1.

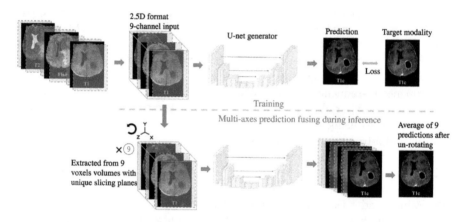

Fig. 1. The used synthesis framework for predicting an exemplary target sequence, e.g., T1-C from input sequences, i.e., T1-N, T2-W, and T2-F

2.1 Dataset

The BraSyn-2023 dataset is based on the RSNA-ASNR-MICCAI BraTS 2021 dataset [5], which includes collections of brain tumor MRI scans from various institutions and annotated tumor subregions. For training data, 1251 scans with four complete image sequences along with their respective segmentation labels are available, i.e., i) pre-contrast T1-weighted (T1-N), ii) post-contrast T1-weighted (T1-C), iii) T2-Weighted (T2-W), and iv) T2 fluid-attenuated inversion recovery (T2-F). In the validation and test sets (including 219 and 570 scans, respectively), a single sequence out of the four sequences will be randomly omitted with the objective of being synthesized. All BraSyn scans have undergone standardized pre-processing according to [5].

2.2 Networks

Synthesis (Generator) Network. Due to promising results of U-net style networks in literature [3], we adapted an architecture from [10] where we used 8 layers of 3 × 3 convolutions with stride 2, each followed by Mish activation function and finally a CeLU activation function for the output layer.

Assuming all MRI sequences are co-registered and after applying appropriate normalization (as detailed in Sect. 2.3), we adapted a multi-slice training procedure in which the input images are arranged in the format of a stack of 2.5D slices, along either the axial, sagittal, or coronal planes (cf. Sect. 2.3). 2.5D input slices, unlike processing 2D slices, provide some additional spatial information and context from the 3D brain. To create the 2.5D input images for each "slice of interest" in all three available MRI sequences, three consecutive slices (providing context information from two neighboring slices of the "slice of interest") are considered. After channel-wise stacking, this forms a 9-channel input image. We added zero slices for regions outside of the original volume for edge slices. The 2.5D stack of the three available MRI sequences is fed into the generator to synthesize the corresponding central slice, i.e., the "slice of interest," from the missing sequence (i.e., target). Therefore, we trained four separate networks to synthesize each missing sequence (T1-N, T1-C, T2-W, or T2-F scans).

Models trained using 2.5D image stacks do not fully account for the continuity in a 3D MRI volume. This can lead to specific synthesizing artifacts, which can be spotted by local structure inconsistency or global brightness changes. To alleviate the discontinuity problem in the output of our models, during inference, we incorporated the multi-axes prediction fusing approach mentioned in Sect. 2.4. Also, unlike models operating on full 3D volumes, they need less GPU memory and have more training data available.

We denote the mapping from the input domain X to the target domain Y using the synthesis or generator model by $G : X \rightarrow Y$, where the synthesized output $\hat{y} = G(x)$, $x \in R^{K_1 \times K_2 \times 9}$ and $\hat{y}, y \in R^{K_1 \times K_2}$, and K_1 and K_2 are dimensions of image slices.

Discriminator. In the case of using adversarial training, we also adopted a patch-wise discriminator from PatchGAN in [4] where we used a 5 layer discriminator with additional series of spectral normalization [8] to stabilize the training further. The discriminator is trained with the mean square loss function. As the discriminator is meant to distinguish between the synthesized and real images of the target, it takes two input slices of the target and synthesized images. We denote the discriminator function as D.

2.3 Training

Being provided by a training set for the challenge (cf. Sect. 2.1), we further split the training set into *train* subset of 1125 scan series for model training and *development* subset of 126 scan series for monitoring the training. We applied a histogram standardization [9] on all scans. For each sequence, the training set is used to find the intensity landmarks. Furthermore, on each set of input voxel series (i.e., 3 voxels) and the target (to be predicted) voxel, MinMax intensity scaling has also been applied to re-scale the range of the input voxel sets and target voxels to intensity range of $[0, 1]$ separately. During the inference, the normalization scale applied to the input series is used to re-scale the normalized predicted scans to the original intensity range, i.e., $[0, \inf]$.

To augment the training data, we sliced the scans in axial, sagittal, and corona planes, which, after removing all-zero slices, resulted in $502,971$ *training* and $56,270$ *development* slices. Furthermore, we also applied online random cropping to 256×256 (after initially zero-padding all slices to 288×288), random horizontal flipping (with a probability of $p = 0.5$), and random rotations in the range of $[-15, 15]$ degrees (with $p = 0.5$).

Our models are trained using the ADAM optimizer with $beta_1 = 0.5$, $beta_2 = 0.99$, an initial learning rate of 0.0001, and a batch size of 64. We reduced the learning rate by a factor of two every 10 epochs and trained the networks for a total of 100 epochs, where $400,000$ training images are used in each epoch.

In this work, we investigated the impact of different synthesis loss functions to train networks to predict each missing sequence, where, in the following, the considered loss functions are briefly introduced.

L1 Loss. L1 norm is the commonly used synthesis loss function in which the mean absolute error between the synthesized and target images is computed with the assumption that the images are well (pixel-to-pixel) aligned.

$$\mathcal{L}_1 = \mathbb{E}_{x,y} |y - G(x)| \tag{1}$$

Masked L1 Loss. $\mathcal{L}_1$ is being computed globally on the whole image (cf. Eq. 1), while one of the problems in brain tumor segmentation is that lesions affect a small portion of the brain. Therefore, for more precise synthesis of tumor regions, the $\mathcal{L}_1$ can be modified to penalize errors in tumor regions and healthy regions of the brain separately, since the segmentation mask for each input series is also available during training. Let M_x^t denote a binary mask around the tumor for each input x. After multiplying $G(x)$ and y by M_x^t and $M_x^h = 1 - M_x^t$, respectively, the corresponding masked tumor and healthy regions are denoted by $G(x)^t$ and y^t and $G(x)^h$ and y^h giving the following loss terms for each region:

$$\mathcal{L}_1^t = \mathbb{E}_{x,y} |y^t - G(x)^t| / |M_x^t|, \tag{2}$$

$$\mathcal{L}_1^h = \mathbb{E}_{x,y} |y^h - G(x)^h| / |M_x^h|, \tag{3}$$

$$\mathcal{L}_1^M = w\mathcal{L}_1^t + (1-w)\mathcal{L}_1^h, \tag{4}$$

where w is the weighting factor to control the contributions of loss terms corresponding to tumor and healthy regions. Here, we used $w = 0.5$.

Adversarial Loss. Adversarial loss has been widely used to improve the overall perceptual quality of synthesized images by overcoming the blurriness produced by L1 norm and capturing high-frequency structures [4]. Adversarial training is achieved through the min-max optimization objective as in [7], where, in practice, the optimal parameters of G and D are approximated using an alternating training procedure. Motivated by the improvement of training stability, in our experiments, we used adversarial training in the least squares GAN (LSGAN) [7] framework resulting in the loss functions:

$$\mathcal{L}_{adv}^{D} = \mathbb{E}_y(D(y) - 1)^2 + \mathbb{E}_x(D(G(x))^2, \quad (5)$$
$$\mathcal{L}_{adv}^{G} = \mathbb{E}_x(D(G(x)) - 1)^2 \quad (6)$$

SSIM Loss. Motivated by considering image structures in the loss function (unlike pixel-wise criterion such as L1 loss) and improving the perceptual quality of synthesized images, SSIM loss has also been introduced and exploited for similar tasks in [13]:

$$\mathcal{L}_{SSIM} = \mathbb{E}_{x,y}|1 - SSIM(y, G(x))| \quad (7)$$

Therefore, in this work, the effectiveness of SSIM loss has also been investigated. For our experiments, we set the kernel size to 11 required for SSIM computation [13].

Perceptual VGG Loss. We also investigated a new variant of the perceptual loss [11], the VGG conv-based perceptual loss [14], which has been reported to be effective in enhancing image synthesis perceptual quality. Here, we used the pre-trained VGG-19 version, and the perceptual loss is defined as

$$\mathcal{L}_{VGG} = \sum_{l \in \{2,7,14,21,28\}} |\lambda_l \left[\phi_l^{\text{conv}}(G(x)) - \phi_l^{\text{conv}}(y)\right]|^2, \quad (3)$$

where $G(x)$ and y are the synthesized and target image, respectively. ϕ_l^{conv} denotes the feature maps of the l-th convolutional layer of the pre-trained VGG-19. λ_l are set to be 0.0002, 0.0001, 0.0001, 0.0002, and 0.0005.

Frequency Loss. Motivated by [3], we also investigated the frequency-based training objective to enhance the image translation process by directly regulating the consistency of information in low and high-frequency domains:

$$\mathcal{L}_{Freq} = \mathbb{E}_{x,y}||\mathcal{F}(y)| \odot M_r - |\mathcal{F}(G(x))| \odot M_r| \\ + \mathbb{E}_{x,y}||\mathcal{F}(y)| \odot \overline{M_r} - |\mathcal{F}(G(x))| \odot \overline{M_r}|, \quad (8)$$

where $|\mathcal{F}(.)|$ denotes the magnitude of discrete Fourier transform. M_r denotes a binary mask such that the circular region around the origin with radius r is set to 1 (capturing low-frequency information) while its inverse (capturing high-frequency information) is denoted as $\overline{M_r} := 1 - M_r$ with $\odot$ denoting the

Hadamard product. Intuitively, the low-frequency components of the loss function are meant to dictate the consistency of information, such as image brightness. On the contrary, the high-frequency components correspond to consistency in sharp edges and more fine-grained details of images [3]. Similarly to [3], we set $r = 21$ in our experiments.

2.4 Inference

Our models synthesize slices of MRI images independently of each other. Therefore, after concatenating the slices to form the 3D volume, strong discontinuities may be observed along different axes, which impairs the entire image synthesis quality. Therefore, we adapt the multi-axes prediction fusing from [1,2] during inference. In multi-axes prediction fusing, the input volume is reformatted into three principal axes (having three different slicing planes) where each is rotated (using interpolation) along two of the principal axes (by 45°) to produce overall 9 volumes with unique slicing planes. The final synthesized image is computed by taking the mean of the 9 reformatted volumes after rotating back to the original acquisition plane [1].

3 Experiments and Results

This section describes the preliminary results obtained using synthesis networks trained under the supervision of multiple losses for different sequence synthesis tasks. Our experiments are structured as follows. First, we investigated the effect of $\mathcal{L}_1$ and $\mathcal{L}_1^M$ on the synthesizing of each sequence. Secondly, we combined $\mathcal{L}_1^M$ with each of the more advanced loss functions such as $\mathcal{L}_{adv}$, $\mathcal{L}_{SSIM}$, $\mathcal{L}_{VGG}$, and $\mathcal{L}_{Freq}$. Finally, we trained on a tuned combined loss $\mathcal{L}_{\text{combined}} = 5\mathcal{L}_1^M + \mathcal{L}_{adv} + \mathcal{L}_{SSIM} + \mathcal{L}_{VGG} + \mathcal{L}_{Freq}$.

For the evaluation of the quality of the synthesized images for each of the four tasks, similar to the evaluation metric used by the challenge organizers, we used the calculated SSIM and PSNR scores in the tumor (denoted as SSIM^t and PSNR^t, respectively) and healthy areas of the brain (denoted as SSIM^h and PSNR^h, respectively). All models are evaluated on our *development* set with 126 scans (which were not used in training). Since the validation phase of the challenge was closed during the submission of the article (because of multiple timeline changes), we cannot report segmentation dice scores or SSIM scores on the validation set. In Sect. 3.3, we report the final test results of the challenge organizers. Due to time constraints, our final submission to the challenge included four models (i.e., one model for each type of sequence) that were trained with $\mathcal{L}_{\text{combined}}$.

3.1 Results and Discussion

In Table 1 the results of training with $\mathcal{L}_1$ or $\mathcal{L}_1^M$ for each sequence are shown. For T1-synN and T2-synW, $\mathcal{L}_1$ performed constantly better than $\mathcal{L}_1^M$ in all four measurements. For T2-synF, $\mathcal{L}_1$ slightly exceeds $\mathcal{L}_1^M$ based on SSIM, but for PSNR it is the other way around. Finally, T1-synC performed better on three

Table 1. Image quality results for training models (i.e., synthesising T1-synN, T1-synC, T2-synF, or T2-synW) with $\mathcal{L}_1$ or $\mathcal{L}_1^M$, The input to each model are always the other three sequences, e.g., for T1-synN, the input contains information from T1-C, T2-W, and T2-F. Bold text highlights the best result for each sequence

Metric \ Loss func.	T1-synN $\mathcal{L}_1$	T1-synN $\mathcal{L}_1^M$	T1-synC $\mathcal{L}_1$	T1-synC $\mathcal{L}_1^M$	T2-synW $\mathcal{L}_1$	T2-synW $\mathcal{L}_1^M$	T2-synF $\mathcal{L}_1$	T2-synF $\mathcal{L}_1^M$
$SSIM^h$	**0.740**	0.723	**0.755**	0.747	**0.619**	0.581	**0.619**	0.607
$SSIM^t$	**0.709**	0.706	0.626	**0.645**	**0.698**	0.691	**0.698**	**0.698**
$PSNR^h$	**17.96**	17.18	22.54	**23.70**	**14.77**	14.43	17.76	**17.90**
$PSNR^t$	**18.74**	17.83	20.96	**21.92**	**17.56**	16.83	**21.16**	21.02

Table 2. Image quality results for training models by combining $\mathcal{L}_1^M$ with $\mathcal{L}_{adv}$, $\mathcal{L}_{SSIM}$, $\mathcal{L}_{VGG}$, or $\mathcal{L}_{Freq}$. Bold text highlights the overall best score for each metric and each image sequence

Metric \ Loss func.	$\mathcal{L}_1^M + \mathcal{L}_{adv}$	$\mathcal{L}_1^M + \mathcal{L}_{SSIM}$	$\mathcal{L}_1^M + \mathcal{L}_{VGG}$	$\mathcal{L}_1^M + \mathcal{L}_{Freq}$
T1-synN				
$SSIM^h$	0.701	0.729	0.736	**0.742**
$SSIM^t$	0.693	0.698	**0.712**	0.710
$PSNR^h$	15.50	16.60	16.29	**17.72**
$PSNR^t$	16.05	17.09	16.79	**17.98**
T1-synC				
$SSIM^h$	0.747	0.759	0.756	**0.768**
$SSIM^t$	0.644	**0.649**	0.643	0.648
$PSNR^h$	23.20	23.12	23.33	**23.92**
$PSNR^t$	21.67	21.38	21.38	**22.04**
T2-synW				
$SSIM^h$	0.591	0.607	0.616	**0.630**
$SSIM^t$	0.698	0.699	0.710	**0.717**
$PSNR^h$	13.86	13.80	**14.25**	14.14
$PSNR^t$	16.29	16.11	**16.47**	16.40
T2-synF				
$SSIM^h$	0.602	0.608	**0.615**	0.607
$SSIM^t$	**0.714**	0.687	0.698	0.703
$PSNR^h$	**17.51**	17.18	16.93	17.37
$PSNR^t$	**21.13**	20.62	20.70	21.04

out of four scores when trained with $\mathcal{L}_1^M$. We choose for our second evaluation to combine $\mathcal{L}_1^M$ with the more advanced loss function, because it helped to improve the results for the tumor regions. The results in Table 2 show that training a model with $\mathcal{L}_1^M + \mathcal{L}_{Freq}$ helped the most to improve our results for T1-synN, T1-synC, and T1-synW. Only for T2-synF, we can see that the combination of $\mathcal{L}_1^M + \mathcal{L}_{adv}$ has the highest overall score.

3.2 Combined Loss and Submitted Solution

We combined all loss functions mentioned in this work and trained four models (i.e., each synthesizing a different sequence) with the results being presented in Table 3. For our final results, we used tuned weights (based on educated guesses) of each loss term to form the combined loss function. We observe that $SSIM^t$ of T1-synC is generally lower than other sequences, suggesting the difficulty of synthesizing T1-C tumor regions. Visually, this is also confirmed by the randomly selected examples in Fig. 2. T1-synC looks overly bright compared to the orig-

Table 3. Image quality results of synthesis networks for predicting different MRI sequences, i.e., T1-synN, T1-synC, T2-synW, and T2-synF, trained under supervision of a combined loss function

Loss func. \ Metric	T1-synN		T1-synC		T2-synW		T2-synF	
	$SSIM^h$	$SSIM^t$	$SSIM^h$	$SSIM^t$	$SSIM^h$	$SSIM^t$	$SSIM^h$	$SSIM^t$
$\mathcal{L}_{combined}$	0.816	0.771	0.761	0.656	0.754	0.790	0.694	0.733

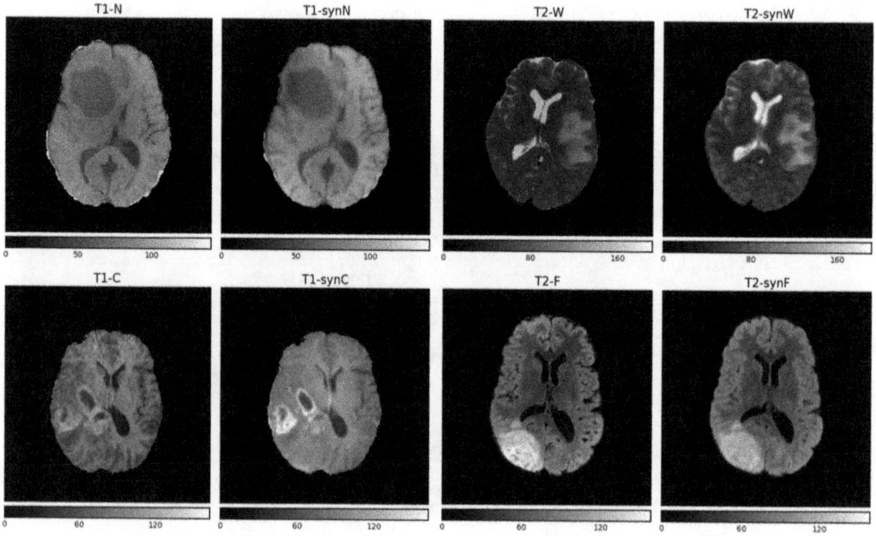

Fig. 2. Randomly selected examples from our *development* set. Each pair (e.g., T1-N and T1-synN) shows the original image and the corresponding synthetic image. All images are histogram normalized and each pair has the same visualisation settings

inal T1-C. However, our model corrected the motion artifacts, which could be advantageous for the downstream segmentation model. For all sequences, we see that $\mathcal{L}_{\text{combined}}$ performed better than the previous results, where we combined two loss functions (cf. Table 2) or trained with a single loss function (cf. Table 2).

3.3 Challenge Results

Figure 3 shows the official results of the segmentation method run on the test set with synthetic volumes. The box plot shows the dice score for each class (i.e., Whole Tumor (WT), Tumor Core (TC), and Enhancing Tumor (ET)). Our winning submission is Team 1. We achieved a median dice of 0.72, 0.78, and 0.44 for ET, TC, and WT, respectively. This was significantly better than the other team. Furthermore, our method had an overall mean SSIM of 0.817 for the test set. The challenge organizers did not provide further stratification of the results.

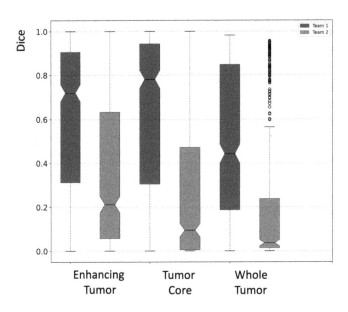

Fig. 3. Dice score results for the test set (reported by challenge organizers). Team 1 is our submitted winning solution

4 Conclusion

Most brain MRI segmentation methods are based on the availability of a certain set of MRI sequences and may fail when one of the MRI sequences is absent. The primary goal of the BraSyn 2023 challenge is to encourage the development of MRI sequence synthesis to estimate the missing sequence for downstream tasks of tumor segmentation. In this work, our aim was to investigate the quality of a deep learning-based MRI synthesis model trained under the supervision of different loss functions. Our preliminary results suggest the importance of choosing the right loss function for the synthesis of the MRI sequences. In the future, we plan to provide a comprehensive comparison between individual and combined loss functions on the quality of image synthesis for each MRI sequence. Furthermore, we plan to release an evaluation framework with improved image quality metrics for synthesized medical images to promote good scientific practice.

References

1. Baltruschat, I.M., et al.: Scaling the U-net: segmentation of biodegradable bone implants in high-resolution synchrotron radiation microtomograms. Sci. Rep. **11**(1), 24237 (2021)
2. Baltruschat, I.M., Janbakhshi, P., Dohmen, M., Lenga, M.: Uncertainty estimation in contrast-enhanced MR image translation with multi-axis fusion (2023)
3. Baltruschat, I.M., Kreis, F., Hoelscher, A., Dohmen, M., Lenga, M.: fRegGAN with k-space loss regularization for medical image translation. arXiv preprint arXiv:2303.15938 (2023)
4. Isola, P., Zhu, J.Y., Zhou, T., Efros, A.A.: Image-to-image translation with conditional adversarial networks. In: Proceedings of the IEEE Conference on Computer Vision and Pattern Recognition, pp. 1125–1134 (2017)
5. Li, H.B., Conte, G.M., Anwar, S.M., Kofler, F., et al.: The brain tumor segmentation (BraTS) challenge 2023: brain MR image synthesis for tumor segmentation (BraSyn) (2023)
6. Liu, J., Pasumarthi, S., Duffy, B., Gong, E., Datta, K., Zaharchuk, G.: One model to synthesize them all: multi-contrast multi-scale transformer for missing data imputation. IEEE Trans. Med. Imaging **42**, 2577–2591 (2023)
7. Mao, X., Li, Q., Xie, H., Lau, R.Y., Wang, Z., Paul Smolley, S.: Least squares generative adversarial networks. In: Proceedings of the IEEE International Conference on Computer Vision, pp. 2794–2802 (2017)
8. Miyato, T., Kataoka, T., Koyama, M., Yoshida, Y.: Spectral normalization for generative adversarial networks. arXiv preprint arXiv:1802.05957 (2018)
9. Nyúl, L.G., Udupa, J.K., Zhang, X.: New variants of a method of MRI scale standardization. IEEE Trans. Med. Imaging **19**(2), 143–150 (2000)
10. Ronneberger, O., Fischer, P., Brox, T.: U-net: convolutional networks for biomedical image segmentation. In: Navab, N., Hornegger, J., Wells, W.M., Frangi, A.F. (eds.) MICCAI 2015. LNCS, vol. 9351, pp. 234–241. Springer, Cham (2015). https://doi.org/10.1007/978-3-319-24574-4_28
11. Simonyan, K., Zisserman, A.: Very deep convolutional networks for large-scale image recognition. arXiv preprint arXiv:1409.1556 (2014)
12. Yu, B., Zhou, L., Wang, L., Shi, Y., Fripp, J., Bourgeat, P.: Ea-GANs: edge-aware generative adversarial networks for cross-modality MR image synthesis. IEEE Trans. Med. Imaging **38**(7), 1750–1762 (2019)
13. Zhao, H., Gallo, O., Frosio, I., Kautz, J.: Loss functions for image restoration with neural networks. IEEE Trans. Comput. Imaging **3**(1), 47–57 (2016)
14. Zhou, P., Xie, L., Ni, B., Liu, L., Tian, Q.: HRinversion: High-resolution GAN inversion for cross-domain image synthesis. IEEE Trans. Circuits Syst. Video Technol. **33**, 2147–2161 (2022)

Previous Datasets Performance for Brain Tumor Segmentation of BraTS 2023 Current Dataset

Agus Subhan Akbar[1]($^{\boxtimes}$)[iD], Ahmad Hayam Brilian[2][iD], Chastine Fatichah[3][iD], and Nanik Suciati[3][iD]

[1] Universitas Islam Nahdlatul Ulama Jepara, Jepara, Jawa Tengah, Indonesia
agussa@unisnu.ac.id
[2] Dinas Komunikasi dan Informatika Bojonegoro, Bojonegoro, Jawa Timur, Indonesia
ahayambr@gmail.com
[3] Institut Teknologi Sepuluh Nopember, Surabaya, Indonesia
{chastine,nanik}@if.its.ac.id
https://www.unisnu.ac.id/

Abstract. Automated brain tumor segmentation continues to be an exciting challenge. The BraTS 2023 challenge comes with nine tasks, one of which is brain tumor segmentation, with an increasing amount of training data by 1251 data for training and 219 data for validation data. Training using large amounts of data will undoubtedly improve model performance but requires more significant resources and a longer time to train segmentation models. In this study, the author proposes using models trained with previous versions of training datasets, including BraTS 2018, BraTS 2019, and BraTS 2020. The models used in this study include Shallow Dilated with Attention UNet2.5D (SDA-UNet2.5D), Single Level UNet3D, and UNet3D. Each model was tested to segment the BraTS 2023 validation dataset. The best dice segmentation performance supported by the best hausdorff95 performance was achieved by the Single Level UNet3D model, which was trained with the BraTS 2020 training dataset. However, the lesionwise dice performance achieved by the Single Level UNet3D model, a new metric, still needs improvement. The pattern of decreased lesionwise dice performance from ET to TC and WT also needs further research on the causes and ways to treat them.

Keywords: Single Level UNet3D · Brain tumor segmentation · SDA-UNet2.5D

1 Introduction

Efforts to segment brain tumors automatically with the help of computer computing are continuing with the BraTS Challenge. The BraTS Challenge itself has been held from 2012 to 2023. This challenge will likely continue to be held to get the best segmentation algorithm results. So that the segmentation architecture/algorithm with the best performance and can generalize to the latest tumor image data can be obtained.

The BraTS 2023 challenge is held with nine tasks, and the data in the provided dataset increases. One of the existing tasks, Adult Glioma, continues previous years' challenges. The dataset provided contains 3D MRI images of patients with four modalities which include T1, T1c, T2, and T2 Flair. Furthermore, for the challenge, the datasets provided include training, validation, and testing datasets. This year's training dataset provided amounted to 1251 data containing four modalities and one ground truth data for training purposes. This year's validation dataset totaled 219 pieces of data without the ground truth data. So to find out the correctness of the segmentation, it needs to be sent to the online validation tools available on the https://synapse.org site. While the testing dataset, the same as the validation dataset, which only contains four modalities without ground truth data, will be available at the end of the challenge [8–11,13].

Table 1 displays the number of datasets for each version since 2018. Based on the information available at https://synapse.org the BraTS 2021 and BraTS 2023 share the same training and validation data. However, the testing dataset for BraTS 2023 has been enhanced with additional routinely-acquired clinical MRI scans, which were not present in the BraTS 2021 dataset.

Table 1. Dataset statistics on brats challenge

BraTS Year	Training Dataset	Validation Dataset
2018	285	66
2019	335	125
2020	369	125
2021	1251	219
2023	1251	219

From the data statistics in the Table 1, the question arises whether the models trained with the BraTS dataset versions 2018, 2019, and 2020 can be used to segment the BraTS 2023 dataset with performance that can still be maintained.

Researchers have made numerous attempts to obtain the best model for the Brats Challenge. These efforts have resulted in the development of various models, including segmentation and patient survival prediction models. Research on brain tumor segmentation has led to the publication of several models, as has research on predicting patient survival (a task in BraTS 2018, BraTS 2019, and BraTS 2020 challenge only). Proposed segmentation models include Simple MyUNet3D [2], SDA-Unet 2.5D [4], Single Level UNet3D [5], UNet3D [6], and Yaru3DFPN [7]. Published models for predicting patient survival can be found in [3,12,14].

The SDA-Unet 2.5D [4], Single Level UNet3D [5], and UNet3D [6] models have been trained using the BraTS 2018, BraTS 2019, and BraTS 2020 datasets and tested with the respective version validation datasets respectively. Each model has been tested with good performance. The results of their performance can be seen in their respective published manuscripts. For this year, the author wants to test the reliability of each model to segment the BraTS 2023 validation dataset. The best performance results from the three models will be used for segmentation testing of the BraTS 2023 dataset testing.

2 Methods

The dataset used in this study was the BraTS 2023 dataset. Segmentation testing was carried out on the BraTS 2023 validation dataset, which totaled 219 patients. The difference between the segmentation targets for 2023 and previous years is in the label value used to mark the segmentation results. In previous years, the segmentation target consisted of the Nec/Net area represented with a value of 1, the Edema Area with a value of 2, and the Enhanced Tumor area with a value of 4. Meanwhile, in 2023 there will be a difference in marking. The label for the Nec/Net area and edema in 2023 is the same as in previous years, expressed with values 1 and 2, respectively. In comparison, the label for the Enhanced Tumor area is expressed with a value of 3. A value of 0 labels areas outside the nec/net area, edema, and enhanced tumor.

The BraTS 2018, BraTS 2019, and BraTS 2020 datasets are used to train three architectures that will be used to segment the BraTS 2023 validation dataset. The weight of each model from the training results using these three datasets is used to segment the BraTS 2023 validation dataset. In other words, the pre-trained weight from the previous training dataset is used to segment the BraTS 2023 validation dataset.

The architecture used to segment the BraTS 2023 validation dataset consists of SDA-Unet2.5D [6], Single Level UNet3D [4], and UNet3D [5]. Each architecture has been trained using the BraTS 2018, BraTS 2019, and BraTS 2020 training datasets. The training used a 5-fold cross-validation strategy to produce 1 model for each fold. Hyperparameters used during training are set as stated in the respective manuscript. Each version segments the BraTS 2023 validation dataset using the ensemble method to produce one segmentation output. The ensemble is done by averaging method.

For the conversion of segmentation results that are different from the previous version, the final output used to express the area of the enhanced tumor is coded differently. Initially, the conversion results for enhanced tumors were expressed with a value of 4. Currently, the segmentation results for enhanced tumors are expressed with a value of 3.

The complete sequences of segmentation steps are stated in the Fig. 1. The description of the steps as follows:

1. Stack, Crop, Norm, and Form
   The four modalities T1n, T1c, T2w, and T2f of each patient in the 2023 BraTS validation dataset were arranged in the order [T2f, T1n, T2w, T1c]. This stack is $4 \times 240 \times 240 \times 155$ in size. This stack is cropped to a certain size so that only the object containing the brain is present, while the background

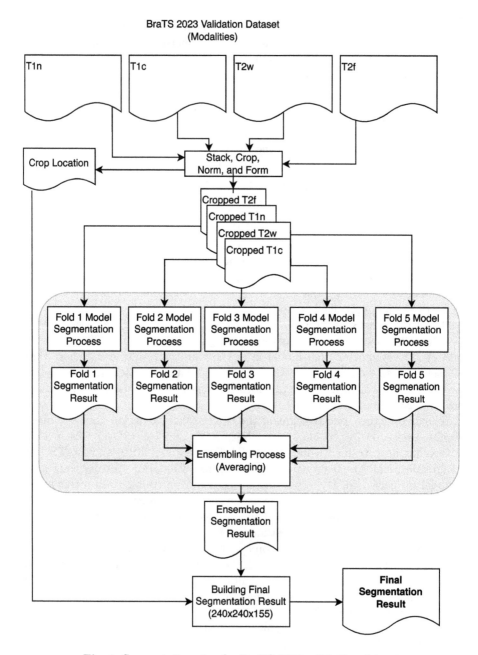

Fig. 1. Segmentation step for BraTS 2023 validation dataset

is cropped as much as possible. The cropping positions are recorded for use during the final shaping process. The cropped image is then normalized per channel using Eq. 1, as used in [2].

$$V_{norm} = \frac{V - \mu}{\sigma} \tag{1}$$

where V_{norm} is the normalized cropped image, V the original cropped image, μ and σ are the mean and the standar deviation of V without its zero values. The normalized cropped image (V_{norm}) is then padded with a voxel value of 0 to adjust the input size required by each model. The final size of the truncation is $4 \times (x + padX) \times (y + padY) \times (z + padZ)$.

2. Segmentation Process
   Each model (fold model) resulting from the 5-fold cross-validation training is used to segment the input image. Each fold model uses the weights obtained during training to segment the input image. The output size of each model fold is the same as the input image size except for the first dimension. The first dimension became 3 to represent the target segmentation area, including nec/net, edema, and enhanced tumor area. The segmentation output from each fold model is then sent to the following process.

3. Ensembling Process
   The results of the segmentation process are five vectors with size $3 \times (x + padX) \times (y + padY) \times (z + padZ)$. These five vectors are processed to become one vector with size $3 \times (x + padX) \times (y + padY) \times (z + padZ)$. The aggregation process is carried out by taking the average of the values in each corresponding position. The output of this process is then sent to the following process stage.

4. Building Final Segmentation Result
   The final process of this method is to produce a final output in the form of a vector measuring $240 \times 240 \times 155$. The Input vector from the previous process that is $3 \times (x + padX) \times (y + padY) \times (z + padZ)$ converted to a vector of size $(x + padX) \times (y + padY) \times (z + padZ)$ by translating to segmentation target areas as done in [4–6]. It is just that specifically for the enhanced tumor area. It is encoded with a value of 3. The conversion results, which measure $(x + padX) \times (y + padY) \times (z + padZ)$ are returned to a size of $240 \times 240 \times 155$ by placing it in the position previously recorded in step 1 and filling the area outside the vector size with a value of 0.
   The result of this process is then stored as a segmentation result file in nii.gz format.

All the results in nii.gz format were then sent to online validation tools to get the performance metrics, including dice, sensitivity, specificity, and hausdorff95 for each segmentation target area. This year, there are new metrics returned by the tools. The new metrics include LesionWise (dice, Hausdorff95), True Positif (TP), False Positif (FP), and False Negatif (FN). According to the boards, the LesionWise metric is for understanding the performance of a model at a lesion level and not at an image level. A brief description of the LesionWise can be found at [1].

The steps in Fig. 1 applied to all the models including:

1. SDA-UNet2.5D [4] trained with BraTS 2018 training dataset and 5-fold cross-validation

2. SDA-UNet2.5D [4] trained with BraTS 2019 training dataset and 5-fold cross-validation
3. SDA-UNet2.5D [4] trained with BraTS 2020 training dataset and 5-fold cross-validation
4. Single Level UNet3D [5] with BraTS 2018 training dataset and 5-fold cross-validation
5. Single Level UNet3D [5] with BraTS 2019 training dataset and 5-fold cross-validation
6. Single Level UNet3D [5] with BraTS 2020 training dataset and 5-fold cross-validation
7. UNet3D [6] trained with BraTS 2018 training dataset and 5-fold cross-validation
8. UNet3D [6] trained with BraTS 2019 training dataset and 5-fold cross-validation
9. UNet3D [6] trained with BraTS 2020 training dataset and 5-fold cross-validation

3 Result

3.1 SDA-UNet2.5D Model Performance on BraTS 2023 Validation Dataset

The performance of dice and haussdorf95 from the SDA-UNet2.5D model on the segmentation of the BraTS 2023 validation dataset is as stated in the Table 2. The sensitivity and specificity performance of the SDA-UNet2.5D model are presented in the Table 3. Meanwhile, the performance of the lesionwise dice and hausdorff95 of the SDA-UNet2.5D model is presented in the Table 4.

Table 2. SDA-UNet2.5D model performance in dice and hausdorff95 metrics

Trained with	Dice (%)			Hausdorff95		
	ET	TC	WT	ET	TC	WT
BraTS 2018	74.86	78.61	88.30	152.91	156.77	183.16
BraTS 2019	76.09	79.54	88.61	25.79	17.20	14.12
BraTS 2020	76.89	79.98	88.75	25.14	18.12	15.11

Table 3. SDA-UNet2.5D model performance in Sensitivity and Spesificity metrics

Trained with	Sensitivity (%)			Specificity (%)		
	ET	TC	WT	ET	TC	WT
BraTS 2018	73.97	82.04	87.32	99.98	99.94	99.92
BraTS 2019	74.53	80.83	88.28	99.98	99.95	99.92
BraTS 2020	74.88	80.47	88.72	99.98	99.96	99.91

Table 4. SDA-UNet2.5D model performance in LesionWise dice and Hausdorff95 metrics

Trained with	LesionWise Dice (%)			LesionWise Hausdorff95		
	ET	TC	WT	ET	TC	WT
BraTS 2018	49.30	48.46	46.46	152.91	156.77	183.16
BraTS 2019	54.44	54.07	48.02	130.61	131.80	175.17
BraTS 2020	53.22	52.70	42.20	137.95	138.35	198.91

In general, the dice performance of the SDA-UNet2.5D model increases as the amount of training data in the dataset increases. The highest dice performance was obtained using the SDA-UNet2.5D model, which was trained using the BraTS 2020 training dataset. As stated in the Table 1, the number of training data in the BraTS 2020 dataset is 369, more than the BraTS training dataset 2019 and BraTS 2018.

In the performance of Hausdorff95, sensitivity, specificity, and LessionWise (Dice and Hausdorff95), the SDA-UNet2.5D model trained with the BraTS 2019 training dataset performs best compared to other training data. Judging from the amount of training data, BraTS 2019 has less training data than BraTS 2020.

The performance of Lesionwise, both dice and hausdorff95, tends to decrease from ET to TC and WT. The highest performance is in the ET area, while the lowest is in the WT area.

3.2 Single Level UNet3D Performance on BraTS 2023 Validation Dataset

The performance of dice and haussdorf95 from the Single Level UNet3D model on the segmentation of the BraTS 2023 validation dataset is as stated in the Table 5. The sensitivity and specificity performance of the Single Level UNet3D model are presented in the Table 6. Meanwhile, the performance of the lesionwise dice and hausdorff95 of the Single Level UNet3D model is presented in the Table 7.

Table 5. Single Level UNet3D model performance in dice and hausdorff95 metrics

Trained with	Dice (%)			Hausdorff95		
	ET	TC	WT	ET	TC	WT
BraTS 2018	78.55	82.12	89.47	21.62	16.25	11.85
BraTS 2019	79.26	82.28	89.49	23.55	16.01	11.80
BraTS 2020	78.28	82.01	89.57	20.37	13.83	10.48

Table 6. Single Level UNet3D model performance in Sensitivity and Spesificity metrics

Trained with	Sensitivity (%)			Specificity (%)		
	ET	TC	WT	ET	TC	WT
BraTS 2018	77.90	84.49	91.65	99.98	99.95	99.90
BraTS 2019	78.82	86.35	91.93	99.98	99.94	99.90
BraTS 2020	78.04	85.88	92.84	99.98	99.95	99.89

Table 7. Single Level UNet3D model performance in LesionWise dice and Hausdorff95 metrics

Trained with	LesionWise Dice (%)			LesionWise Hausdorff95		
	ET	TC	WT	ET	TC	WT
BraTS 2018	72.77	73.89	61.44	53.17	55.70	124.56
BraTS 2019	73.32	69.24	56.90	56.81	74.21	142.91
BraTS 2020	72.08	73.14	54.94	57.92	55.45	148.92

The highest dice performance of the Single Level UNet3D model was achieved using a model trained with the BraTS 2019 training dataset, in particular for the ET and TC areas. Whereas for the WT area, the model trained with the BraTS 2020 training dataset achieved the highest dice performance. However, from the Hausdorff95 performance side, the dominant best performance was achieved by the model trained with the BraTS 2020 training dataset.

The lesionwise performance of the Single Level UNet3D model, both dice and hausdorff95, has a downward trend from the ET to TC and WT areas. This descending pattern is evenly distributed in all versions of the training data used.

3.3 UNet3D Performance on BraTS 2023 Validation Dataset

The performance of dice and hausdorff95 from the UNet3D model on the segmentation of the BraTS 2023 validation dataset is as stated in the Table 8. The sensitivity and specificity performance of the UNet3D model are presented in the Table 9. Meanwhile, the performance of the lesionwise dice and hausdorff95 of the UNet3D model is presented in the Table 10.

Table 8. UNet3D model performance in dice and hausdorff95 metrics

Trained with	Dice (%)			Hausdorff95		
	ET	TC	WT	ET	TC	WT
BraTS 2018	74.57	78.73	87.72	26.52	16.67	20.55
BraTS 2019	77.32	81.24	88.38	28.32	15.71	15.98
BraTS 2020	76.23	80.11	88.10	28.98	17.45	17.59

Table 9. UNet3D model performance in Sensitivity and Spesificity metrics

Trained with	Sensitivity (%)			Specificity (%)		
	ET	TC	WT	ET	TC	WT
BraTS 2018	71.98	78.77	90.96	99.98	99.96	99.88
BraTS 2019	78.23	84.33	92.03	99.97	99.95	99.87
BraTS 2020	79.28	82.32	91.20	99.97	99.96	99.88

Table 10. UNet3D model performance in LesionWise dice and Hausdorff95 metrics

Trained with	LesionWise Dice (%)			LesionWise Hausdorff95		
	ET	TC	WT	ET	TC	WT
BraTS 2018	64.81	62.41	40.90	79.74	95.42	205.92
BraTS 2019	61.81	63.87	41.07	103.55	96.66	205.03
BraTS 2020	62.04	62.30	46.87	101.37	98.28	181.75

The best dice performance from the UNet3D model was obtained from a model trained using the BraTS 2019 training dataset. The hausdorff95 performance of the model also showed the best results when trained with the BraTS 2019 training dataset. The pattern of decreasing dice and hausdorff95 performance was also experienced by the UNet3D model in the ET area to TC and WT. This pattern of performance degradation is uniform for all versions of the training data used.

4 Discussion

The best dice and hausdorff95 performance of the three models used was achieved by the Single Level UNet3D model, which was trained using the BraTS 2020 training dataset. However, the dice performance in the ET and TC areas in this model was best trained with BraTS 2019. However, from the performance of Hausdorff95, the Single Level UNet3D model trained using the BraTS 2020 training dataset remains the best compared to the other two training datasets.

Based on the model performance results from the use of training data, the increase in training data is indeed very influential on performance. Even though the Single Level UNet3D model was not trained with the BraTS 2023 training dataset, it still has high dice and hausdorff95 performance for segmentation of the BraTS 2023 validation dataset, which totals 219 data. Of course, training the Single Level UNet3D model using the BraTS 2023 training dataset will improve its performance.

The performance of lesion dice and lesion hausdorff95 decreases from performance in the ET to TC and WT areas. This decline needs further investigation of the factors that cause it. This low score in performance may be due to the training dataset used or the need to change the model's training strategy to deal with this new performance metric.

References

1. GitHub - rachitsaluja/BraTS-2023-Metrics: Official BraTS 2023 Segmentation Performance Metrics—https://github.com/. https://github.com/rachitsaluja/BraTS-2023-Metrics. Accessed 11 Mar 2024
2. Akbar, A.S., Fatichah, C., Suciati, N.: Simple MyUnet3D for BraTS segmentation. In: ICICoS 2020 - Proceeding: 4th International Conference on Informatics and Computational Sciences (2020). https://doi.org/10.1109/ICICoS51170.2020.9299072
3. Akbar, A.S., Fatichah, C., Suciati, N.: Modified mobilenet for patient survival prediction. In: Crimi, A., Bakas, S. (eds.) BrainLes 2020. LNCS, vol. 12659, pp. 374–387. Springer, Cham (2021). https://doi.org/10.1007/978-3-030-72087-2_33
4. Akbar, A.S., Fatichah, C., Suciati, N.: SDA-UNET2.5D: shallow dilated with attention Unet2.5D for brain tumor segmentation. Int. J. Intell. Eng. Syst. **15**(2), 135–149 (2022). https://doi.org/10.22266/ijies2022.0430.14
5. Akbar, A.S., Fatichah, C., Suciati, N.: Single level UNet3D with multipath residual attention block for brain tumor segmentation. J. King Saud Univ. - Comput. Inf. Sci. **34**(6, Part B), 3247–3258 (2022). https://doi.org/10.1016/j.jksuci.2022.03.022
6. Akbar, A.S., Fatichah, C., Suciati, N.: Unet3D with multiple atrous convolutions attention block for brain tumor segmentation. In: Crimi, A., Bakas, S. (eds.) BrainLes 2021. LNCS, vol. 12962, pp. 182–193 (2022). Springer, Cham. https://doi.org/10.1007/978-3-031-08999-2_14
7. Akbar, A.S., Fatichah, C., Suciati, N., Za'in, C.: Yaru3DFPN: a lightweight modified 3D UNet with feature pyramid network and combine thresholding for brain tumor segmentation. Neural Comput. Appl. (2024). https://doi.org/10.1007/s00521-024-09475-7
8. Baid, U., et al.: The RSNA-ASNR-MICCAI BraTS 2021 benchmark on brain tumor segmentation and radiogenomic classification (2021)
9. Bakas, S., et al.: Segmentation labels for the pre-operative scans of the TCGA-GBM collection (2017)
10. Bakas, S., et al.: Segmentation labels for the pre-operative scans of the TCGA-LGG collection (2017)
11. Bakas, S., et al.: Advancing the cancer genome atlas glioma MRI collections with expert segmentation labels and radiomic features. Sci. Data **4**(1), 170117 (2017)
12. Carver, E., et al.: Automatic brain tumor segmentation and overall survival prediction using machine learning algorithms. In: Crimi, A., Bakas, S., Kuijf, H., Keyvan, F., Reyes, M., van Walsum, T. (eds.) BrainLes 2018. LNCS, vol. 11384, pp. 406–418. Springer, Cham (2019). https://doi.org/10.1007/978-3-030-11726-9_36
13. Menze, B.H., et al.: The multimodal brain tumor image segmentation benchmark (BRATS). IEEE Trans. Med. Imaging **34**(10), 1993–2024 (2015)
14. Yang, H.-Y., Yang, J.: Automatic brain tumor segmentation with contour aware residual network and adversarial training. In: Crimi, A., Bakas, S., Kuijf, H., Keyvan, F., Reyes, M., van Walsum, T. (eds.) BrainLes 2018. LNCS, vol. 11384, pp. 267–278. Springer, Cham (2019). https://doi.org/10.1007/978-3-030-11726-9_24

Enhanced Data Augmentation Using Synthetic Data for Brain Tumour Segmentation

André Ferreira[1,2,3(✉)], Naida Solak[2,6], Jianning Li[2,3,4], Philipp Dammann[7], Jens Kleesiek[3,4,5], Victor Alves[1], and Jan Egger[2,3,4,6]

[1] Center Algoritmi/LASI, University of Minho, 4710-057 Braga, Portugal
[2] Computer Algorithms for Medicine Laboratory, Graz, Austria
[3] Institute for AI in Medicine (IKIM), University Medicine Essen, Girardetstraße 2, 45131 Essen, Germany
id10656@alunos.uminho.pt
[4] Cancer Research Center Cologne Essen (CCCE), University Medicine Essen, Hufelandstraße 55, 45147 Essen, Germany
[5] German Cancer Consortium (DKTK), Partner Site Essen, Hufelandstraße 55, 45147 Essen, Germany
[6] Institute of Computer Graphics and Vision, Graz University of Technology, Inffeldgasse 16, 8010 Graz, Austria
[7] Department of Neurosurgery and Spine Surgery, University Hospital Essen, Essen, Germany

Abstract. Deep Learning is the state-of-the-art technology for segmenting brain tumours. However, this requires a lot of high-quality data, which is difficult to obtain, especially in the medical field. Therefore, our solutions address this problem by using unconventional mechanisms for data augmentation. Generative adversarial networks and registration are used to massively increase the amount of available samples for training three different deep learning models for adult glioma segmentation, the Task 1 of the BraTS 2023 challenge. The first model is the standard nnU-Net, the second is the Swin UNETR and the third is the winning solution of the BraTS 2021 Challenge. The entire pipeline is built on the nnU-Net implementation, except for the generation of the synthetic data. The use of convolutional algorithms and transformers is able to fill each other's knowledge gaps. Our solution achieves the lesion-wise Dice metric of 0.8851, 0.8719, 0.8685 and lesion-wise HD95 of 22.838, 22.974, 16.713 (whole tumour, tumour core and enhancing tumour) on the testing cohort.

Keywords: Generative adversarial networks · Registration · Synthetic data · Brain Tumour segmentation · nnU-Net

---

Supported by organizations University of Minho and Institute for Artificial Intelligence in Medicine.

1 Introduction

Brain tumours originate from different cell types, mainly from glialcells (astrocytes, oligodendrocytes, microglia, ependymal cells) and are then referred to as gliomas. The World Health Organization (WHO) classifies brain tumours into grades 1 to 4 based on histologic features and molecular parameters. Grade 1 tumours are typically slow-growing and benign, and grade 4 tumours, such as glioblastomas (GBMs), are the most aggressive and malignant forms. Indeed, Glioblastomas are among the most deadly types of cancer due to their location and invasive growth. Patients diagnosed with glioblastoma now have a median survival of approximately 16 months with standard treatment (radiotherapy and temozolomide). Despite extensive research to improve diagnosis, characterization and treatment, the mortality rate of GBMs remains high and significant improvements in patient survival have been elusive. Extensive research to improve diagnosis, characterisation and treatment has reduced the mortality rate of this disease [23]. Glioma segmentation is a critical step for tumour evolution, treatment efficacy assessment, survival prediction and treatment planning. Multiple modalities of MRI scans (T1, T2, T1Gd and FLAIR) are usually used for accurate segmentation of the tumour and individual regions [29].

MRI is a medical imaging technique that is often used to detect and assess response to glioma treatment [30]. The development of new therapies for treatment depends on accurate segmentation. Manual segmentation has been used for this purpose, but is very time-consuming and suffers from inter- and intra-examiner variability [7,29]. Efforts have therefore been made to automate this process. Machine learning techniques have been the most advanced methods for performing such segmentation, but they have the disadvantage of requiring large, high-quality datasets for the training process in order to achieve the performance required for clinical purposes [6].

The Brain Tumor Segmentation Challenge (BraTS) [2–5,18,23] provides a large, fully annotated and publicly available dataset for model development and promotes a competition to evaluate the latest state-of-the-art approaches for brain diffuse glioma segmentation. This competition was launched in 2012 and continues to evolve each year, adding more samples and many different tasks. The 2023 competition includes 9 different tasks, the first of which is the traditional segmentation of adult gliomas. The proposed solution refers to Task 1 - Segmentation of adult gliomas.

1.1 State-of-the-Art

Since the challenge of 2014, deep convolutional networks have been the state-of-the-art for brain tumour segmentation [24,28]. Recently, the most advanced strategies are mainly based on deep neural networks (DNNs), due to the rapid development of these tools, the availability of increasingly powerful GPUs and the availability of training data. Most solutions are based on the U-Net [25] which has yielded convincing results. Many architectural changes to the U-Net have been introduced to improve it, e.g., residual connections [14], densely connected layers [22,33] and attention mechanisms [11].

The winners of the last 6 editions all used DNNs. Kamnitsas et al. [15] (2017 winner) explore the ensemble of multiple models and architecture (EMMA), more specifically the 3D convolutional networks DeepMedic [16,17], FCN [20] and U-Net [25]. The use of EMMA seems to reduce the influence of the metaparameters of each model and helps to avoid overfitting.

The winners of the 2020 edition [13], with respect to task 1, propose the use of the nnU-Net [12], a U-Net based architecture, as a baseline and implements some BraTS specific optimisations. These optimizations are: optimising regions rather than individual classes, using a bigger batch size (from 2 to 5), applying a more aggressive data augmentation, replacing the instance normalisation with batch normalisation (which is better with more aggressive data augmentation), using of batch Dice instead of regular Dice, and applying post-processing distinct from the regular nnU-Net.

The winners of 2021 edition [21] also use the nnU-Net as baseline, using the same BraTS-specific optimizations as [12] and new optimizations. They claim that due to the change in the dataset from the 2020 edition (494 cases) to the 2021 edition (1470 cases), [21] decided to use a larger network by doubling the number of filters in the encoder part of the nnU-Net, and increasing the maximum number of filters in the bottleneck to 512, while keeping the decoder intact. Batch normalisation is replaced by group normalisation as it performs better with small batch sizes, allowing the use of batch size 2 instead of 5. Axial attention decoder was also applied but not tested in the final phase of the BraTS challenge, and it did not improve the results in the 5-fold cross validation.

The winners of the 2022 edition [31] achieved the best results by using an ensemble of three different architectures: DeepSeg [32], the improved nnU-Net proposed by [21], and DeepSCAN [22]. The ensemble is created using the Simultaneous Truth and Performance Level Estimation (STAPLE). 2023 Challenge *BraTS-Africa* [1] also uses the STAPLE ensemble of three different models to create the ground truth segmentations.

It is important to note that the same post-processing is done for all three solutions. As explained in detail in [13], there is ground truth without an enhancing tumour (ET) label, so the BraTS evaluation gives the worst possible results for false positive predictions. To mitigate this scenario, when the number of voxels is below a certain threshold, ET is replaced by necrotic (NCR). A threshold of 200 is used in all three experiments. This year (BraTS 2023), however, a new metric is used that requires new post-processing techniques, as will be explained later.

Our approach consists of solving the problem of brain tumour segmentation by increasing the amount of available data, using two different, non-conventional strategies for data augmentation. Furthermore, convolutional neural networks (CNNs) and transformer-based networks are assumed to complement each other, which is why ensemble of these two distinct architectures are also tested.

2 Methods

The machine used for all these tasks is a IKIM cluster node with 6 NVIDIA RTX 6000, 49 GB of VRAM, 1024 GB of RAM, and AMD EPYC 7402 24-Core Processor.

2.1 Data

The Task 1 dataset consists of 1470 patients, each of which contains 4 modalities (T1, T1Gd, T2 and FLAIR). 1251 cases have the corresponding ground truth, so this subset is used for training, and the remaining (219 cases) that do not contain a freely available ground truth form the subset for evaluation. The test set in this year's (2023) edition contains many more routine clinical multi-parametric MRI scans. All MRI scans were pre-processed as follows: were co-registered to the same anatomical template, interpolated to the same resolution (1 mm3), and skull-striped. The scans have the shape $240 \times 240 \times 155$.

The ground truth of the subset of evaluation is hidden from the participants, being only possible to access the Dice scores and 95% Hausdorff distance through the participation platform. The evaluation is performed by sub-region and not by individual label. The sub-regions are the ET represented by the value 3, the tumour core (TC) represented by the values 1 and 3 (NCR and ET), and the whole tumour (WT) represented by the values 1, 2 and 3 (NCR, peritumoral edematous/invaded tissue and ET). In previous BraTS challenges the ET was represented by the value 4, however, this year (BraTS 2023), the value 4 was replaced by the value 3. The naming convention has also changed from the previous challenges.

2.2 Data Augmentation

Data Augmentation via Registration. Inspired by the winning solution for the AutoImplant Challenge 2020 [8], a larger dataset was built via registration. The idea of registration in general is to combine features (shape and 'content') for each pair of scans, meaning that for each pair in n samples we can compute a transformation that describes the relation between those 2 samples and generate 2 additional new samples (n^2 in total).

Usually, one (first) image is used as the moving image, and the other (second) one as the fixed image - meaning that the moving image is warped into the fixed image space by applying the computed transformation, and also the inverse transformation in order to warp the fixed image into the moving image space, as shown in Fig. 1. Advanced Normalization Tools (ANTs) [2] package is used to perform this registration. It is a software package used for normalizing data to a template, and it provides different scripts (such as antsRegistrationSyNQuick.sh) that enable applying different transformations on the images, such as rigid, affine, non-linear and all of them combined.

Only the training set was used to create new samples via registration, since it is the only one that contains the ground truth. The transformation and inverse transformation matrix are computed for each case and applied to each scan (including the ground truth). After creating a reasonable amount of registered data (23049 samples, 92000 MRI scans and 23049 ground truths), all data were converted to integer, as the results of registering creates floats. This process took around 2 weeks. Figure 2 presents a sample.

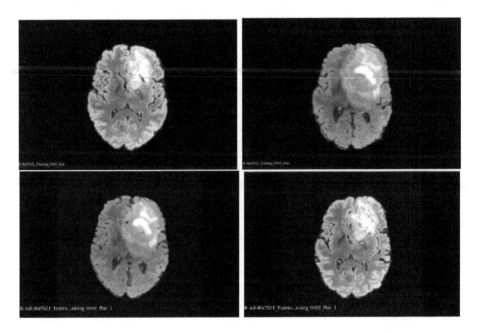

Fig. 1. The non-linear registration is computed between the brain images of the Subject 0000 (top left) and the Subject 0002 (top right). As a result, we have two additional scans: on the bottom left image, we can see an artificially generated brain MRI scan with a similar shape as the Subject 0000 (top left), and similar 'content' as the Subject 0002 (top right); on the bottom right image, the newly created brain MRI scan has a shape similar to the Subject 0002 and 'content' similar to the Subject 0000

Data Augmentation with GANs. Generative adversarial networks (GANs) are known for their ability to generate realistic data. Ferreira et al. [9] presents an overview of the generation of realistic volumetric data. In this systematic review, it can be seen that a large number of works use GANs for various tasks, e.g. denoising, classification, segmentation, image translation, reconstruction and others. In many cases, synthetic data generated by GANs is even used to increase the amount of data available for training deep learning models, i.e. for data augmentation.

In this work, a GAN is used to randomly place tumours in the healthy parts of the provided training set of scans to reduce the class imbalance between the

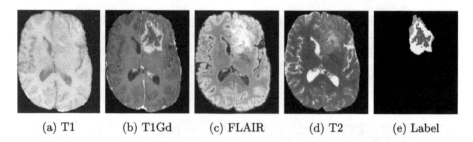

Fig. 2. All four modalities of the sample BraTS-GLI-00000-000 and respective ground-truth registered with the sample BraTS-GLI-00003-000 (a, b, c, d, e) from the BraTS 2023 dataset

tumour labels and the healthy brain tissue. The GAN architecture consists of a generator and a discriminator. The generator uses the MONAI [27] implementation of the Swin UNETR [11], with parameters: img_size = (96, 96, 96), in_channels = 4, out_channels = 1, and feature_size = 48. The discriminator is a CNN based on [10], with increased number of layers (one more 3D convolution at the end, with stride 1, kernel size 3, padding 0 and no spectral normalisation), and sigmoid before the output.

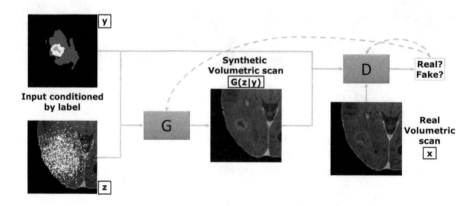

Fig. 3. The training pipeline of the **GliGAN**. The noise scan (z) and the label (y) are concatenated and fed into the generator (G). The discriminator (D) assesses the realism of a real scan and the reconstruction

The input of the generator is created as follows: Each scan is cropped with centre in the tumour volume (size 96 × 96 × 96), normalised between $[-1, 1]$, added noise and normalised between $[-1, 1]$ again, resulting in a noisy scan as can be seen in Fig. 3 (z). Voxels with a tumour label different from 0 are replaced by Gaussian noise, as is the surrounding tissue, with the probability of the voxel value being replaced by noise decreasing with distance from the tumour centre, creating a spherical effect. This strategy allows for more realistic generation, as it is harder to detect the edges of the noise. Square noise has been tested but produces unrealistic results, as shown in Fig. 4 (first row). This GAN is referred to as **GliGAN**.

The loss functions of the generator (G) and discriminator (D) are:

$$L_D = \mathbb{E}_{y,z}[\log D(G(z|y))] - \mathbb{E}_{x,y}[\log D(x|y)] \tag{1}$$

$$L_G = -\lambda_1 \mathbb{E}_{y,z}[\log D(G(z|y))] + \lambda_2 \mathbb{E}_{x,y,z} \|x - G(z|y)\|_{MAE} \tag{2}$$

The training is divided into two steps. The first step uses $\lambda_1 = 1$ and $\lambda_2 = 5$ for 200000 iterations. After performing the first step, it was found that the tissue visible to the generator (voxels without noise) was noisy, but the tumour volume was realistic. To solve this problem, the network was trained for another 1000 epochs, linearly increasing the weight of the mean absolute error (MAE) component (λ_2). This allowed for a realistic surrounding tissue and tumour with realistic texture and overall appearance, as shown in Fig. 4 (second row). The baseline uses only the MAE component as the loss function.

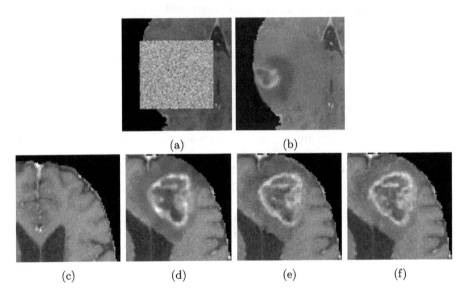

Fig. 4. Differences in terms of the realism of the tumours produced. If using a square shaped noise: a) Crop of a real scan (T1Gd) with squared noise b) Reconstruction using GANs; or spherical noise: c) Healthy crop d) baseline e) first step training f) second step training

Two approaches were tested for the creation of new scans with inserted fake tumours in order to create two data sets. In the first datasets, for each real case in the training dataset, 30 random labels (from the remaining dataset) were selected and randomly placed in a healthy part of the scan. From the total set, 23049 cases were randomly selected. This dataset is referred to as **pG**. The second dataset was created using a random label generator, i.e. another GAN based on [10] was trained to generate new labels and these labels are then used as input to the **GliGAN**. This dataset is referred to as **rG**. To allow a fair comparison between all data augmentation strategies, 23049 cases were generated for each strategy.

Pre-procesing: Pre-processing is performed by the nnU-Net pipeline. Before the training step, the brain voxels of each scan are normalised using z-score normalisation, keeping the background at zero.

Networks: Multiple networks were tested to determine which network (or ensemble) provided better results. Each network was implemented in the newer version of the nnU-Net (V2) to take advantage of the pre-processing and data augmentation pipeline provided by this framework.

Baseline (B): The fully automated framework nnU-Net [12] was used as a baseline (3D full resolution), without any configuration changes. The input is random patches of the shape $128 \times 160 \times 112$. Batch size 5, region-based training, and deep supervised.

Swin UNETR (S): The Swin UNETR [11] is a U-Net like network in which the convolutional encoder is replaced by Swin transformer blocks. This encoder is, therefore, capable of capturing long-range information, as opposed to fully convolutional networks. The Swin Transformer uses shifted windows, allowing the use of high resolution images, as is the case of the BraTS dataset (by having linear computational complexity regarding the image size [19]).

The architecture of the Swin UNETR is described in [11]. The input are random patches of shape $128 \times 128 \times 128$, and the remaining pre-processing, including regular data augmentation, is applied by the nnU-Net pipeline. Since this network is heavier, a batch size of 4 is used, as well as deep supervision.

We hypothesise that a transformer-based architecture is complementary to the fully convolutional nnU-Net architecture, as found by [34].

2021 winner (L): The winners of the 2021 edition [21] use the framework provided by nnU-Net and implemented some improvements over the nnU-Net solution proposed in 2020 [13]. [13] purposes the use of a more aggressive data augmentation than the provided by default in the nnU-Net pipeline, and therefore to use batch normalisation instead of instance normalisation, as this seems to produce better results with a very aggressive data augmentation. Since the dataset used for training includes samples generated by our own data augmentation strategies as well as those explained in [13], we believe that batch normalisation gives better results than any other normalisation. Batch Dice is also used for gradient computation instead of sample Dice [13]. In addition, Luu et al. [21] double the number of filters in the encoder and increases the size of the bottleneck to 512. They also use group normalisation as they claim it is better for small batch sizes. However, we were able to use a batch size of 5, so batch normalisation would be the best option.

2.3 Selection Criteria

As mentioned by [13], the BraTS challenge follows a "rank and then aggregate" approach for ranking the proposed solutions, as it is well suited for the using of different segmentation metrics. This ranking method works as follows: each participant is ranked for each of the testing cases (X); each case includes 3 regions, the metrics used are the Dice similarity coefficient (DSC) and the 95% Hausdorff distance (HD95); this makes $X \times 3 \times 2$; the final ranking is the average of all these rankings normalised by the number of participants, from 0 (best) to 1 (worst). In situations where the baseline data does not have a specific label, false positives are strongly penalised by assigning the worst possible value for each metric (DSC 0 and HD95 374) and the best possible result when the model outputs an empty label (DSC 1 and HD95 0).

This year (BraTS 2023), two new performance metrics are used, the lesion-based Dice score and the lesion-based Hausdorff distance-95. With these metrics, the evaluation is done at the lesion level rather than at the scan level. These new metrics can be used to assess how well the model can detect multiple tumours in the same case. Therefore, for each case, the DSC and HD95 are calculated for each lesion and averaged per patient. Thus, the results are heavily penalised by the segmentation of non-existent tumours (FP) and the lack of segmentation (FN). FNs are almost impossible to avoid in a post-processing step, but FP can be reduced by using a suitable threshold to remove some segmentations, although this comes with a slight increase in the number of FNs.

Therefore, selecting the solution with the best DSC and/or HD95 is not the best approach for an optimal performance on the BraTS 2023 competition. For this choice, an implementation based on the ranking strategy of the BraTS competition is used, in order to select the best solution.

2.4 Ensemble Strategy

Sawant et al. [26] claim that the maximum success of ensembles is only achieved when the number of models used is between 60 and 70. However, training and inference of more than 60 models makes the segmentation task too difficult and heavy. Therefore, it was decided to train one model for each architecture and for each data augmentation strategy, giving a total of $3 \times 3 = 9$ models. Each model was trained with a 5-fold cross-validation resampling method, i.e. a total of $9 \times 5 = 45$ models were trained.

In order to get the best out of all the models and find the best solution, several ensemble methods were tested:

– Averaging: averaging the probabilities of all 45 models;
– STAPLE: Application of the STAPLE algorithm to each label provided by each network (after averaging the 5-fold probability map and converting to integers);

- CNN: Training a CNN to produce the final labels using the probability maps of each network as input (after averaging the 5-folds probability maps);
- Weighting: Similar to the previous method, but instead of convolutions, a learnable parameter is used that learns how much weight each region of each individual probability mask of each network should have.

3 Results

We refer to our solutions using the following abbreviations:

- **B**: Baseline network, explained in Sect. 2.2.
- **S**: Swin UNETR, explained in Sect. 2.2.
- **L**: Architecture based on BraTS2021 winner, explained in Sect. 2.2.
- **pG**: Synthetic data generated by the GliGAN, explained in Sect. 2.2.
- **rG**: Synthetic data generated by the random label generator and GliGAN, explained in Sect. 2.2.
- **R**: Synthetic data generated by registration, explained in Sect. 2.2.

Since, in this edition of BraTS a new metric was introduced that takes into account the number of tumours in the ground-truth and predictions, penalising the FPs and FNs, Table 1 presents both legacy (old metric) and new metric for the training set. Each solution if formally defined as S_M^{DA} where S is the solution, M the model and DA the data augmentation strategy. E.g., the solution which uses the baseline network **B** and the synthetic dataset **pG** is represented as S_B^{pG}. For ensembles, several model and data represented are used, e.g., $S_{B,S}^{pG,rG}$. Table 2 shows the results (using the new metric) of the online validation platform. This evaluation is performed online as the participants have no access to the ground-truth. Only ensembles were submitted to the platform as they produced the better results and the number of submissions is limited. The results of the 3 model ensembles help to evaluate how good each data augmentation strategy is. The solution presented for the test phase was the ensemble of all trained models using thresholds of 250, 150 and 100 voxels for the WT, TC and ET respectively.

4 Discussion

From Table 1 we can conclude that the best solution is the ensemble (average of the probability maps of each model and rounded to an integer). However, if we compare the old results with the results of the new metric, we can also deduce that our solution is heavily penalised by the existence of FP and FN. Therefore, post-processing based on a threshold is performed to remove some small tumours that are detected but are not actually tumours. For this purpose, several values were tested for each region (WT, TC and ET). It was found that the best thresholds for the training set are $WT_{250}TC_{100}ET_{50}$ (for DSC) and $WT_{250}TC_{50}ET_{50}$ (for HD96). However, for the test in the validation set, the best values are $WT_{250}TC_{150}ET_{100}$ (for both DSC and HD95).

Table 1. Results of the training set. The best results are in **bold** and the second best underlined. The "All" is defined as $S_{B,L,S,B,L,S,B,L,S}^{pG,pG,pG,rG,rG,rG,R,R,R}$

Solutions	Legacy (DSC)				New metric (DSC)			
	WT	TC	ET	Mean	WT	TC	ET	Mean
S_B^{pG}	0.9388	0.9204	0.8833	0.9142	0.8326	0.8690	0.8168	0.8395
S_S^{pG}	0.9378	0.9148	0.8787	0.9104	0.7855	0.8533	0.8010	0.8133
S_L^{pG}	0.9377	0.9183	0.8846	0.9136	0.8332	0.8673	0.8207	0.8404
S_B^{rG}	0.9405	0.9213	0.8819	0.9146	0.8265	0.8774	0.8224	0.8421
S_S^{rG}	0.9397	0.9165	0.8797	0.9120	0.7627	0.8569	0.8057	0.8084
S_L^{rG}	0.9400	0.9188	<u>0.8873</u>	0.9154	0.8525	0.8669	0.8160	0.8451
S_B^{R}	0.9380	0.9180	0.8742	0.9101	0.8423	0.8731	0.8118	0.8424
S_S^{R}	0.9357	0.9085	0.8680	0.9041	0.8013	0.8415	0.7889	0.8106
S_L^{R}	0.9387	0.9139	0.8830	0.9119	0.8401	0.8664	0.8183	0.8416
$S_{B,L,S}^{pG,pG,pG}$	0.9409	0.9211	**0.8879**	0.9166	0.8526	0.8742	0.8249	0.8505
$S_{B,L,S}^{rG,rG,rG}$	<u>0.9428</u>	<u>0.9215</u>	0.8866	<u>0.9170</u>	0.8583	0.8790	<u>0.8268</u>	<u>0.8547</u>
$S_{B,L,S}^{R,R,R}$	0.9405	0.9186	0.8783	0.9124	0.8531	<u>0.8809</u>	0.8196	0.8512
All	**0.9432**	**0.9229**	0.8861	**0.9174**	**0.8663**	**0.8839**	**0.8291**	**0.8598**

Several other combinations of ensembles and thresholds were tested in the validation set, and it was always found that the validation set required larger thresholds than the training set. It was also found that disabling the data augmentation option during inference yielded better results in the validation set, which also allows the use of more models for the ensemble, as "fast" inference is up to 8 times faster than normal inference.

Table 2 shows the extension of the influence of large values of threshold. Two different thresholds are given for each ensemble. The first is the threshold with the best results in the training set (using the ranking system) and the second adjustments after analysing the results provided by the platform after running the first. It can be seen that larger thresholds are required for the validation set than for the training set. However, it is important to note that we cannot increase the threshold too much, as this could increase the number of FNs. The last row of the table shows the best overall results, however a value of 1450 voxels for the threshold of the WT might be too high for the test group. Therefore, the first solution is chosen for the test phase.

The results of our solution on the test cohort is presented in Table 3. All reported values were provided by the challenge organizers. Our method took first place in the BraTS 2023 Adult Glioma competition. In the test set, our method demonstrates superior performance in DSC for both TC and Enhancing Tumor (ET) regions compared to the validation set. However, the segmentation of WT exhibits a lower DSC. When assessing the HD95 metric, it becomes evident that our approach yields worse values for WT and TC, but better value for

Table 2. Validation set results computed by the validation platform (new metric). The values between parentheses are the threshold value used for (WT, TC, ET) respectively. The "All" is defined as $S_{B,L,S,B,L,S,B,L,S}^{pG,pG,pG,rG,rG,rG,R,R,R}$

Solutions	Thresholds			DSC				HD95			
	WT	TC	ET	WT	TC	ET	Mean	WT	TC	ET	Mean
$S_{B,L,S}^{pG,pG,pG}$	100	50	100	0.8867	0.8575	**0.8537**	0.8660	19.322	18.807	**17.321**	18.483
$S_{B,L,S}^{pG,pG,pG}$	300	200	200	0.8969	0.8660	<u>0.8528</u>	0.8719	15.798	16.397	19.470	17.222
$S_{B,L,S}^{rG,rG,rG}$	100	50	50	0.8918	0.8565	0.8347	0.8610	17.201	19.352	23.880	20.144
$S_{B,L,S}^{rG,rG,rG}$	250	150	100	0.8972	**0.8686**	0.8527	0.8728	15.510	**14.420**	<u>17.643</u>	15.858
$S_{B,L,S}^{R,R,R}$	100	50	50	0.8874	0.8564	0.8269	0.8569	19.637	19.090	23.794	20.840
$S_{B,L,S}^{R,R,R}$	250	150	100	0.8990	0.8606	0.8350	0.8648	15.121	18.275	21.049	18.148
All	250	150	100	<u>0.9005</u>	<u>0.8673</u>	0.8509	<u>0.8729</u>	<u>14.940</u>	<u>14.467</u>	17.699	<u>15.702</u>
All	1450	150	100	**0.9101**	<u>0.8673</u>	0.8509	**0.8761**	**11.113**	<u>14.467</u>	17.699	**14.426**

Table 3. Test set results computed by the organizers (new metric). The values between parentheses are the threshold value used for (WT, TC, ET) respectively. The "All" is the submitted solution, defined as $S_{B,L,S,B,L,S,B,L,S}^{pG,pG,pG,rG,rG,rG,R,R,R}$ using thresholds of 250, 150 and 100 voxels for the WT, TC and ET respectively

	DSC			HD95		
	WT	TC	ET	WT	TC	ET
mean	0.8851	0.8719	0.8685	22.838	22.974	16.713
std	0.1698	0.2357	0.1821	59.871	75.842	63.104
25quantile	0.8983	0.9102	0.8534	1.000	1.000	1.000
median	0.9555	0.9631	0.9331	2.000	1.414	1.000
75quantile	0.9775	0.9816	0.9655	5.605	3.345	2.236

ET. These findings suggest that employing different thresholds could potentially enhance overall results, yet it is noteworthy that the performance of ET remains consistently strong across both validation and test sets.

We can also conclude that the data augmentation with GliGAN gives the better DSC and HD95 for the ET. Furthermore, the ensemble of all available models gives the best solution using the ranking system (as explained in [13]) both in the training and validation set.

The other ensemble strategies were also tested but produced worse results than regular averaging, so they are not presented here. Although, these strategies have the potential to improve results, since the focus of our solution is on the use of synthetic data, most of the effort has gone into improving the synthetic data rather than improving the ensemble strategy.

Acknowledgements. André Ferreira thanks the Fundação para a Ciência e Tecnologia (FCT) Portugal for the grant 2022.11928.BD. This work has been supported by FCT within the R&D Units Project Scope: UIDB/00319/2020 and this work received funding from enFaced (FWF KLI 678), enFaced 2.0 (FWF KLI 1044) and KITE (Plattform für KI-Translation Essen, EFRE-0801977) from the REACT-EU initiative (https://kite.ikim.nrw/).

References

1. Adewole, M., et al.: The Brain Tumor Segmentation (BraTS) Challenge 2023: Glioma Segmentation in Sub-Saharan Africa Patient Population (BraTS-Africa). arXiv preprint arXiv:2305.19369 (2023)
2. Baid, U., et al.: The RSNA-ASNR-MICCAI BraTS 2021 benchmark on brain tumor segmentation and radiogenomic classification. arXiv preprint arXiv:2107.02314 (2021)
3. Bakas, S., et al.: Segmentation labels and radiomic features for the pre-operative scans of the TCGA-GBM collection. The cancer imaging archive (2017). https://doi.org/10.7937/K9/TCIA.2017.KLXWJJ1Q
4. Bakas, S., et al.: Segmentation labels and radiomic features for the pre-operative scans of the TCGA-LGG collection. The cancer imaging archive (2017). https://doi.org/10.7937/K9/TCIA.2017.GJQ7R0EF
5. Bakas, S., et al.: Advancing the cancer genome atlas glioma MRI collections with expert segmentation labels and radiomic features. Sci. Data **4**(1), 1–13 (2017). https://doi.org/10.1038/sdata.2017.117
6. Egger, J., et al.: Medical deep learning—a systematic meta-review. Comput. Methods Programs Biomed. **221**, 106874 (2022)
7. Egger, J., et al.: GBM volumetry using the 3D Slicer medical image computing platform. Sci. Rep. **3**(1), 1364 (2013)
8. Ellis, D.G., Aizenberg, M.R.: Deep learning using augmentation via registration: 1st place solution to the autoimplant 2020 challenge. In: Li, J., Egger, J. (eds.) AutoImplant 2020. LNCS, vol. 12439, pp. 47–55. Springer, Cham (2020). https://doi.org/10.1007/978-3-030-64327-0_6
9. Ferreira, A., Li, J., Pomykala, K.L., Kleesiek, J., Alves, V., Egger, J.: GAN-based generation of realistic 3D volumetric data: a systematic review and taxonomy. Med. Image Anal. **93**, 103100 (2024)
10. Ferreira, A., Magalhães, R., Mériaux, S., Alves, V.: Generation of synthetic rat brain MRI scans with a 3D enhanced alpha generative adversarial network. Appl. Sci. **12**(10), 4844 (2022)
11. Hatamizadeh, A., Nath, V., Tang, Y., Yang, D., Roth, H.R., Xu, D.: Swin UNETR: swin transformers for semantic segmentation of brain tumors in MRI images. In: Crimi, A., Bakas, S. (eds.) BrainLes 2021. LNCS, vol. 12962, pp. 272–284. Springer, Cham. https://doi.org/10.1007/978-3-031-08999-2_22
12. Isensee, F., Jaeger, P.F., Kohl, S.A., Petersen, J., Maier-Hein, K.H.: nnU-Net: a self-configuring method for deep learning-based biomedical image segmentation. Nat. Methods **18**(2), 203–211 (2021)
13. Isensee, F., Jäger, P.F., Full, P.M., Vollmuth, P., Maier-Hein, K.H.: nnU-Net for brain tumor segmentation. In: Crimi, A., Bakas, S. (eds.) BrainLes 2020. LNCS, vol. 12659, pp. 118–132. Springer, Cham (2021). https://doi.org/10.1007/978-3-030-72087-2_11

14. Jiang, Z., Ding, C., Liu, M., Tao, D.: Two-stage cascaded U-Net: 1st place solution to BraTS challenge 2019 segmentation task. In: Crimi, A., Bakas, S. (eds.) BrainLes 2019. LNCS, vol. 11992, pp. 231–241. Springer, Cham (2020). https://doi.org/10.1007/978-3-030-46640-4_22
15. Kamnitsas, K., et al.: Ensembles of multiple models and architectures for robust brain tumour segmentation. In: Crimi, A., Bakas, S., Kuijf, H., Menze, B., Reyes, M. (eds.) BrainLes 2017. LNCS, vol. 10670, pp. 450–462. Springer, Cham (2018). https://doi.org/10.1007/978-3-319-75238-9_38
16. Kamnitsas, K., Chen, L., Ledig, C., Rueckert, D., Glocker, B., et al.: Multi-scale 3D convolutional neural networks for lesion segmentation in brain MRI. Ischemic Stroke Lesion Segmentation **13**, 46 (2015)
17. Kamnitsas, K., et al.: Efficient multi-scale 3D CNN with fully connected CRF for accurate brain lesion segmentation. Med. Image Anal. **36**, 61–78 (2017)
18. Karargyris, A., et al.: Federated benchmarking of medical artificial intelligence with MedPerf. Nat. Mach. Intell. **5**(7), 799–810 (2023)
19. Liu, Z., et al.: Swin transformer: hierarchical vision transformer using shifted windows. In: Proceedings of the IEEE/CVF International Conference on Computer Vision, pp. 10012–10022 (2021)
20. Long, J., Shelhamer, E., Darrell, T.: Fully convolutional networks for semantic segmentation. In: Proceedings of the IEEE Conference on Computer Vision and Pattern Recognition, pp. 3431–3440 (2015)
21. Luu, H.M., Park, SH.: Extending nn-UNet for brain tumor segmentation. In: Crimi, A., Bakas, S. (eds.) BrainLes 2021. LNCS, vol. 12963, pp. 173–186. Springer, Cham (2022). https://doi.org/10.1007/978-3-031-09002-8_16
22. McKinley, R., Meier, R., Wiest, R.: Ensembles of densely-connected CNNs with label-uncertainty for brain tumor segmentation. In: Crimi, A., Bakas, S., Kuijf, H., Keyvan, F., Reyes, M., van Walsum, T. (eds.) BrainLes 2018. LNCS, vol. 11384, pp. 456–465. Springer, Cham (2019). https://doi.org/10.1007/978-3-030-11726-9_40
23. Menze, B.H., et al.: The multimodal brain tumor image segmentation benchmark (BraTS). IEEE Trans. Med. Imaging **34**(10), 1993–2024 (2014). https://doi.org/10.1109/TMI.2014.2377694
24. Pereira, S., Pinto, A., Alves, V., Silva, C.A.: Brain tumor segmentation using convolutional neural networks in MRI images. IEEE Trans. Med. Imaging **35**(5), 1240–1251 (2016)
25. Ronneberger, O., Fischer, P., Brox, T.: U-Net: convolutional networks for biomedical image segmentation. In: Navab, N., Hornegger, J., Wells, W.M., Frangi, A.F. (eds.) MICCAI 2015. LNCS, vol. 9351, pp. 234–241. Springer, Cham (2015). https://doi.org/10.1007/978-3-319-24574-4_28
26. Sawant, S., et al.: Comparing ensemble methods combined with different aggregating models using micrograph cell segmentation as an initial application example. J. Pathol. Inform. **14**, 100304 (2023)
27. The MONAI Consortium: Project MONAI (2020). https://doi.org/10.5281/zenodo.4323059
28. Urban, G., Bendszus, M., Hamprecht, F., Kleesiek, J.: Multi-modal brain tumor segmentation using deep convolutional neural networks. In: MICCAI BraTS (Brain Tumor Segmentation) Challenge. Proceedings, Winning Contribution, pp. 31–35 (2014)
29. Visser, M., et al.: Inter-rater agreement in glioma segmentations on longitudinal MRI. NeuroImage: Clin. **22**, 101727 (2019)
30. Vollmuth, P., et al.: Automated quantitative tumour response assessment of MRI in neuro-oncology with artificial neural networks (2019)

31. Zeineldin, R.A., Karar, M.E., Burgert, O., Mathis-Ullrich, F.: Multimodal CNN networks for brain tumor segmentation in MRI: a BraTS 2022 challenge solution. arXiv preprint arXiv:2212.09310 (2022)
32. Zeineldin, R.A., Karar, M.E., Coburger, J., Wirtz, C.R., Burgert, O.: DeepSeg: deep neural network framework for automatic brain tumor segmentation using magnetic resonance FLAIR images. Int. J. Comput. Assist. Radiol. Surg. **15**, 909–920 (2020)
33. Zhao, Y.-X., Zhang, Y.-M., Liu, C.-L.: Bag of tricks for 3D MRI brain tumor segmentation. In: Crimi, A., Bakas, S. (eds.) BrainLes 2019. LNCS, vol. 11992, pp. 210–220. Springer, Cham (2020). https://doi.org/10.1007/978-3-030-46640-4_20
34. Zhou, H.Y., Guo, J., Zhang, Y., Yu, L., Wang, L., Yu, Y.: nnFormer: interleaved transformer for volumetric segmentation. arXiv preprint arXiv:2109.03201 (2021)

Attention-Enhanced Hybrid Feature Aggregation Network for 3D Brain Tumor Segmentation

Ziya Ata Yazıcı[1]✉, İlkay Öksüz[1], and Hazım Kemal Ekenel[1,2]

[1] Department of Computer Engineering, Istanbul Technical University, Istanbul, Turkey
{yaziciz21,oksuzilkay,ekenel}@itu.edu.tr
[2] Department of Computer Science and Engineering, Qatar University, Doha, Qatar
hekenel@qu.edu.qa

Abstract. Glioblastoma is a highly aggressive and malignant brain tumor type that requires early diagnosis and prompt intervention. Due to its heterogeneity in appearance, developing automated detection approaches is challenging. To address this challenge, Artificial Intelligence (AI)-driven approaches in healthcare have generated interest in efficiently diagnosing and evaluating brain tumors. The Brain Tumor Segmentation Challenge (BraTS) is a platform for developing and assessing automated techniques for tumor analysis using high-quality, clinically acquired MRI data. In our approach, we utilized a multi-scale, attention-guided and hybrid U-Net-shaped model – GLIMS – to perform 3D brain tumor segmentation in three regions: Enhancing Tumor (ET), Tumor Core (TC), and Whole Tumor (WT). The multi-scale feature extraction provides better contextual feature aggregation in high resolutions and the Swin Transformer blocks improve the global feature extraction at deeper levels of the model. The segmentation mask generation in the decoder branch is guided by the attention-refined features gathered from the encoder branch to enhance the important attributes. Moreover, hierarchical supervision is used to train the model efficiently. Our model's performance on the validation set resulted in 92.19, 87.75, and 83.18 Dice Scores and 89.09, 84.67, and 82.15 Lesion-wise Dice Scores in WT, TC, and ET, respectively. The code is publicly available at https://github.com/yaziciz/GLIMS.

Keywords: Brain Tumor Segmentation · Vision Transformer · Deep Learning · Hybrid · Attention · BraTS

1 Introduction

Glioblastoma is a type of brain tumor that falls under high-grade gliomas (HGG), which are aggressive and malignant tumors originating from brain glial cells.

These tumors proliferate rapidly and often require surgery, radiotherapy, and have a poor prognosis in terms of survival [19]. Magnetic Resonance Imaging (MRI) has emerged as a crucial diagnostic tool for brain tumor analysis, providing detailed information about tumor location, size, and morphology. To comprehensively evaluate glioblastoma, multiple complimentary 3D MRI modalities, including T1, T1 with contrast agent (T1c), T2, and Fluid-attenuated Inversion Recovery (FLAIR), are utilized to highlight different tissue properties and areas of tumor spread [7]. With the advent of AI in healthcare, there is an increasing demand for AI-driven intervention strategies in diagnosing and preliminary evaluating brain tumors from MRI scans. The accurate segmentation and characterization of glioblastoma using AI techniques has the potential to significantly improve treatment planning and patient outcome predictions. In medical imaging research, the BraTS challenge promotes innovation and collaboration in tumor segmentation. The challenge provides high-quality, clinically-acquired, 3D multimodal and multi-site MRI scans with their ground truth masks annotated by radiologists [1].

The hybrid approaches in medical image segmentation tasks have been previously proposed [4,6,17,20]. These approaches involve integrating transformers, attention modules and convolutional layers to leverage the advantages of these structures; however, their implementation on the brain tumor segmentation task is limited. The utilization of Vision Transformer [8] (ViT) models, a sequence-to-sequence feature extractor, has greatly improved medical image segmentation tasks [9,10]. These models have demonstrated their advantages over Convolutional Neural Network (CNN)-based models in terms of their global feature extraction ability and segmentation performance when a large number of available data exists. On the contrary, CNN models excel in extracting local features, which is particularly advantageous in region-based segmentation tasks, where overlapping regions require clear edge segmentation.

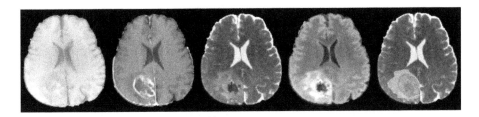

Fig. 1. A sample MRI scan displayed in four modalities – T1, T1c, T2, FLAIR – and the corresponding segmentation mask, left to right. NCR is represented by green, ET by red, and ED by yellow (Color figure online)

With this motivation, we propose a U-Net-shaped [18] **A**ttention-**G**uided **LI**ghtweight **M**ulti-**S**cale Hybrid Network (GLIMS) for 3D brain tumor segmentation, encompassing depth-wise multi-scale feature aggregation modules in a transformer-enhanced network. To improve the fine-grained segmentation mask prediction, we refine the encoder features via the channel and spatial-wise attention blocks as guidance on a skip connection. Furthermore, the model is supervised with multi-scale segmentation outputs, including the deeper decoder levels. With this approach, we participated in the Adult Glioblastoma Segmentation Task (Task 1) of the BraTS 2023 challenge, and our implementation ranked within the top 5 best-performing approaches in the validation phase.

2 Dataset

The dataset provided in BraTS 2023 consists of 1,251 multi-institutional 3D brain MRI scans in four modalities – T1, T1c, T2, and FLAIR – with the tumor segmented masks in four regions – necrotic tumor core (NCR), peritumoral edematous tissue (ED), enhancing tumor (ET) and the background (Fig. 1) [1–3,13,16]. The cross-sectional images of each modality are properly registered and the skull is removed from the images. The slices have a high-resolution isotropic voxel size of $1 \times 1 \times 1$ mm^3, and each MRI scan has a size of $240 \times 240 \times 155$ voxels in height, width, and depth. To comply with the ranking rules of the challenge, the given mask labels were converted into new label groups: Whole Tumor (WT) (NCR + ED + ET), Tumor Core (TC) (NCR + ET), and Enhancing Tumor (ET). A validation set with 219 cases without ground truth labels is also provided to evaluate the model performances through the official servers of BraTS 2023.

3 Methods

In the following sections, the architecture of GLIMS, pre- and post-processing approaches, the deep supervision technique, the evaluation metrics and the implementation details are given.

3.1 Model Overview

Our model's overall architecture is illustrated in Fig. 2, which utilizes **D**epth-**W**ise **M**ulti-**S**cale **F**eature Extraction (DMSF) modules and **D**epth-**W**ise **M**ulti-**S**cale **U**psampling (DMSU) modules in encoder and decoder branches, respectively. In each module, two consecutive **D**ilated Feature **A**ggregator **C**onvolutional **B**locks (DACB) are located. Depending on the branch, the convolutional blocks are followed with dilated $2 \times 2 \times 2$ convolution layer to downsample or transposed convolution to upsample. Each dilated convolutional layer in DACB is concatenated together, and two $1 \times 1 \times 1$ point-wise convolutions are applied sequentially to weight further the important features more and reduce the channels gradually, as shown in Fig. 3. The resulting output is added to the input scan for the next layer to prevent gradient-vanishing. By this proposed module, the fine-grained features of the regions could be extracted in different resolutions, which provides robustness in both local and global feature extraction compared to the standalone convolution and transformer networks. The

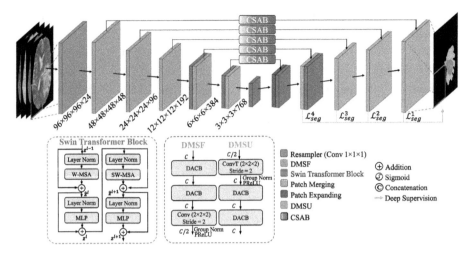

Fig. 2. The proposed architecture of 3D segmentation model, GLIMS. Each color represents a unique module (Color figure online)

lower levels of the proposed model are designed as a hybrid combination of convolutions and transformer blocks to enhance the contextual and global feature extraction together. The main motivation behind the hybrid design was to utilize the locality of convolutions and globality of the transformer layers to benefit both overall and region-wise tumor segmentation. The Swin Transformer layers were used in the deeper layers, which utilize the shifted-window self-attention approach to reduce the trainable parameters and, therefore, the model's complexity. Finally, the refined features via the **C**hannel and **S**patial-Wise **A**ttention **B**locks (CSAB) (Fig. 3) from the encoder branch were fused to the decoder branch with skip connections. The CSAB module refines input feature maps, y_l, by selectively enhancing or inhibiting features in the channel and spatial dimensions separately. After obtaining the refined features, $\hat{y}_l$, the decoder leverages them to guide the mask predictions.

The proposed model was designed to work efficiently on small graphical processing units due to its patch-based nature. A random patch from the whole input scan is sampled and processed with the model in each iteration. By this method, the training process requires less memory and benefits from a random-sampling augmentation process. Accordingly, the input size of the model is selected as $X \in \mathbb{R}^{H \times W \times D \times S}$, where H, W, and D are chosen as 96. The initial input is resampled with a $1 \times 1 \times 1$ point-wise convolutional layer to have a depth of S as 24. In each layer of the encoder branch, the spatial resolution of the feature matrix is halved and the channel resolution is doubled. The Swin Transformer block is used in the network's deeper encoder, decoder, and bottleneck parts for a hybrid approach. The input features to the transformer blocks are first partitioned with a patch size of $2 \times 2 \times 2$ to create tokens of $\left[\frac{H}{2}\right] \times \left[\frac{W}{2}\right] \times \left[\frac{D}{2}\right]$. The created patches are added with learnable positional embeddings in the shape of $\left[\frac{H}{2}\right] \times \left[\frac{W}{2}\right] \times \left[\frac{D}{2}\right] \times C$, where C is the hidden size of the current layer. Self-attention modules are applied to non-overlapping embedding windows for efficient processing. To perform the attention at transformer level l, we equally partition 3D tokens into $\left[\frac{H'}{M}\right] \times \left[\frac{W'}{M}\right] \times \left[\frac{D'}{M}\right]$, where $M \times M \times M$ is the window resolution; H', W' and D' are the current shape of the feature matrix in height, width, and depth, respectively. In the following layer $l+1$, the patches are shifted to capture local context and improve the model's ability to capture fine-grained local details. By shifting the patches, each patch can attend to its neighboring patches, allowing it to gather information from the surrounding local context. The shifting operation ensures that the receptive fields of the patches overlap, enabling the model to integrate the local feature relations effectively. To achieve this, the windows are shifted by $\left(\left[\frac{M}{2}\right], \left[\frac{M}{2}\right], \left[\frac{M}{2}\right]\right)$ voxels. The outputs of layers l and $l+1$ are found as shown in Eq. 1.

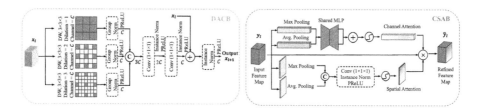

Fig. 3. The proposed DACB and CSAB modules from left to right, respectively

$$\begin{aligned}
\hat{z}_l &= \text{W-MSA}(\text{LN}(z_{l-1})) + z_{l-1} \\
z_l &= \text{MLP}(\text{LN}(\hat{z}_l)) + \hat{z}_l \\
\hat{z}_{l+1} &= \text{SW-MSA}(\text{LN}(z_l)) + z_l \\
z_{l+1} &= \text{MLP}(\text{LN}(\hat{z}_{l+1})) + \hat{z}_{l+1}
\end{aligned} \qquad (1)$$

In Eq. 1, W-MSA, SW-MSA, LN, and MLP represent windowed and shifted window multi-head self-attention modules, layer normalization, and multi-layer perceptron, respectively. The patches are shifted after every W-MSA layer using cyclic-shift [15]. This ensures that the number of windows for self-attention remains the same and the complexity does not increase. Finally, GLIMS has 72.30G FLOPs and 47.16M trainable parameters, making it comparably lightweight to the previous studies.

3.2 Data Pre-processing

Each MRI scan has a NIfTI format with separate modalities and a segmentation mask in three classes. In the scope of the challenge, the segmentation results should be evaluated in modified sub-regions such as WT, TC, and ET. Therefore, the label modifications and augmentations were applied on the fly during training by using the MONAI [5] framework. To implement the patch-based training technique, a randomly cropped volume with a size of 96 × 96 × 96 is taken from a 3D MRI scan. Each cropped region was flipped in X-Y-Z axes with an equal probability of 0.5. Z-normalization was applied to the scans and each normalization was performed independently between the modalities. The normalized intensities were scaled and shifted to simulate the different scanner properties with a factor of 0.2 and a probability of 0.2. To make the model robustly generalize the unseen data, the contrast of the cropped volumes was changed with a gamma value between $[0.5, 4.5]$ and a probability of 0.2. Additionally, Gaussian noise was added with $\sigma = 0.2$, $\mu = 0$, and Gaussian smoothing was applied with a varying σ value in X-Y-Z axes between $[0.25, 1.15]$ with a probability of 0.2.

3.3 Evaluation Metrics and Loss Function

The segmentation performance of the models was evaluated with Dice Score and Hausdorff95 (HD95) distance metrics. Compared to the previous BraTS challenges, two new evaluation metrics were introduced this year: Lesion-wise Dice Score and Lesion-wise HD95. These metrics provide insights into how well models detect and segment multiple individual lesions within a scan, addressing the importance of identifying large and small lesions in clinical practice. For the Lesion-wise metrics, the ground truth masks undergo a $3 \times 3 \times 3$ mm^3 dilation before calculating the Dice Score and HD95. Following the process, connected component analysis is performed on the predictions to compare the lesions with the ground truth labels by counting the number of True Positive (TP), False Positive (FP), True Negative (TN), and False Negative (FN) predicted voxels.

The models were optimized with the combination of Dice Loss (Eq. 2) and Cross-Entropy Loss (Eq. 3) as shown in Eq. 4.

$$\mathcal{L}_{Dice} = \frac{2}{K} \sum_{k=1}^{K} \frac{\sum_{i=1}^{N} y_{i,k} p_{i,k}}{\sum_{i=1}^{N} y_{i,k}^2 + \sum_{i=1}^{N} p_{i,k}^2} \tag{2}$$

$$\mathcal{L}_{CE} = \sum_{k=1}^{K} \sum_{i=1}^{N} y_{i,k} \log(p_{i,k}) \tag{3}$$

$$\mathcal{L}_{Seg} = 1 - \alpha \mathcal{L}_{Dice} - \beta \mathcal{L}_{CE} \tag{4}$$

where K represents the total number of classes, N represents the number of voxels, y refers to the ground truth labels, and p refers to the predicted one-hot classes. The weights of α and β were selected as 0.5 to calculate the total loss.

3.4 Deep Supervision

Deep supervision [21] is a technique of computing the loss function, $\mathcal{L}_{DS}$, from the last layer and incorporating the deeper layers of the decoder. It involves training CNNs with multiple intermediate supervision signals, allowing for better performance and improved segmentation results. Traditionally, the network is trained end-to-end with a single mask output, making it difficult to identify and correct errors at different stages of the network. However, by introducing intermediate supervision, additional loss functions are applied at multiple network layers, enabling the network to learn more discriminative and informative features. The utilized loss function can be seen in Eq. 5, where each $L_{seg}^i, i \in \{1,2,3,4\}$ represents the loss values corresponding to the combination of $\mathcal{L}_{Dice}$ and $\mathcal{L}_{CE}$ for level i. While shallower layers have the highest weight, the given weight decreases for the deeper layers.

$$\mathcal{L}_{DS} = \mathcal{L}_{seg}^1 + \frac{1}{2}\mathcal{L}_{seg}^2 + \frac{1}{4}\mathcal{L}_{seg}^3 + \frac{1}{8}\mathcal{L}_{seg}^4 \tag{5}$$

3.5 Post-processing

The post-processing of the predicted region masks could improve the metric results significantly, as experimented by the previous studies [12,14]. Especially in the cases where no ground truth class occurs in a specific slice, eliminating false positive predictions increases the Dice Score from 0 to 100. Thus, to advance the model's performance more, three post-processing steps were considered to be applied in our approach:

- **Region Removal:** Small regions with # of voxels less than ψ with mean confidence less than θ are removed from the predictions. This is applied to eliminate the false positive predictions of the scans with no ground truth label to increase the Dice Score from 0 to 100.
- **Threshold Modification:** The models are optimized to perform thresholding at 0.5 while selecting the hard labels from the region probabilities. However, adjusting the confidence level during inference could be beneficial to eliminate exceeding region borders or including border voxels to the region.
- **Center Filling:** To improve the segmentation performance of class ET and TC, the center voxels of the ET components are replaced with NCR. This could improve ET and TC Dice Scores.

3.6 Implementation Details

Our model, GLIMS, was implemented in PyTorch framework v2.0.1 by using the MONAI library v1.2.0. The experiments were performed on a single NVIDIA 3090 GPU with 24 GB VRAM for 800 epochs in a 5-fold cross-validation approach. The learning rate was set to 0.001 and the cosine annealing scheduler was used to update the learning rate. The parameters were updated with the AdamW optimizer. The batch size was selected as two, and a sliding window approach with a 0.8 inference overlap was applied using 96 × 96 × 96 patch size. The model parameters were saved for the highest Dice Scores on the internal validation set, and the experiments were performed on the best model states.

4 Results

The performance of the proposed model was compared with the nnU-net [11] architecture as a baseline, which was among the top-performing models of the previous years. The experiments were conducted using the same training dataset and data distribution for both models. We maintained consistency in all implementation details while conducting the experiments. The results in Table 1 show that our method performed better by 0.88% in the overall performance in terms of the Lesion-wise Dice Score.

Table 1. The experimental results of 5-fold cross-validation in Legacy Dice Scores (%) without post-processing is applied

Model	Fold 1	Fold 2	Fold 3	Fold 4	Fold 5	Average ↑
nnU-net [11]	90.12	90.80	91.45	91.75	90.42	90.91
Ours	**91.19**	**91.52**	**92.74**	**92.21**	**91.27**	**91.79**

The experiments were extended to the validation set to select the best-performing settings. These studies cover post-processing and ensemble approaches with varying parameter selection. We first observed the influence of the post-processing techniques on the validation set performance. The results in Table 2 show the improvement of the methods as they were applied to the predicted segmentation masks. As the post-processing techniques were applied, the average Lesion-wise Dice Score improvement was observed as 15.5% for Fold 0. The removal of small false positive predictions in the slices without true positive ground truth labels increased the individual Dice Scores from 0 to 100.

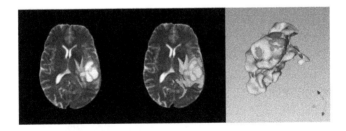

Fig. 4. The prediction result of Case ID: 208 in the validation set. Left: The T2 image of the slice. Middle: The segmented output. Right: 3D rendered visualization of the tumor. The yellow, red, and green colors represent ED, ET, and NCR regions (Color figure online)

Based on the experiments, the best settings were selected as the removal of the ET and NCR regions smaller than 75mm^3 and ED regions smaller than

Table 2. The experimental results on the online validation set with different post-processing and ensemble approaches. The results are given in the Lesion-wise metrics and were obtained through the submission system of BraTS 2023. *RR*: Region Removal, *TM*: Threshold Modification, *CF*: Center Filling. [a]The TC threshold was set to 0.6. [b]The ET threshold was set to 0.6

Model	Method			HD95 (mm) ↓			Dice Score (%) ↑			
	RR	TM	CF	ET	TC	WT	ET	TC	WT	Avg.
Fold 0				91.49	70.59	107.07	66.66	73.13	66.20	68.66
Fold 1				141.51	112.12	133.34	54.56	62.32	59.38	58.75
Fold 0	✓			25.63	33.10	19.07	81.85	81.76	87.98	83.86
Fold 0[a]	✓	✓		25.63	29.42	19.07	81.85	82.57	87.98	84.13
Fold 0[a]	✓	✓	✓	25.63	29.42	18.43	81.85	82.57	88.12	84.18
Fold 2[a]	✓	✓	✓	26.34	23.75	17.35	82.04	83.91	88.56	84.84
Fold 3[a]	✓	✓	✓	28.76	34.30	16.47	80.91	80.87	88.49	83.42
Fold 2+4[ab]	✓	✓	✓	**25.16**	**20.75**	**15.80**	**82.15**	**84.67**	**89.09**	**85.30**

$500\,\text{mm}^3$ if the model's average confidence is less than 0.9. For the threshold modification method, threshold levels between 0.5 and 0.7 were tested. It was observed that changing the threshold of ET and TC from 0.5 to 0.6 was the most effective approach, which reduced the false positive TC predictions. Lastly, after a connected component analysis in 3D, the voxels inside the ET regions were replaced as NCR voxels. This approach improved the TC segmentation performance as well as WT if any unassigned voxels occurred. The ensemble methods also improved the results; thus, our submission was based on the combination of post-processed Fold 2 and Fold 4 models, as it yielded the highest Lesion-wise Dice Score. Lastly, as a qualitative result of the approach, a sample mask prediction and a 3D-rendered tumor output from the validation set can be seen in Fig. 4.

Table 3. The segmentation performance of the proposed approach in Lesion-wise metrics on the online validation and test sets. The scores are retrieved from the official submission system of BraTS 2023

Data Split	HD95 (mm) ↓				Dice Score (%) ↑			
	ET	TC	WT	Avg.	ET	TC	WT	Avg.
Validation	25.16	20.75	15.80	20.57	82.15	84.67	89.09	85.30
Test	26.01	34.68	28.50	29.73	83.67	82.90	85.97	84.18

The approach that yielded the best validation result was also evaluated on the blinded test set. Compared to the validation split, the MRI samples in the testing set are sampled from a different patient cohort and multi-institutional sensors compared to the training set. According to the post-challenge results on the testing data, our model had a slight decrease in the mean Lesion-wise Dice Score and an increase in Lesion-wise HD95 metrics by 1.12% and 9.16 mm, achieving an average of 84.18% Dice Score and 29.73 mm HD95 in lesion-wise performance, as shown in Table 3.

5 Discussion and Conclusions

In this study, we proposed a U-net-shaped hybrid 3D MRI segmentation model for the BraTS 2023 challenge. We utilized depth-wise multi-scale feature extraction blocks and attention modules to perform fine-grained region-based segmentation tasks with high Lesion-wise performance. To reduce the number of trainable parameters; transformer blocks were incorporated in the bottleneck, the convolutional layers were converted to perform depth-wise operations and the sliding window inference technique was used. An attention guidance method was implemented to support tumor region prediction by utilizing important features from the encoder branch. Additionally, the impact of the post-processing techniques on the segmentation performance was examined. Although the Legacy Dice Score was less affected by post-processing techniques; removing small false positive regions from the outputs, adjusting the prediction threshold, and filling the center of the connected components significantly improved the Lesion-wise Dice Score. On the online validation set, GLIMS achieved a Lesion-wise Dice Score of 0.8909, 0.8467, and 0.8215 for WT, TC, and ET classes, respectively, placing it among the top 5 best-performing approaches in the validation phase. In the testing phase, as the data distribution changed compared to the training set, our approach achieved 84.18% Lesion-wise Dice Score by a decrease of 1.12%, and 29.73 mm Lesion-wise HD95 by an increase of 9.16 mm compared to the validation result.

The results represent our model's enhanced performance on the 3D brain tumor segmentation task and the robustness of the post-processing techniques. As a slight performance decrease occurred in the test set, we could diversify the representation of the patients and the sensors in the training dataset by synthetically generating healthy and diseased MRI scans. Therefore, as a further study, synthetic data generation techniques could be employed to improve the model's generalizability on unseen data by introducing MRI samples in wider settings. Additionally, to reduce the possible defects in the predicted masks further, new post-processing methods could be employed by integrating the field knowledge of the physicians. Moreover, the proposed models should be further optimized to run efficiently on the end-user side. Although increasing the model size generally improves the segmentation performance, it becomes challenging to deploy and use effectively. Thus, in the future, we aim to investigate the impact of the synthetic data, reduce the model complexity more by utilizing lightweight yet robust modules, and perform better optimization techniques.

Acknowledgements. This study has been partially funded by Istanbul Technical University, Department of Computer Engineering and Turkcell via a Research Scholarship grant provided to Ziya Ata Yazıcı.

References

1. Baid, U., et al.: The RSNA-ASNR-MICCAI BraTS 2021 Benchmark on Brain Tumor Segmentation and Radiogenomic Classification. arXiv preprint arXiv:2107.02314 (2021). https://doi.org/10.48550/arXiv.2107.02314
2. Bakas, S., et al.: Segmentation Labels and Radiomic Features for the Pre-operative Scans of the TCGA-GBM Collection. The Cancer Imaging Archive (2017). https://doi.org/10.7937/K9/TCIA.2017.KLXWJJ1Q
3. Bakas, S., et al.: Segmentation Labels and Radiomic Features for the Pre-Operative Scans of the TCGA-LGG Collection. The Cancer Imaging Archive (2017). https://doi.org/10.7937/K9/TCIA.2017.GJQ7R0EF
4. Bao, H., Zhu, Y., Li, Q.: Hybrid-scale contextual fusion network for medical image segmentation. Comput. Biol. Med. **152**, 106439 (2023). https://doi.org/10.1016/j.compbiomed.2022.106439
5. Cardoso, M.J., et al.: MONAI: An Open-Source Framework for Deep Learning in Healthcare. arXiv preprint arXiv:2211.02701 (2022). https://doi.org/10.48550/arXiv.2211.02701
6. Chen, Q., et al.: MixFormer: mixing features across windows and dimensions. 2022 IEEE/CVF Conference on Computer Vision and Pattern Recognition (CVPR) (2022). https://doi.org/10.1109/cvpr52688.2022.00518
7. van Dijken, B.R., van Laar, P.J., Smits, M., Dankbaar, J.W., Enting, R.H., van der Hoorn, A.: Perfusion MRI in treatment evaluation of glioblastomas: clinical relevance of current and future techniques. J. Magn. Reson. Imaging **49**(1), 11–22 (2018). https://doi.org/10.1002/jmri.26306
8. Dosovitskiy, A., et al.: An image is worth 16×16 words: transformers for image recognition at scale. arXiv preprint arXiv:2010.11929 (2020). https://doi.org/10.48550/arXiv.2010.11929
9. Hatamizadeh, A., Nath, V., Tang, Y., Yang, D., Roth, H.R., Xu, D.: Swin UNETR: swin transformers for semantic segmentation of brain tumors in MRI images. In: Crimi, A., Bakas, S. (eds.) BrainLes 2021. LNCS, vol. 12962, pp. 272–284. Springer, Cham (2022). https://doi.org/10.1007/978-3-031-08999-2_22
10. Heidari, M., et al.: HiFormer: hierarchical multi-scale representations using transformers for medical image segmentation. In: 2023 IEEE/CVF Winter Conference on Applications of Computer Vision (WACV) (2023). https://doi.org/10.1109/wacv56688.2023.00614
11. Isensee, F., Jaeger, P.F., Kohl, S.A., Petersen, J., Maier-Hein, K.H.: nnU-Net: a self-configuring method for deep learning-based biomedical image segmentation. Nat. Methods **18**(2), 203–211 (2021). https://doi.org/10.1038/s41592-020-01008-z
12. Jabareen, N., Lukassen, S.: Segmenting brain tumors in multi-modal MRI scans using a 3D SegNet architecture. In: Crimi, A., Bakas, S. (eds.) BrainLes 2021. LNCS, vol. 12962, pp. 377–388. Springer, Cham (2022). https://doi.org/10.1007/978-3-031-08999-2_32
13. Karargyris, A., et al.: Federated benchmarking of medical artificial intelligence with MedPerf. Nat. Mach. Intell. **5**(7), 799–810 (2023). https://doi.org/10.1038/s42256-023-00652-2

14. Kotowski, K., Adamski, S., Machura, B., Zarudzki, L., Nalepa, J.: Coupling nnU-Nets with expert knowledge for accurate brain tumor segmentation from MRI. In: Crimi, A., Bakas, S. (eds.) BrainLes 2021. LNCS, vol. 12963, pp. 197–209. Springer, Cham (2022). https://doi.org/10.1007/978-3-031-09002-8_18
15. Liu, Z., et al.: Swin transformer: hierarchical vision transformer using shifted windows. In: 2021 IEEE/CVF International Conference on Computer Vision (ICCV) (2021). https://doi.org/10.1109/iccv48922.2021.00986
16. Menze, B.H., et al.: The multimodal brain tumor image segmentation benchmark (BraTS). IEEE Trans. Med. Imaging **34**(10), 1993–2024 (2015). https://doi.org/10.1109/tmi.2014.2377694
17. Oktay, O., et al.: Attention U-Net: learning where to look for the pancreas. In: Medical Imaging with Deep Learning (2022). https://doi.org/10.48550/arXiv.1804.03999
18. Ronneberger, O., Fischer, P., Brox, T.: U-Net: convolutional networks for biomedical image segmentation. In: Navab, N., Hornegger, J., Wells, W., Frangi, A. (eds.) MICCAI 2015. LNCS, vol. 9351, pp. 234–241. Springer, Cham (2015). https://doi.org/10.1007/978-3-319-24574-4_28
19. Thakkar, J.P., et al.: Epidemiologic and molecular prognostic review of glioblastoma. Cancer Epidemiol. Biomark. Prev. **23**(10), 1985–1996 (2014). https://doi.org/10.1158/1055-9965.epi-14-0275
20. Yuan, F., Zhang, Z., Fang, Z.: An effective CNN and transformer complementary network for medical image segmentation. Pattern Recogn. **136**, 109228 (2023). https://doi.org/10.1016/j.patcog.2022.109228
21. Zhu, Q., Du, B., Turkbey, B., Choyke, P.L., Yan, P.: Deeply-supervised CNN for prostate segmentation. In: 2017 International Joint Conference on Neural Networks (IJCNN) (2017). https://doi.org/10.1109/ijcnn.2017.7965852

3D ST-Net: A Large Kernel Simple Transformer for Brain Tumor Segmentation

Jiahao Zheng and Liqin Huang[✉]

Institute of Bioengineering, Fuzhou University, Fuzhou, China
hlq@fzu.edu.cn

Abstract. Glioblastoma is the most common primary malignant brain tumor, necessitating precise depiction through magnetic resonance (MR) imaging for effective treatment. Due to the tumor's heterogeneous and elusive boundaries, appearance, and shape, automated segmentation remains a complex task. With the emergence of deep learning, researchers have significantly improved brain tumor segmentation using convolutional neural networks. In this article, we propose a novel volume-based 3D Simple Transformation Network (ST-Net), which utilizes large convolutional kernels ($7 \times 7 \times 7$) to map the original three-dimensional images into a lower-dimensional latent space, and employ depthwise convolutional scaling (DCS) to separate spatial and channel dimensions, reducing memory parameters and computational load while enlarging the receptive field. To enhance segmentation performance, our loss function combines cross-entropy and Dice loss. Through online validation, the enhanced Dice scores for Enhancing Tumor (ET), Tumor Core (TC), and Whole Tumor (WT) are 0.776, 0.790, and 0.880, respectively, while the Hausdorff distance measures are 36.7, 35.3, and 18.2.

Keywords: Brain tumor segmentation · convolutional neural network · Simple Transformer

1 Introduction

Glioblastoma is one of the most common and fatal primary brain tumors in adults. It exhibits a high degree of invasiveness and is prone to spreading to other tissues, making complete resection a formidable challenge. The goal of surgical removal is to excise the tumor while preserving neurological function and minimizing damage. The heterogeneity of gliomas presents uncertainties in terms of their appearance, morphology, and histology, affecting prognosis.

Magnetic resonance imaging (MRI) plays a pivotal role in the diagnosis of brain tumors. Tumor segmentation forms the foundation of tumor treatment. Describing and segmenting the tumor and its respective subregions is a complex and time-consuming task requiring the expertise of medical image annotators. Accurate prediction of tumor regions in medical images is crucial for the diagnosis and treatment management of glioblastoma.

The BraTS (Brain Tumor Segmentation) challenge offers a platform for participants to evaluate their models utilizing the BraTS 2023 dataset and compare their findings with other teams [1–4,12]. In the realm of brain tumor segmentation, the U-Net [15] framework and its variant networks performance in addition to strong segmentation capabilities [6,7,13,19,20]. An extended iteration of nn-UNet was proposed during BraTS 2021 and won the Challenge Championship. They performed various enhancements on nn-UNet, including using larger networks, using group normalization instead of batch normalization, and integrating axial attention in the decoder. Through 5-fold cross-validation and evaluation within the organizers, they demonstrated the effectiveness of their method [11]. The team led by Wang Wenxuan has proposed TransBTS, a breakthrough innovation in 3D CNN. For the first time, the Transformer model is applied in tumor segmentation of MRI brain scans. TransBTS still adopts the encoder-decoder U-shaped framework, utilizing 3D CNN as the feature extractor and incorporating the Transformer model to capture global contextual information. The decoder integrates the feature embeddings from the Transformer model and achieves accurate segmentation images through progressive upsampling at each layer. [17]. Ali Hatamizadeh et al. proposed Swin UNETR, reformulating the task of 3D brain tumor semantic segmentation as a sequence-to-sequence prediction problem. They map multi-modal input data into one-dimensional embedding sequences as inputs for a layered Swin Transformer encoder. The Swin Transformer encoder employs shifted windows for self-attention computation, extracting features at various resolutions and connecting them with skip connections to a decoder based on Fully Convolutional Neural Networks (FCNN) [8]. Additionally, Zhaopei Li et al. proposed a U-Net-based segmentation network with the inclusion of multi-scale feature extraction and recalibration modules to achieve improved segmentation performance. This approach utilizes the structure of U-Net to extract features at each scale and enhance feature expressiveness through recalibration modules [10].

In this passage, we propose a segmentation model called the Simple Transformer Network for automating semantic segmentation of different subregions of brain tumors in the BraTS 2023 challenge. This network employs convolutional modules with large kernels to achieve a wider receptive field, thereby enhancing its understanding of image structures and texture information at various scales, ultimately improving segmentation accuracy. To address the issue of class imbalance in brain tumor segmentation tasks, we introduce weighted coefficients in the loss terms, including cross-entropy and Dice loss. This balanced consideration helps to focus attention on minority classes, enriching the overall quality of the segmentation results. Experimental results are obtained through evaluation on the 2023 BraTS Glioma Challenge dataset, with Dice coefficients of 88.05% for whole tumor (WT), 79.02% for tumor core (TC), and 77.69% for enhanced tumor(ET).

2 Method

In the subsequent section, namely Sect. 2.1, we elaborate on the complete network framework. Subsequently, in Sect. 2.2, we present the Simple Transformer and delve into a detailed elucidation of both DCONV and DCT. Section 2.3 further elucidates the structure of the decoder. Finally, in Sect. 2.4, we offer a comprehensive exegesis of the loss function.

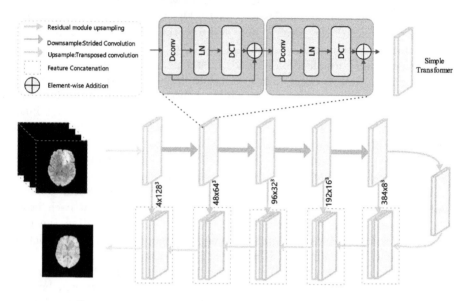

Fig. 1. The overall network architecture.

2.1 Network Architecture

In general, Our network architecture adheres to a U-shaped structure similar to the 3D U-Net encoder-decoder. The encoder part consists of four simplistic transformer modules and four downsampling modules. These downsampling modules effectively reduce the size of feature maps, capturing feature information at various scales. The decoder part comprises four upsampling layers and residual modules intertwined with four basic blocks. Upsampling layers restore the size of the feature maps from the encoder to match the input size, enabling refinement and reconstruction of the target. The residual modules learn the residual information of the features, enhancing and merging them before concatenation [9]. The complete architecture of the 3D simplistic transformer is illustrated in Fig. 1, providing a better understanding of the structure and information flow of the model.

2.2 Simple Transformer Encoder

The encoder component utilizes large convolutional modules as feature extractors, taking in image data of volume $C \times H \times W \times D$ and performing convolutional operations with a large kernel size of $7 \times 7 \times 7$. This generates an output feature map with 48 channels and spatial dimensions halved compared to the input. To reduce computation and enhance generalization capability, deep convolutional modules (DCONV) and layer normalization (LN) operations are employed. The output of layer L and layer L+1 are defined as:

$$\begin{aligned} Z^{L'} &= DCONV(Z^{L-1}) \\ Z^L &= DCT(LN(Z^{L'})) + Z^{L'} \\ Z^{(L+1)'} &= DCONV(Z^L) \\ Z^{L+1} &= DCT(LN(Z^{(L+1)'})) + Z^{(L+1)'} \end{aligned} \quad (1)$$

Z(L′) and Z(L+1′) are the outputs from DCONV layers at different depths, used for inter-channel information exchange. LN represents layer normalization operation, while DCT represents nonlinear transformation. The DCT module begins by expanding the number of channels to four times the input channel count in the depthwise convolutional scaling(DCS). It is then passed through the GELU and Global Response Normalization(GRN) [18]. Finally, the depthwise convolutional scaling module restores the channel count to match the input channel count. The DCT structure is illustrated as shown in Fig. 2(a).

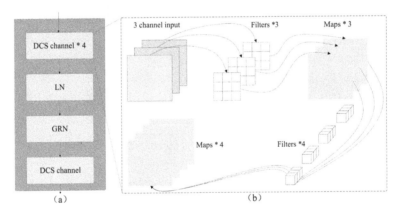

Fig. 2. The diagram in (a) illustrates the structure of the DCT module, while (b) shows the simplified structure of DCS.

The GRN layer enhances feature competition among channels in convolutional neural networks, making the model more expressive and better at generalization. DCS primarily consists of two components: Depthwise Convolution and Pointwise Convolution. Its advantage lies in reducing the number of parameters and computational load. In the Depthwise Convolution stage, each channel only needs to learn one convolution kernel without considering the correlation between multiple channels, effectively reducing the number of parameters. Additionally, Pointwise Convolution can effectively reduce the number of channels, further reducing the overall computational load. Its structure is depicted in Fig. 2(b).

By employing standard convolution blocks with dimensions of $2 \times 2 \times 2$, the resolution of the features is reduced by a factor of 2, with a stride of 2. Through stages 2, 3, and 4, the same process is iteratively repeated, resulting in resolutions of $\frac{H}{4} \times \frac{W}{4} \times \frac{D}{4}$, $\frac{H}{8} \times \frac{W}{8} \times \frac{D}{8}$, and $\frac{H}{16} \times \frac{W}{16} \times \frac{D}{16}$ respectively, gradually decreasing in scale. The number of feature channels continuously increases, with quantities of 48, 96, 192, and 384. This design enhances the expressive and learning capabilities of the model, by incorporating more contextual information and reducing redundancy. Alongside the decrease in resolution, computational complexity is also reduced, leading to improved computational efficiency.

2.3 Decoder

At each stage of the encoder, the multi-scale outputs are passed through residual modules and connected to the decoder. The residual modules consist of two post-normalized $3 \times 3 \times 3$ convolutional layers to enhance feature representation and learning capability. In the decoder, transpose convolutional layers are used for upsampling operations to restore feature maps to the size of the original input. The output of the skip connection from the residual network is concatenated with the feature map of the previous layer for feature fusion and enhancement. This decoder structure facilitates the fusion of low-level information, thereby enhancing the network's feature representation and information transmission capability.

2.4 Loss

The formula for the Total Weighted Loss function is as follows:

$$L_T(B, \hat{B}) = \frac{1}{N} \sum_{i=1}^{N} [L_{CE}(B_i, \hat{B}_i) + L_{DSC}(B_i, \hat{B}_i)] \quad (2)$$

The L_T is a combination of category-weighted cross-entropy (CE) loss and category Dice loss [5]. Through this overall weighted loss function, both the category-weighted cross-entropy loss and category Dice loss are taken into account simultaneously, enabling a comprehensive evaluation of the differences between the model predictions and the ground truth. This facilitates optimization and training. B_i represents the i-th ground truth of a batch of input images, while $\hat{B}_i$ represents the i-th Mask predicted from the batch. N is the total number of pixels in the input slices of a batch. L_{DSC} refers to the Dice loss, which is defined by the following formula:

$$L_{DSC}(B, \hat{B}) = \frac{1}{C} \sum_{i=1}^{C} W_C (1 - \frac{2|B_i \cap \hat{B}_i|}{B_i + \hat{B}_i}) \quad (3)$$

In this context, C refers to the number of categories in the classification, with a total of four categories (GD-enhancing tumor, peritumoral edema/invasive tissue, necrotic tumor core, and background). Wc represents the weight of the Dice loss for each category, B is the ground truth of a batch input image, and B_i is the predicted Mask of a batch. Furthermore, L_{CE} stands for class-weighted cross-entropy loss, which can be expressed as follows:

$$L_{CE}(B, \hat{B}) = \frac{1}{C} \sum_{i=1}^{C} W_C \sum_{j=1}^{P} [P_{cj} \log \hat{P_{cj}} + (1 - P_{cj}) \log (1 - \hat{P_{cj}})] \quad (4)$$

p_{cj} is the j-th basic true value pixel of class c. p_{cj} refers to the corresponding prediction probability. Wc represents the weight of each categorys Dice loss.

3 Experiments

In this section, we will present the datasets used in the experiments outlined in Sect. 3.1, while elucidating the evaluation metrics employed in Sect. 3.2. Subsequently, the preprocessing and postprocessing techniques adopted will be described in Sects. 3.3 and 3.4, respectively.

3.1 Dataset

The 2023 BraTS Glioma Challenge dataset is divided into a training set, validation set, and test set. Each data includes multi-modal MRI images, including native (T1), post-contrast T1-weighted (T1Gd), T2-weighted (T2), and T2 fluid-attenuated inversion recovery (T2-FLAIR). These imaging datasets have been manually annotated and labeled using the same annotation protocol, and have been reviewed by experienced neuro-radiologists. The annotations include gadolinium-enhanced tumor (ET - label 3), peritumoral edema/infiltration (ED - label 2), and necrotic tumor core (NCR - label 1). TC (Tumor Core) entails the label 3, WT (Whole Tumor) entails the TC and label 2, as illustrated in Fig. 3. The ground truth data were created after preprocessing, which involved co-registering them to a common anatomical template and interpolating them to the same resolution ($1\,\text{mm}^3$.), while excluding the skull. The validation set consists of 219 cases, with annotations withheld from the participants. The test set, on the other hand, is not publicly available to the participants for the final evaluation of their models.

3.2 Metrics

The Dice similarity coefficient measures the similarity between predicted segmentation results and true segmentation. The range of the Dice coefficient is from 0 to 1, where a higher value indicates increased overlap between the projected and labeled regions. On the other hand, the Hausdorff distance (HD) is used to assess the proximity of the segmentation result to the actual segmentation boundary. In the field of segmentation tasks, the Hausdorff distance can be

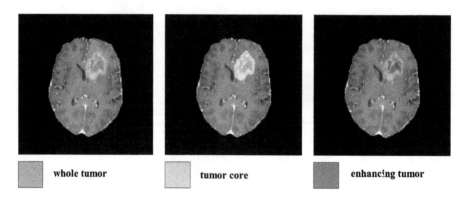

Fig. 3. Tumors and their respective subregions

utilized to evaluate the consistency between the projected boundaries and the ground truth.

Unlike the BraTS 2021 challenge, the BraTS 2023 challenge incorporates the LesionWise_Dice and LesionWise_Hausdorff95, which are specifically designed for evaluating the segmentation performance in the presence of damage. Unlike Dice and HD, these two metrics are highly sensitive to the false positive rate. Blindly improving the segmentation performance may increase the false positive rate and consequently lower the values of these metrics. Therefore, the LesionWise_Dice and LesionWise_Hausdorff95 offer more comprehensive measures.

3.3 Data Preprocessing and Augmentation

In order to reduce the computational complexity and enhance overall performance during the training process, a series of data preprocessing [16] steps were undertaken. The following are the adopted preprocessing steps:

Data normalization: All input images were standardized through zero mean and unit standard deviation normalization, ensuring uniformity in their processing. Spatial cropping: Images were center cropped from $240 \times 240 \times 155$ voxels to $128 \times 128 \times 128$ voxels, reducing the computational resources required during the training phase. This cropping process selectively removed irrelevant information at the image edges while preserving crucial tumor and brain tissue structures. Multimodal data concatenation: Four MRI modalities (T1N, T2F, T2W, and T1C) were concatenated and used as inputs to the neural network. This approach aids in extracting various spatial features during the training process, thereby enhancing the overall segmentation effectiveness for brain tumors.

Data augmentation: Various data augmentation techniques were employed to expand the training dataset. These techniques included cropping, rotation, flipping, adding Gaussian noise, altering contrast, and enhancing brightness. Through these augmentation techniques, a more diverse set of training samples was generated, improving the model's robustness to different transformations and noise. These preprocessing steps play a crucial role in reducing computational complexity, enhancing performance, and diversifying the training data, thus optimizing the training process for brain tumor segmentation models.

3.4 Postprocessing

To minimize the false positive rate, we employ post-processing on the predicted results by selecting the largest connected component. Finally, the maximum connected 3D segmentation graph is obtained. Additionally, we adhere to the requirements set by the BraTS 2023 challenge in terms of standardizing the origin and file naming format.

4 Result

Our experiment was conducted in PyTorch [14]. During training, the number of epochs was set to 60, and the batch size was set to 1. We utilized stochastic gradient descent (SGD) as the optimizer, with a learning rate of 1e−4, momentum of 0.9, and weight decay of 5e−4. Cosine annealing of the learning rate is a commonly used method for adjusting the learning rate. In the first 10 epochs, the learning rate gradually increased from the minimum value of 0.002 to the maximum value of 0.004. During the subsequent training process, the learning rate was decayed according to the cosine function, gradually decreasing it. Our experiment was conducted on a Tesla P100 with 16 GB GPU memory. The figure showcases some examples of the training data, ground truth, and predicted values.

For the validation set results, we conducted both quantitative and qualitative analyses. In terms of quantitative analysis, Table 1 and the box plots in Fig. 4 demonstrate our model's average LesionWise_Dice scores of 81.97%, 83.85%, and 88.22% in the ET, TC, and WT regions, respectively, along with LesionWise_Hausdorff95 scores of 25.96, 24.11, and 17.12. As for the qualitative analysis results, they are presented in Fig. 5.

Table 1. The proposed approach yields a LW_Dice score and LW_HD95 on the validation set.

	LW_Dice (%)			LW_HD95 (mm)		
	ET	TC	WT	ET	TC	WT
mean	77.69	79.02	88.05	36.79	35.37	18.25
std	27.64	27.14	14.85	94.90	88.03	47.99
25 quantile	79.42	75.95	88.58	1	1.41	2
median	88.89	91.77	93.41	2	4.12	3.60
75 quantile	94.12	95.93	93.41	6.54	10.04	6.63

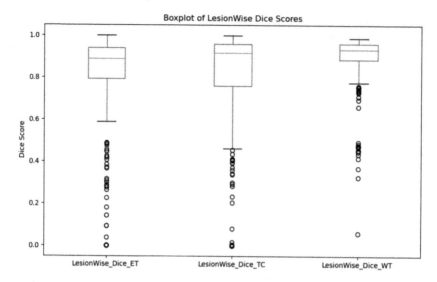

Fig. 4. The box-and-whisker plots represent the distribution of LesionWise_Dice scores for the Validation Phase Results, showcasing the minimum, lower quartile, median, upper quartile, and maximum values for each tumor class

Table 2 presents the performance of the model in the test cohort. Our model achieved average LesionWise_Dice scores of 78.90%, 80.50%, and 85.99% in the ET, TC, and WT regions, respectively, along with LesionWise_Hausdorff95 scores of 40.44, 39.36, and 25.71.

Table 2. The proposed approach yields a LW_Dice score and LW_HD95 on the test set.

	LW_Dice (%)			LW_HD95 (mm)		
	ET	TC	WT	ET	TC	WT
mean	78.90	80.50	85.99	40.44	39.36	25.71
std	25.76	27.80	18.16	95.46	93.73	62.06
25quantile	76.29	80.64	86.32	1	1	1.41
median	90.42	94.05	93.16	1.41	3	4.12
75quantile	95.04	96.96	96.43	6.11	8.87	9.87

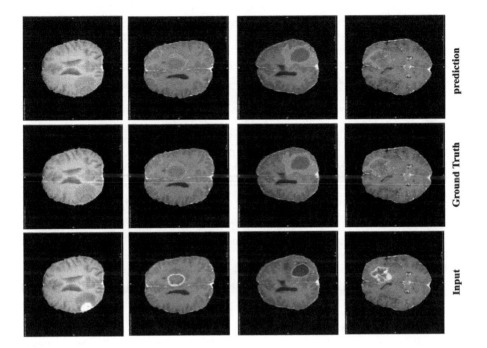

Fig. 5. Comparison between predicted results and ground truth (The bottom is the input image, the middle is the real value, and the top is the predicted result)

5 Discussion and Conclusion

We propose a streamlined volumetric convolutional neural Network, 3D ST-Net, for brain tumor segmentation. By utilizing larger convolutional kernels, we are able to capture a more extensive receptive field, facilitating better integration of contextual information and explicit modeling of global features. Experimental evaluation on the BraTS 2023 test dataset and validation set demonstrates the effectiveness of 3D ST-Net.

Acknowledgement. This work was supported by the National Natural Science Foundation of China (62271149), and the Fujian Provincial Natural Science Foundation projects (2021J02019, 2021J01578).

References

1. Baid, U., et al.: The RSNA-ASNR-MICCAI BraTS 2021 benchmark on brain tumor segmentation and radiogenomic classification. arXiv preprint arXiv:2107.02314 (2021)
2. Bakas, S., et al.: Segmentation labels and radiomic features for the pre-operative scans of the TCGA-GBM collection (2017). https://doi.org/10.7937/K9/TCIA.2017.KLXWJJ1Q
3. Bakas, S., et al.: Segmentation labels and radiomic features for the pre-operative scans of the TCGA-LGG collection. Cancer Imaging Arch. **286** (2017)

4. Bakas, S., et al.: Advancing the cancer genome atlas glioma MRI collections with expert segmentation labels and radiomic features. Sci. Data **4**(1), 1–13 (2017)
5. Bertels, J., et al.: Optimizing the dice score and Jaccard index for medical image segmentation: theory and practice. In: Shen, D., et al. (eds.) MICCAI 2019. LNIP, vol. 11765, pp. 92–100. Springer, Cham (2019). https://doi.org/10.1007/978-3-030-32245-8_11
6. Bi, W.L., et al.: Artificial intelligence in cancer imaging: clinical challenges and applications. CA: Cancer J. Clin. **69**(2), 127–157 (2019)
7. Haque, I.R.I., Neubert, J.: Deep learning approaches to biomedical image segmentation. Inform. Med. Unlocked **18**, 100297 (2020)
8. Hatamizadeh, A., Nath, V., Tang, Y., Yang, D., Roth, H.R., Xu, D.: Swin UNETR: swin transformers for semantic segmentation of brain tumors in MRI images. In: Crimi, A., Bakas, S. (eds.) BrainLes 2021. LNCS, vol. 12962, pp. 272–284. Springer, Cham (2021). https://doi.org/10.1007/978-3-031-08999-2_22
9. Lee, H.H., Bao, S., Huo, Y., Landman, B.A.: 3D UX-Net: a large kernel volumetric convnet modernizing hierarchical transformer for medical image segmentation. arXiv preprint arXiv:2209.15076 (2022)
10. Li, Z., Shen, Z., Wen, J., He, T., Pan, L.: Automatic brain tumor segmentation using multi-scale features and attention mechanism. In: Crimi, A., Bakas, S. (eds.) BrainLes 2021. LNCS, vol. 12962, pp. 216–226. Springer, Cham (2022). https://doi.org/10.1007/978-3-031-08999-2_17
11. Luu, H.M., Park, S.H.: Extending nn-UNet for brain tumor segmentation. In: Crimi, A., Bakas, S. (eds.) BrainLes 2021. LNCS, vol. 12963, pp. 173–186. Springer, Cham (2022). https://doi.org/10.1007/978-3-031-09002-8_16
12. Menze, B.H., et al.: The multimodal brain tumor image segmentation benchmark (BRATS). IEEE Trans. Med. Imaging **34**(10), 1993–2024 (2014)
13. Oktay, O., et al.: Attention U-Net: learning where to look for the pancreas. arXiv preprint arXiv:1804.03999 (2018)
14. Paszke, A., et al.: PyTorch: an imperative style, high-performance deep learning library. Adv. Neural Inf. Process. Syst. **32** (2019)
15. Ronneberger, O., Fischer, P., Brox, T.: U-Net: convolutional networks for biomedical image segmentation. In: Navab, N., Hornegger, J., Wells, W., Frangi, A. (eds.) MICCAI 2015. LNCS, vol. 9351, pp. 234–241. Springer, Cham (2015). https://doi.org/10.1007/978-3-319-24574-4_28
16. Simonyan, K., Zisserman, A.: Very deep convolutional networks for large-scale image recognition. arXiv preprint arXiv:1409.1556 (2014)
17. Wang, W., Chen, C., Ding, M., Yu, H., Zha, S., Li, J.: TransBTS: multimodal brain tumor segmentation using transformer. In: de Bruijne, M., et al. (eds.) MICCAI 2021. LNIP, vol. 12901, pp. 109–119. Springer, Cham (2021). https://doi.org/10.1007/978-3-030-87193-2_11
18. Woo, S., et al.: ConvNeXt V2: co-designing and scaling convnets with masked autoencoders. In: Proceedings of the IEEE/CVF Conference on Computer Vision and Pattern Recognition, pp. 16133–16142 (2023)
19. Xiao, X., Lian, S., Luo, Z., Li, S.: Weighted Res-UNet for high-quality retina vessel segmentation. In: 2018 9th International Conference on Information Technology in Medicine and Education (ITME), pp. 327–331. IEEE (2018)
20. Zhou, Z., Rahman Siddiquee, M.M., Tajbakhsh, N., Liang, J.: UNet++: a nested U-Net architecture for medical image segmentation. In: Stoyanov, D., et al. (eds.) DLMIA 2018, ML-CDS 2018. LNIP, vol. 11045, pp. 3–11. Springer, Cham (2018). https://doi.org/10.1007/978-3-030-00889-5_1

Multimodal Brain Tumor Segmentation Using Modified 3D UNet3+ Architecture

Xiao Yang and Shaohua Zheng(✉)

Intelligent Image Processing and Analysis Laboratory, Fuzhou University, Fuzhou, China
sunphen@fzu.edu.cn

Abstract. Glioma is a type of tumor that originates in the glial cells of the brain or the spinal cord, which is the most common and aggressive malignant primary tumor of the central nervous system in adults. Magnetic resonance imaging (MRI) is an efficient way of detection for brain tumors, it contains precise knowledge about the location of the tumor and its component. Manual tumor labeling is a tedious and time-consuming task, hence accurate automatic segmentation has important clinical significance in the diagnosis, and deep learning shows great power on it. In this paper, we propose an improved 3D U-Net3 + segmentation network. We adopt the residual structure in the encoder part to address the challenge of diminishing gradient problem, as well as to enhance the encoder's capability for feature extraction, thereby facilitating comprehensive feature fusion during up-sampling within the network. Meanwhile, we add a critic network at the end of the U-Net3+, that contributes to the generation of segmentation results that are more authentic and dependable from the segmentation network. We trained and evaluated the architecture on the BraTS 2023 dataset, and achieved Lesion-Wise_Dice of 88.22%, 83.85%, 81.97% for the whole tumor, tumor core and enhancing tumor, respectively.

Keywords: Brain tumor segmentation · Unet3+ · Full-scale skip connection

1 Introduction

Brain tumors, such as glioblastoma, are among the most challenging and devastating diseases affecting the central nervous system. With their unpredictable behavior and potentially life-threatening consequences, brain tumors pose significant diagnostic and therapeutic challenges to medical professionals and researchers worldwide. Some certain occupations, environmental carcinogens, and diet have been reported to be associated with an elevated risk of glioma [11], but the only environmental factor clearly associated with an increased risk of brain tumors is therapeutic X-ray exposure.

The clinical manifestations of brain tumors can vary widely depending on their location, size, and the specific brain regions affected. Common symptoms include persistent headaches, seizures, cognitive impairments, and focal neurological deficits. Early diagnosis and accurate characterization of brain tumors play a crucial role in determining the appropriate treatment strategy and improving patient outcomes, and accuracy tumor segmentation can significantly improve the therapeutic effect.

Over the years, imaging techniques such as magnetic resonance imaging (MRI) have played a pivotal role in the detection and evaluation of brain tumors. These imaging modalities have provided valuable information regarding tumor size, location, and morphology. However, accurately distinguishing between different tumor types and assessing their aggressiveness remains a formidable task. In recent years, the advent of artificial intelligence has shown promising potential in addressing the challenges associated with brain tumor diagnosis and treatment. Advanced computational techniques, including image segmentation, feature extraction, and classification algorithms, have paved the way for the development of automated and accurate tumor detection and segmentation systems. To this end, The Brain Tumor Segmentation Challenge (BraTS) serves as a platform for participants to assess their models and compare their outcomes with those of other teams by using The BraTS 2023 dataset [1–5]. The BraTS 2023 has more tasks, including segmentation and synthesis. In this work, we focus on the segmentation task on Adult Glioma.

The advancement of medical image segmentation has been significantly boosted by the adoption of Fully Convolutional Neural Networks (FCNs) [6]. One of the significant research directions is the enhancement of the benchmark network based on the fully convolutional network (FCN) or the U-Net [7] to create an improved model [8, 9]. Simultaneously, the Network variation [14–16] based on the U-Net framework has demonstrated exceptional performance in the segmentation of brain tumors, as evidenced by its remarkable results in the BraTS challenge. For example, Jiang et al. [10] introduced an image reconstruction branch based on VAE (Variational Autoencoder) to the U-Net benchmark network. This entailed integrating a variable auto-encoding branch into the decoder structure, thereby providing a conditional constraint for segmentation. Ahmad et al. [12] devised a context-aware 3D U-Net architecture that leverages densely connected blocks in both the encoder and decoder paths. This approach enables the extraction of multi-contextual information by incorporating the concept of feature reusability. Himashi et al. [13] proposed a straightforward yet impactful approach for enhancing the training of 3D U-Net through reciprocal adversarial learning. Despite achieving satisfactory results in brain tumor segmentation, these methods lacked the ability to capture information from multiple scales, indicating the need for further enhancements.

In this paper, we propose an improved 3D U-Net3+ network with residual structure in the encoder part to tackle the issue of diminishing gradient problem and bolster the encoder's feature extraction capabilities, thereby facilitating comprehensive feature fusion during up-sampling within the network. In addition, inspired by the adversarial learning strategy proposed by Himashi et al. [13], we introduced the critic network at the output of 3D U-Net3+ to activate the segmentation network to produce more realistic results closer to GT. Furthermore, to solve the class imbalance issue associated with brain tumors, we integrate the cross entropy (CE) loss and dice (DSC) loss. This is achieved by introducing weighted coefficients to the loss components, allowing for a more comprehensive and balanced loss function. We evaluated the proposed method on brain tumor segmentation (BraTS) Challenge 2023. Experiment results have shown the effectiveness of our method.

2 Method

In the following, we begin with detailing the overall network architecture on Sect. 2.1 (Fig. 1). Then the full-scale skip connection part of 3D U-Net3+ is specified on Sect. 2.2. Finally, we elaborate on the loss functions used for segmentation network and critic network on Sect. 2.3.

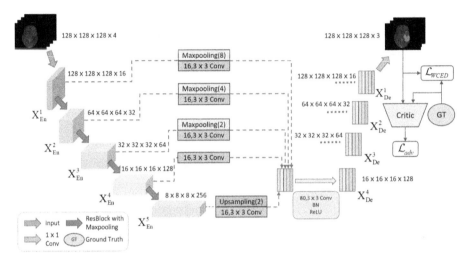

Fig. 1. The overall network architecture.

2.1 Network Architecture

In general, the network we utilized consists of two parts, namely the U-net3+ as the segmentation network, followed with a critic network. The U-Net3+ is an enhanced version of the U-Net architecture, which combines the encoder-decoder structure of U-Net with novel modifications [17]. Its framework follows the basic U-Net architecture, consisting of an encoder and decoder connected by skip connections for feature concatenation. The encoder comprises five residual blocks, which we used for the vanishing gradient problem caused by the increasing in network depth, and enhancing the feature extraction ability of the encoder which is instrumental in full feature fusion when up-sampling in the network [18]. The residual blocks are interleaved with four down-sampling layers with a kernel size of 2 and the stride of 2, the number of feature maps in the five blocks are 16, 32, 64, 128, 256, respectively. While the decoder also includes four up-sampling layers interleaved with four residual blocks for feature decoding and recovery of spatial details.

In addition to enhancing the encoder component, skip connections have garnered significant attention. For instance, the U-Net++ architecture features nested and dense skip connections built upon the U-Net framework [19]. Nevertheless, Huang et al. [17] thought that U-Net++ lacks adequate information from diverse scales. To address this concern, they introduce full-scale skip connections that combine high-level and low-level semantics from various scales in the U-Net3+, aiming to furnish more extensive information for the up-sampling process. The detail of full-scale skip connections is illustrated in Fig. 2.

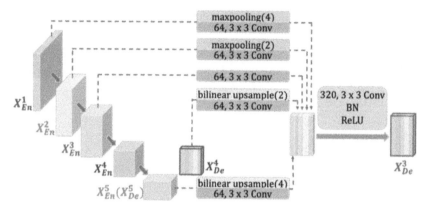

Fig. 2. An example of constructing decoder with Full-Scale skip connection

The critic network is designed as a fully convolutional adversarial network, containing four convolution layers with a kernel size of 3, integrated with batch normalization and leaky ReLU activation function [13]. Depicting Markovian PatchGAN architecture [20], it constructively imposes the segmentation network to predict segmentation masks that are more similar to ground truth masks by producing confidence scores for prediction masks to provide uncertainty information to the segmentation network. Similar to PatchGAN, the network is implemented with a cubic size of $1 \times 1 \times 1$.

2.2 Full-Scale Skip Connection

Figure 2 gives an example of how to structure a X_{De}^n feature map for the decoder, where the X_{De}^3 feature map structure is elucidated, which bears resemblance to the U-Net architecture by directly receiving feature maps X_{En}^3 from the corresponding scale encoder layer. However, unlike U-Net, multiple skip connections are present. Among these connections, two of them perform pooling down-sampling on the lower-level encoder layers X_{En}^1 and X_{En}^2 using distinct max pooling operations to transmit low-level semantic information. Another purpose of this down-sampling is to standardize the resolution of the feature map. As depicted in Fig, X_{En}^1 needs to reduce its resolution by a factor of four while X_{En}^2 requires a reduction by a factor of two. The subsequent two skip connections employ bilinear interpolation for up-sampling X_{En}^4 and X_{En}^5 in the decoder to enhance the resolution of the feature map. From the figure, it can be observed that X_{En}^5 necessitates a quadruple increase in resolution while X_{En}^4 requires doubling its resolution. After aligning all feature maps' sizes, unifying their channel numbers becomes essential as well. By applying 3×3 convolution followed by concatenation along the channel dimension, we achieve feature fusion resulting in generating a new feature map. Finally, Conv followed with Batch Normalization and ReLU activation yields our desired output X_{De}^3.

2.3 Loss Function

To address the issue of class imbalance, we employ a combination of weighted cross-entropy (WCE) and dice (DSC) loss functions, referred to as WCED, for our segmentation network. The WCE loss is utilized to mitigate pixel-level imbalance, while the DSC loss helps alleviate region-level imbalances.

Specifically, the WCE loss is defined as follows:

$$\mathcal{L}_{\text{WCE}}(P_i, \hat{P}_i) = -\frac{1}{S}\sum_{s=1}^{S}\omega_s\sum_{j=1}^{M}P_{js}\log\hat{P}_{js} \quad (1)$$

The DSC loss can be represented by:

$$\mathcal{L}_{DSC}(P_i, \hat{P}_i) = \sum_{j=1}^{M}\left(1 - \frac{2|P_j \cap \hat{P}_j|}{P_j + \hat{P}_j}\right) \quad (2)$$

where S denotes the total number of classes (four in our case), P_j and $\hat{P}_j$ represents the jth predicted result and the corresponding ground truth, P_{js} represents the jth ground truth pixel of class S, and $\hat{P}_{js}$ with a hat corresponds to its predicted probability. Additionally, ω_s signifies the weighted coefficient for class S and M refers to the total number of pixels in a batch.

The weighted cross-entropy and dice loss for brain tumor segmentation (WCED) is formulated as:

$$\mathcal{L}_{\text{WCED}}(P, \hat{P}) = \frac{1}{N}\sum_{i=1}^{N}\left(\theta\mathcal{L}_{\text{WCE}}(P_i, \hat{P}_i) + (1-\theta)\mathcal{L}_{DSC}(P_i, \hat{P}_i)\right) \quad (3)$$

where θ controls the contribution of the WCE loss and DSC loss to the total loss. P_i is the ith ground truth of a batch of input images, and $\hat{P}_i$ is the ith predicted mask of a batch of predictions. N denotes the labeled images within a minibatch. In general, the WCED loss is a weighted combination of class weighted cross-entropy loss and class-weighted dice loss.

For the critic network, in accordance with Himashi et al. [13], the normalized loss of the critic for prediction distribution is defined as follows:

$$\mathcal{L}_{adv}(P, \hat{P}) = -\sum_{a\in H}\sum_{b\in W}\{(1-\eta)\log(\psi(P)[a, b]) + \eta\log(\psi(\hat{P})[a, b]\} \quad (4)$$

where η is set to 0 when the sample is generated by the segmentation network, and 1 when it is drawn from the ground truth labels. By incorporating this adversarial loss, the segmentation network aims to deceive the critic by generating predictions that are more holistically similar to ground truth masks.

Finally, the total loss is formulated as:

$$\mathcal{L}_{total} = \alpha\mathcal{L}_{WCED} + (1-\alpha)\mathcal{L}_{adv} \quad (5)$$

3 Experiments

In this section, we show the dataset we used in our experiment first on Sect. 3.1, and then explain the new evaluation metrics on Sect. 3.2, as well as the detailed procedure of pre-processing and post-processing methods on Sect. 3.3 and Sect. 3.4, respectively. Finally, the implementation details are specified on Sect. 3.5.

3.1 Dataset

The datasets we have used in this study are the BraTS 2023 Training dataset and the BraTS 2023 validation dataset, and they are the same as the dataset used in BraTS 2021, while the testing dataset has been updated with many more routine clinically-acquired multi-parametric MRI (mpMRI) scans. They were obtained from ample multi-institutional routine clinically-acquired mpMRI scans of glioma.

The training dataset contains 1251 patient data with four modalities, T1, T1Gd, T2, and T2-Flair, accompanied by the corresponding annotations. Segmentation labels are divided into four values, that is a value of 1 indicating necrotic tumor core, 2 representing edema, a value of 3, compared to 4 in previous BraTS Challenges, indicating enhancing tumor, and 0 for non-tumor and background. In the basis above, the whole tumor (WT) class includes all labels (1, 2, 3), while the tumor core (TC) class is a union of label 1 and label 3. The labels provided are annotated manually by one to four raters and are checked and approved by experienced neuro-radiologists.

While the validation dataset with 219 cases of MRI does not come with labels. So the segmentation results must be validated online by submitting it to the provided online validation site to obtain the correctness of labeling.

3.2 Metrics

The previous BraTS challenge adopted the Dice similarity coefficient (DSC) and Hausdorff95 (95%HD) for quantitatively evaluation. DSC calculates the similarity between the ground truth and the prediction, that the spatial overlap between the prediction results of brain tumor segmentation and the label. DSC is sensitive to the segmented internal filling. While 95%HD measures how far two subsets of a metric space are from each other, which is defined as the longest distance between a point set A and the most adjacent point of set B. 95%HD is sensitive to the segmented boundary. Different from the above, LesionWise_Dice and LesionWise_Hausdorff95 were introduced in the BraTS 2023 challenge. The two indexes are quite sensitive to false positive (FP) predictions, high score on DSC may result in low score on LesionWise_Dice because of some FP predictions. So how to reduce FP predictions attaches great importance to the results in BraTS 2023 challenge.

3.3 Preprocessing

The NIfTI file format is utilized to provide the BraTS 2023 dataset, wherein the MRI volumes exhibit inconsistencies in intensities that can be attributed to various factors such as patient movements during examinations, diverse acquisition devices from different manufacturers, and variations in sequences and parameters employed for image acquisition. To ensure consistency across all volumes, we implemented min-max normalization and subsequently adjusted the intensity values. Furthermore, during training the images were center cropped to a patch size of 128 × 128 × 128 to cut unnecessary background pixels for learning more features of the region of interest.

3.4 Postprocessing

Lesionwise_Dice and LesionWise_Hausdorff95 are very demanding for low FP predictions due to the new metrics adopted in this challenge, so we also performed the operation of maximum connected domain by removing the isolated part in the 3D space on each class after obtaining the predicted label. In addition, for three labels, ET, TC and WT, we set the threshold values after some trial to improve the accuracy of the prediction.

3.5 Implementation Details

The experiment is conducted in PyTorch [21] and trained without pre-training. We use the Adam optimizer [22] with standard back-propagation, and the learning rate of 2e−4. The network is trained over 100 epochs with a batch size of 1. Our experiments are run on a NVIDIA A5000 with 24G GPU memory.

4 Results

We present the evaluation of our model's performance on the BraTS 2023 dataset below. The initial results, obtained from the validation set, are reported first. The final results will be obtained after evaluating our proposed model on the test set.

4.1 Evaluation Results on Validation Phase

For evaluation on the validation set, we trained our model on the entire training set and submitted the segmentation results to the challenge website to obtain segmentation performance metrics. The quantitative and qualitative results during the validation phase for our proposed approach are shown in Table 1 and Fig. 3. Through training, our model achieved the average LesionWise_Dice of 81.97%, 83.85%, 88.22% and LesionWise_Hausdorff95 of 25.96, 24.11, 17.12 in the ET, TC, and WT regions, respectively. It is worth noting that our proposed framework successfully identifies fine predictions.

4.2 Evaluation Results on Test Phase

For evaluation on the test set, we made a ML Cube and submitted it to the challenge website to obtain segmentation performance metrics. The results for our proposed approach are shown in Table 2. Our model achieved the average LesionWise_Dice of 81.30%, 81.22%, 85.46% and LesionWise_Hausdorff95 of 30.27, 37.48, 26.45 in the ET, TC, and WT regions, respectively. Meanwhile, sensitivity and specificity of each class are given in the table.

Table 1. Quantitative results on BraTS 2023 Validation set (LW is short for LesionWise).

Class	LW_Dice	LW_HD95	Num_TP	Num_FP
Enhanced Tumor (ET)	81.97%	25.96	0.8767	0
Tumor Core (TC)	83.85%	24.11	0.9863	0.0137
Whole Tumor (WT)	88.22%	17.12	1	0.0046

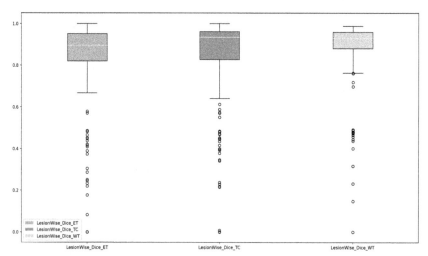

Fig. 3. The box and whisker plots of the distribution of the LesionWise_Dice for Validation Phase Results. It shows the minimum, lower quartile, median, upper quartile and maximum for each tumor class.

Table 2. Quantitative results on BraTS 2023 Test set (LW is short for LesionWise).

Class	LW_Dice	LW_HD95	Sensitivity	Specificity
Enhanced Tumor (ET)	81.30%	30.27	0.8750	0.9997
Tumor Core (TC)	81.22%	37.48	0.8725	0.9995
Whole Tumor (WT)	85.46%	26.45	0.9090	0.9992

4.3 The Effectiveness of Reducing FP

Below in the Fig. 4 we give an example where our post-processing has achieved remarkable improvements in the poor results, in which the red box on the left is the FP prediction, and we have removed it in the right.

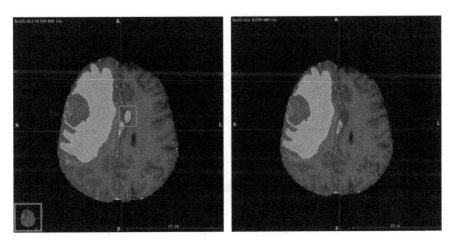

Fig. 4. Comparison before (Left) and after (Right) post-processing. We use red for ET, blue for TC, and green for WT. (Color figure online)

5 Conclusion

In this paper, we presented an improved 3D U-Net3+ architecture for brain tumor segmentation which improving the False Positive judging ability compare to the previous version. Our proposed model includes a 3D U-Net3+ network for segmentation and a critic network to optimize the segmentation results. By incorporating multi-scale features and skip connections, the 3D U-Net3+ architecture effectively captures both local and global context information, enabling precise segmentation of tumor sub-regions. Experimental results on BraTS 2023 dataset have demonstrated promising results in accurately delineating tumor regions. However, there is still room for improvement in the proposed approach to improve the performance of the model, such as data pre-processing and post-processing, data augmentation, model complexity and so on. Overall, our study emphasizes the effectiveness of leveraging 3D U-Net3+ architecture for accurate brain tumor segmentation and we hope that our findings contribute to the ongoing advancements in medical image analysis.

Acknowledgement. This work was supported by the National Natural Science Foundation of China (62271149), and the Fujian Provincial Natural Science Foundation project (2021J02019, 2021J01578).

References

1. Baid, U., et al.: The RSNA-ASNR-MICCAI BraTS 2021 Benchmark on Brain Tumor Segmentation and Radiogenomic Classification. arXiv:2107.02314 (2021)
2. BH Menze 2015 The multimodal brain tumor image segmentation benchmark (BRATS) IEEE Trans. Med. Imaging 34 10 1993 2024 https://doi.org/10.1109/TMI.2014.2377694
3. S Bakas 2017 Advancing the cancer genome atlas glioma MRI collections with expert segmentation labels and radiomic features Nat. Sci. Data 4 170117 https://doi.org/10.1038/sdata.2017.117
4. S Bakas 2017 Segmentation labels and radiomic features for the pre-operative scans of the TCGA-GBM collection Cancer Imaging Arch. https://doi.org/10.7937/K9/TCIA.2017.KLXWJJ1Q
5. Bakas, H., et al.: Segmentation labels and radiomic features for the pre-operative scans of the TCGA-LGG collection. Cancer Imaging Arch. (2017). https://doi.org/10.7937/K9/TCIA.2017.GJQ7R0EF
6. Long, J., Shelhamer, E., Darrell, T.: Fully convolutional networks for semantic segmentation. IEEE Trans. Pattern Anal. Mach. Intell. **39**, 640–651 (2015)
7. Ronneberger, O., Fischer, P., Brox, T.: U-Net: convolutional networks for biomedical image segmentation. In: Navab, N., Hornegger, J., Wells, W., Frangi, A. (eds.) MICCAI 2015. LNIP, vol. 9351, pp. 234–241. Springer, Cham (2015). https://doi.org/10.1007/978-3-319-24574-4_28
8. Oktay, O., et al.: Attention U-Net: learning where to look for the pancreas. arXiv preprint arXiv:1804.03999 (2018)
9. Xiao, X., Lian, S., Luo, Z., Li, S.: Weighted Res-UNet for high-quality retina vesselsegmentation. In: 2018 9th International Conference on Information Technology in Medicine and Education (ITME), pp. 327–331. IEEE (2018)
10. Jiang, Z., Ding, C., Liu, M., Tao, D.: Two-stage cascaded U-Net: 1st place solution to BraTS challenge 2019 segmentation task. In: Crimi, A., Bakas, S. (eds.) BrainLes 2019. LNCS, vol. 11992, pp. 231–241. Springer, Cham (2020). https://doi.org/10.1007/978-3-030-46640-4_22
11. H Ohgaki P Kleihues 2005 Epidemiology and etiology of gliomas Acta Neuropathol. 109 1 93 108
12. Ahmad, P., Qamar, S., Shen, L., Saeed, A.: Context aware 3D UNet for braintumor segmentation. In: Crimi, A., Bakas, S. (eds.) BrainLes 2020. LNCS, vol. 12658, pp. 207–218. Springer, Cham (2021). https://doi.org/10.1007/978-3-030-72084-1_19
13. Peiris, H., Chen, Z., Egan, G., Harandi, M.: Reciprocal adversarial learning for brain tumor segmentation: a solution to BraTS challenge 2021 segmentation task. In: Crimi, A., Bakas, S. (eds.) BrainLes 2021. LNCS, LNCS, vol. 12962, pp. 171–181. Springer, Cham (2022). https://doi.org/10.1007/978-3-031-08999-2_13
14. Li, Z., Shen, Z., Wen, J., He, T., Pan, L.: Automatic brain tumor segmentation using multiscale features and attention mechanism. In: Crimi, A., Bakas, S. (eds.) BrainLes 2021. LNCS, vol. 12962, pp. 216–226. Springer, Cham (2021). https://doi.org/10.1007/978-3-031-08999-2_17
15. Yang, H., Shen, Z., Li, Z., Liu, J., Xiao, J.: Combining global information with topological prior for brain tumor segmentation. In: Crimi, A., Bakas, S. (eds.) BrainLes 2020. LNCS, vol. 12962, pp. 204–215. Springer, Cham (2021). https://doi.org/10.1007/978-3-031-08999-2_16
16. Akbar, A.S., Fatichah, C., Suciati, N.: UNet3D with multiple atrous convolutions attention block for brain tumor segmentation. In: Crimi, A., Bakas, S. (eds.) BrainLes 2021. LNCS, vol. 12962, pp. 182–193. Springer, Cham (2021). https://doi.org/10.1007/978-3-031-08999-2_14

17. Huang, H., Lin, L., Tong, R., et al.: UNet 3+: a full-scale connected UNet for medical image segmentation. In: ICASSP 2020-2020 IEEE International Conference on Acoustics, Speech and Signal Processing (ICASSP), pp. 1055–1059. IEEE (2020)
18. He, K., Zhang, X., Ren, S., et al.: Deep residual learning for image recognition. In: IEEE Conference on Computer Vision and Pattern Recognition, Las Vegas, NV, USA, pp. 770–778 (2016)
19. Zhou, Z., Siddiquee, M.M.R., Tajbakhsh, N.: UNet++: a nested U-Net architecture for medical image segmentation. In: Stoyanov, D., et al. (eds.) DLMIA 2018, ML-CDS 2018. LNIP, vol. 11045, pp. 3–11. Springer, Cham (2018). https://doi.org/10.1007/978-3-030-00889-5_1
20. Isola, P., Zhu, J.Y., Zhou, T., Efros, A.A.: Image-to-image translation with conditional adversarial networks. In: Proceedings of IEEE Conference on Computer Vision and Pattern Recognition (CVPR), pp. 1125–1134 (2017)
21. A Paszke 2019 PyTorch: an imperative style, high-performance deep learning library Adv. Neural Inf. Process. Syst. 32 8026 8037
22. Kingma, D.P., Ba, J.: Adam: a method for stochastic optimization. arXiv preprint arXiv:1412.6980 (2014)

Enhancing Encoder with Attention Gate for Multimodal Brain Tumor Segmentation

Yi Li[1], Zhirui Fang[1], Di Li[2], Xin Xie[1], and Yanqing Guo[1] (✉)

[1] Dalian University of Technology, Dalian, China
guoqy@dlut.edu.cn
[2] Dalian Municipal Central Hospital, Dalian, China

Abstract. Magnetic Resonance Imaging (MRI) is widely applied to diagnose malignant brain tumors like glioblastoma (GBM). Recent deep network based brain tumor segmentation algorithms have facilitated automatic and accurate segmentation on MRI data, benefiting the clinical diagnosis with efficiency. However, existing methods most work on certain datasets but suffer from performance degradation when tested on unseen out-of-sample datasets. In this paper, we integrate the encoder-decoder network structure with attention gate and Variational Autoencoders (VAE) to achieve promising segmentation results across different situations. Considering there are four modalities in each brain MRI sample, an encoder based on 3D convolution is employed to capture the local correlation among both spatial and modal neighbors. Then the extracted volumetric feature maps are fed into a decoder, finally generating the segmentation results with attention gate module. To facilitate better segmentation, we further adopt VAE as an auxiliary decoder to improve the performance of the encoder.

Keywords: Brain Tumor Segmentation · Variational Autoencoders · Attention Gate · Federated Evaluation · FeTS Challenge

1 Introduction

Glioblastomas (GBM) are deemed as the most aggressive and heterogeneous adult brain tumor [16], with the median survival of approximately 15 months [15]. In practice, magnetic resonance imaging (MRI) offers an applicable choice for routine clinical diagnosis in GBM. There are usually four modalities in each MRI sample, including T1-weighted (T1), contrast-enhanced T1-weighted (T1c), T2-weighted (T2), and Fluid Attenuated Inversion Recovery (FLAIR) images. Since these modalities provides different pathology clues, it is of great importance to learn them comprehensively for better segmentation performance.

1.1 Medical Image Segmentation

With the rise of deep learning, Convolutional Neural Networks (CNN) based approaches have achieved remarkable progress in medial image segmentation. Among them, the Fully Convolutional Network (FCN) [12] is an epochal work that produces impressive segmentation results with an end-to-end network. It afterward is usually used as the feature extractor for medical image analysis. Another representative architecture in medical image segmentation is U-Net [18] which builds connections between the encoder layer and the corresponding decoder layer via feature map duplication. With these connections that skip the network bottleneck, lower level details are sent to the decoder for delicate segmentation outputs. Later literatures [8,14,28] continue to improve the U-Net architecture from different points of view. However, these methods are inevitably limited by the inductive locality bias of convolution, the reason coming from the marginal scale of the receptive field. Therefore, how to model the long-range dependencies becomes one of the breakthroughs in medical image segmentation.

1.2 Self-attention

Arising from natural language processing, the attention mechanism helps networks to capture long-range dependencies in feature maps. Many works [19,24] have explored to combine the advantages of CNN and the attention mechanism. Recently, the transformer framework [22] is proposed and achieves the fantastic performance on sequence-to-sequence translation. The essence of the transformer is multiple self-attention layers, which can capture interactions between all pairs of elements in the input sequence regardless of their relative position. Now the transformer is also applied to computer vision tasks successfully. For example, it is introduced to image classification [1,7,9], 3-Dimensional video grounding [20,21,26], object detection [6,27] and style Transfer [11,25]. Despite the excellent and convincing results, the computational complexity of the transformer based approaches increase exponentially. The issue becomes even more serious in medical image analysis, because the qualified data can be very scarce for uncommon diseases like GBM. Therefore, how to balance the parameter scale of the transformer and the training data is an important problem to be solved.

1.3 The Generalization Problem

Although the approaches based on neural networks have witnessed great progresses in medical image segmentation, they still face challenges in practical scenarios, including "AI chasm". "AI chasm" refers to the performance discrepancy of an AI algorithm in research environments and real-life applications. Algorithms based on networks are essentially data-driven and tend to be limited by the diversity of the training data. Existing methods are usually trained and tested on the subset of a dataset, sliding over the data discrepancy in practice. When evaluated on unseen out-of-sample datasets from various institutions that did not contribute data on the training set like the FeTS Challenge does, most deep learning models will experience performance deterioration. To measure the generalization ability, in the FeTS Challenge, the segmentation models are evaluated across different medical institutions, MRI scanners, image acquisition parameters and populations. Therefore, it has practical significance to tackle the distribution shift between the training and the test sets and thus raise the generalization ability of the model.

1.4 Method Motivation

On the basis of the above considerations, we summarize that an advanced method for multimodal brain tumor segmentation should have the following characters.

- Taking both encoded and decoded information in the medical image into account
- Exploiting the effective collaboration among different modalities of MRI
- Tackling the distribution discrepancy between the training and the test sets
- Producing accurate segmentation results with affordable computation cost

Inspired by the recent progress [2–5,10,13,23] in multimodal brain tumor segmentation, we implement a typical encoder-decoder structure. As in [23], instead of using 2D convolution to process the MRI sample slice-by-slice, a 3D CNN is employed to learn different modalities of MRI as a whole, which can capture the local features within as well as across MRI modalities. Different from [23], we further utilize an auxiliary VAE to enhance the ability of encoder in feature extraction. Besides, attention gates are used to conduct the skip connections for obtaining more accurate segmentation, which mitigates the over-fitting risk and benefits the model generalization ability.

2 Method

2.1 Overview

Figure 1 (a) presents an illustration of the designed network consisting of roughly four components. It essentially follows the encoder-decoder structure, whereas the 3D CNN builds up the enhanced encoder together and there are two branches of decoder during training. Given an MRI sample $I \in \mathbb{R}^{C \times H \times W \times D}$, the 3D CNN first embeds the input into a feature map F, to capture the local knowledge within and across different modalities. Specifically, C refers to the number of modalities, $H \times W$ is the spatial resolution of the medical image, and D is the depth (or number of slices) of the medial image. Then the segmentation result is output by the chief decoder (the upper decoder in Fig. 1) (a) with a series of deconvolution layers. The auxiliary VAE (the lower decoder in Fig. 1 (a) is employed to help with the parameter learning of the 3D CNN during training. Following the U-Net structure, there are also skip connections through attention gates between the corresponding layers in the encoder and the decoder.

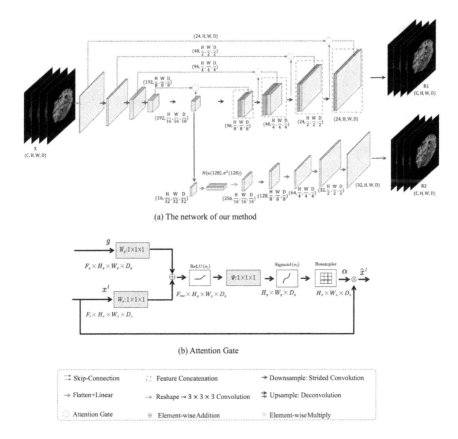

Fig. 1. Overview of the designed network.

2.2 3D CNN

For the encoder component, we employ residual blocks, with each individual block comprising two convolutional layers accompanied by normalization and Rectified Linear Unit (ReLU) activation. Following this, an additive identity skip connection is incorporated. To achieve this, we utilize convolution operations employing a kernel size of 3 × 3 × 3. This step allows for a gradual reduction in the dimensions of the image by a factor of 2, progressively integrating the nearby context into a feature map denoted as F within the real-number space $\mathbb{R}^{192 \times \frac{H}{16} \times \frac{W}{16} \times \frac{D}{16}}$. Moreover, we apply Batch Normalization (BatchNorm) as the chosen normalization technique, which in turn leads to enhanced performance outcomes. By subjecting the input data to the 3D Convolutional Neural Network (CNN), we not only acquire more intricate local details, but we also alleviate the computational burden. This is due to the fact that the necessity to individually process each component or modality is obviated.

2.3 Attention Gate

Like [14], we utilize the attention gates (AGs) to alleviate feature loss through skip connections. The attention gate block is illustrated in Fig. 1 (b). The input features (x^l) undergo scaling using attention coefficients (α) computed within the AG module. Spatial regions are chosen by analyzing both the activations and contextual information derived from the gating signal (g), which is acquired from a more coarse-grained level. Resampling of attention coefficients on a grid is accomplished through trilinear interpolation. In this paper, we adopt multi-dimensional AGs where we extract and blend complementary information to establish the output of the skip connection. To alleviate the burden of excessive trainable parameters and the computational intricacy associated with AGs, we execute linear transformations without involving spatial support (utilizing $1 \times 1 \times 1$ convolutions). Moreover, we downsample the input feature-maps to match the resolution of the gating signal. This strategic approach ensures that attention units across various scales possess the capacity to influence responses encompassing a broad spectrum of foreground content within the images. Consequently, we proactively prevent the reconstruction of dense predictions solely from minute subsets of skip connections.

2.4 Decoder

The segmentation result $R_1 \in \mathbb{R}^{C \times H \times W \times D}$ is produced by the decoder with the intermediate feature F as the input. There are two decoders in the network shown in Fig. 1 (a), the upper being the chief decoder while the lower being the auxiliary decoder. The chief decoder is the U-Net architecture with the skip connections and holds individual parameters. Different from the chief decoder, the auxiliary decoder is the VAE network, sampling from the Gaussian distribution $N(\mu(128), \sigma^2(128))$. Hence the function of them differs from each other, the chief decoder aims at better segmentation results while the auxiliary one is to prevent the latent feature loss, which means encoder can better capture the tumor information. For the loss functions, we use the softmax Dice loss which can be calculated by

$$\mathcal{L}_{dice} = 1 - Dice(g_j^c, p_j^c) = 1 - \frac{2\sum_{c=1}^{M}\sum_{j=1}^{N_c} g_j^c p_j^c}{\sum_{c=1}^{M}\sum_{j=1}^{N_c}(g_j^c)^2 + \sum_{c=1}^{M}\sum_{j=1}^{N_c}(p_j^c)^2} \quad (1)$$

where g_j^c is a binary variable that indicates whether c is the correct label for position j, p_j^c is the predicted probability of label c at position j, M refers to the number of labels, and N_c represents the voxel number of label c in the sample. Since there are usually three types of regions to be concerned (including enhancing tumor region (ET), tumor core region (TC), and the whole tumor region (WT)), the total loss varies in the range of $[0, 3]$ theoretically.

Besides, we use the typical cross entropy loss to further promise the segmentation accuracy:

$$\mathcal{L}_{cross} = -\sum g_j^c \log(p_j^c) \quad (2)$$

Table 1. The network details of our method.

Component	Block	Operation	Output size
Encoder: 3D CNN	InitConv	$\begin{bmatrix} Conv3, BN, ReLU \\ Conv3, BN, ReLU \end{bmatrix}$	$24 \times 160 \times 160 \times 128$
	DownSample i	Maxpool(kernel2)	$(24 \times 2^i) \times (160 \times 2^{-i}) \times$
	EncBlock i	$\begin{bmatrix} Conv3, BN, ReLU \\ Conv3, BN, ReLU \end{bmatrix}$	$(160 \times 2^{-i}) \times (128 \times 2^{-i})$
	(i = 1, 2, 3)		
	DownSample	Maxpool(kernel2)	$192 \times 10 \times 10 \times 8$
	EncBlock	$\begin{bmatrix} Conv3, BN, ReLU \\ Conv3, BN, ReLU \end{bmatrix}$	
Decoder: Chief	AttentionBlock i	AttentionLayer	$(192 \times 2^{-i}) \times (10 \times 2^i) \times$
	DeBlock i	$\begin{bmatrix} Conv3, BN, ReLU \\ Conv3, BN, ReLU \end{bmatrix}$	$(10 \times 2^i) \times (8 \times 2^i)$
	(i = 1, 2, 3)		
	AttentionBlock	AttentionLayer	$24 \times 160 \times 160 \times 128$
	DeBlock	$\begin{bmatrix} Conv3, BN, ReLU \\ Conv3, BN, ReLU \end{bmatrix}$	
	EndConv	$Conv3$	$4 \times 160 \times 160 \times 128$
Decoder: Auxiliary	Decoder	$\begin{bmatrix} GN, ReLU \\ Conv3, Dense \end{bmatrix}$	256×1
	Sample	Sample $\sim$ $\begin{bmatrix} N(\mu(128), \sigma^2(128)) \end{bmatrix}$	128×1
	UpBlock	$\begin{bmatrix} Dense, ReLU \\ Conv1, Uplinear \end{bmatrix}$	$256 \times 10 \times 10 \times 8$
	DeBlock i	Conv3, UpLinear	$(256 \times 2^{-i}) \times (10 \times 2^i) \times$
	(i = 1, 2, 3)	$\begin{bmatrix} GN, ReLU, Conv3 \\ GN, ReLU, Conv3 \end{bmatrix}$ AddId	$(10 \times 2^i) \times (8 \times 2^i)$
	DeBlock	Conv3, UpLinear $\begin{bmatrix} GN, ReLU, Conv3 \\ GN, ReLU, Conv3 \end{bmatrix}$ AddId	$32 \times 160 \times 160 \times 128$
	EndConv	$Conv3$	$4 \times 160 \times 160 \times 128$

The term $\mathcal{L}_{L_2}$ corresponds to an L_2 loss applied to the output $R_2 \in \mathbb{R}^{C \times H \times W \times D}$ of the VAE branch, with the objective of aligning it with the input data X. This loss mechanism operates by quantifying the Euclidean distance between the generated VAE output and the original input, fostering an optimization process that aims to minimize the dissimilarity between the two representations.

$$\mathcal{L}_{L_2} = \|R_2 - X\|_2^2 \tag{3}$$

$\mathcal{L}_{KL}$ stands for the conventional penalty term utilized in a variational autoencoder (VAE) framework. It quantifies the Kullback-Leibler (KL) divergence between the estimated normal distribution $N(\mu, \sigma^2)$ and a predefined prior distribution $N(0, 1)$. Notably, this term plays a crucial role in regulating the latent space during the VAE training process. Its closed-form expression is an essential feature of VAEs and contributes to the overall effectiveness of the model.

$$\mathcal{L}_{KL} = \frac{1}{N} \sum \mu^2 + \sigma^2 - \log \sigma^2 - 1 \tag{4}$$

The total loss function is:

$$\mathcal{L} = (1 - \alpha) \times \mathcal{L}_{cross} + \mathcal{L}_{dice} \times \alpha + \alpha_1 \times \mathcal{L}_{L2} + \alpha_2 \times \mathcal{L}_{KL} \tag{5}$$

where $\alpha, \alpha_1, \alpha_2$ are the hyper-parameters to balance each loss item.

3 Results

3.1 Data and Implementation

Data used in this publication are provided by the FeTS Challenge, and were obtained as part of the RSNA-ASNR-MICCAI Brain Tumor Segmentation (BraTS) Challenge project through Synapse ID (syn28546456) [2,16,17]. The training set contains 1000 samples each with four modalities of T1, T1ce, T2 and FLAIR while the valid set contains 200 samples. Every modality of a sample is presented with a volume of 240 × 240 × 155 which is randomly cropped to 160 × 160 × 128. Although the validation set is also provided but without the ground truth. Therefore we divide the training data into two parts without overlap, and use about 1/4 data merely for model evaluation and result analysis. We use the classical Dice score (the higher the better) as the metric, calculated in regions of ET, TC and WT respectively. For the loss weights, we set $\alpha = 0.5$, $\alpha_1 = 0.5$ and $\alpha_2 = 0.5$.

Based on the open source of [23], the network is implemented under the Pytorch framework. We train it with one NVIDIA A100 GPUs (each has 80GB memory) from scratch using a batch size of 1. The initial learning rate is $4 \times e^{-4}$. For more training details including learning rate decay and data augmentation strategies, please refer to [23]. The network details are provided in Table 1. $Conv3$ denotes a convolutional layer with the kernel size of 3 × 3 × 3, BN is short for Batch Normalization, GN is short for Group Normalization, $UpLinear$ means 3D linear spatial upsampling, $Dense$ stands for full connections and $AddId$ represents addition of identity skip connection.

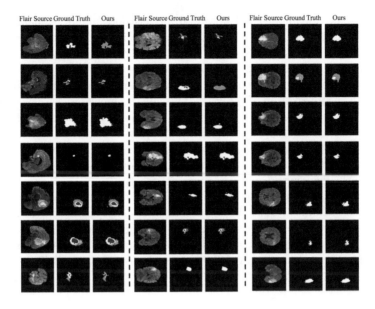

Fig. 2. The segmentation results of our method.

3.2 Discussion

Following the acquisition of the segmentation outcomes, we proceed with an evaluation encompassing per-class Dice coefficients, Hausdorff distances.

Dice coefficient, often denoted as D, is a common metric used for assessing the overlap between two sets. It is defined as:

$$\mathcal{D} = \frac{2 \times |X \cap Y|}{|X| + |Y|} \tag{6}$$

where X represents the ground truth segmentation mask and Y represents the predicted segmentation mask. $|\cdot|$ denotes the cardinality of a set, and $|\cdot \cap \cdot|$ represents the intersection of two sets.

Hausdorff distance, denoted as H, is a measure of the maximum distance between the points of two sets. Specifically, the Hausdorff distance between sets X and Y is defined as:

$$H(X, Y) = \{sup_{x \in X} \ inf_{y \in Y} d(x, y), sup_{y \in Y} \ inf_{x \in X} d(x, y)\} \tag{7}$$

where $d(x, y)$ represents the distance between point x in set X and point y in set Y. The Hausdorff distance measures the similarity between two sets by capturing the maximum distance of a point in one set to the closest point in the other set.

Besides, two innovative performance metrics referred to as lesion-wise Dice scores and lesion-wise Hausdorff distances at the 95th percentile (HD95). These were developed to evaluate segmentation performance at a lesion level rather than at the whole study level. By evaluating segmentation performance at the lesion level we can understand how well models detect and segment multiple individual lesions within a single patient. Traditional performance metrics used in prior BraTS are biased for large lesions. The results of this evaluation are presented in both Table 2 and Table 3. A comparison against models with a single decoder branch highlights a noticeable enhancement in segmentation performance with the integration of the VAE. This enhancement serves as a compelling testament to the efficacy of our proposed methodology. For enhanced clarity, we visually represent the segmentation outcomes in Fig. 2. In contrast to the quantitative metrics, these visual depictions offer a more intuitive assessment of segmentation quality. Across most scenarios, our outcomes closely resemble the ground truth, demonstrating the promising practical applicability of our approach. However, it is acknowledged that certain shortcomings persist within the segmentation results, such as the occasional omission of small, scattered regions. We proceed with a comprehensive examination of the convergence within our network. We present the curves depicting the variation in loss across training iterations in Fig. 3, providing a visual representation of the model's convergence dynamics. Notably, a rapid reduction in loss is evident during the initial 50 iterations.

Table 2. Dice score and Hausdorff distance-95 (HD95) measurements of the proposed segmentation method. EN - enhancing tumor core, WT - whole tumor, TC - tumor core.

Method	Dice Score (%) ↑			HD95 Score ↓		
	ET	WT	TC	ET	WT	TC
Attention+VAE	75.5	80.2	70.8	26.49	13.17	31.73
Attention	72.9	78.7	69.4	31.31	15.14	40.22

Table 3. Lesion-wise dice score and lesion-wise Hausdorff distance-95 measurements of the proposed segmentation method.

Method	LesionWise Dice (%) ↑			LesionWise HD95 ↓		
	ET	WT	TC	ET	WT	TC
Attention+VAE	62.6	72.4	62.8	95.11	59.39	85.37
Attention	59.7	71.9	56.5	109.78	63.92	106.26

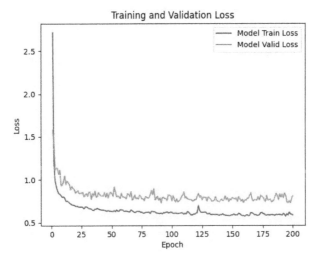

Fig. 3. The loss decline trend of the model in train and valid datasets.

4 Conclusion

In this paper, we have taken steps to elevate the capabilities of the encoder within the encoder-decoder network architecture by incorporating 3D convolutions and attention gates. This augmentation has resulted in remarkable brain tumor segmentation outcomes when applied to MRI samples. This enhancement offers a threefold advantage: (1) Exploiting 3D Convolution: The integration of 3D convolution goes beyond capturing local correlations within individual modalities of MRI. It extends its reach across all four modalities, comprehensively enhancing our ability to decipher intricate patterns. (2) Harnessing Attention Gates: Our implementation of attention gates has proven to be a pivotal advancement. These gates facilitate superior feature fusion through skip connections, effectively thwarting the risk of detail leakage. (3) Empowering Encoder with VAE: We have also integrated a Variational Autoencoder (VAE) as an auxiliary decoder, effectively bolstering the capabilities of the encoder to capture complex features. The entire network has been meticulously trained and validated using MRI data provided by the esteemed Federated Tumor Segmentation (FeTS) 2023 Challenge. Notably, our approach excels in producing convincing and promising segmentation outcomes in the Federated Evaluation phase, firmly underscoring the remarkable generalization prowess of our proposed methodology.

Acknowledgements. This work is supported in part by the National Natural Science Foundation of China (No. 62106037, No. 62076052), in part by the Major Program of the National Social Science Foundation of China (No.19ZDA127), and in part by the Fundamental Research Funds for the Central Universities (No. DUT22YG205).

References

1. Arnab, A., Dehghani, M., Heigold, G., Sun, C., Lučić, M., Schmid, C.: ViViT: a video vision transformer. In: IEEE International Conference on Computer Vision (ICCV), pp. 6836–6846 (2021)
2. Baid, U., et al.: The RSNA-ASNR-MICCAI BraTS 2021 benchmark on brain tumor segmentation and radiogenomic classification. arXiv preprint arXiv:2107.02314 (2021)
3. Bakas, S., et al.: Segmentation labels and radiomic features for the pre-operative scans of the TCGA-GBM collection (2017). https://doi.org/10.7937/K9/TCIA.2017.KLXWJJ1Q
4. Bakas, S., et al.: Segmentation labels and radiomic features for the pre-operative scans of the TCGA-LGG collection. Cancer Imaging Arch. **286** (2017)
5. Bakas, S., et al.: Advancing the cancer genome atlas glioma MRI collections with expert segmentation labels and radiomic features. Sci. Data **4**(1), 1–13 (2017)
6. Carion, N., Massa, F., Synnaeve, G., Usunier, N., Kirillov, A., Zagoruyko, S.: End-to-end object detection with transformers. In: Vedaldi, A., Bischof, H., Brox, T., Frahm, JM. (eds.) ECCV 2020. LNIP, vol. 12346, pp. 213–229. Springer, Cham (2020). https://doi.org/10.1007/978-3-030-58452-8_13
7. Chen, M., et al.: Generative pretraining from pixels. In: International Conference on Machine Learning, pp. 1691–1703. PMLR (2020)
8. Çiçek, Ö., Abdulkadir, A., Lienkamp, S.S., Brox, T., Ronneberger, O.: 3D U-Net: learning dense volumetric segmentation from sparse annotation. In: Ourselin, S., Joskowicz, L., Sabuncu, M., Unal, G., Wells, W. (eds.) MICCAI 2016. LNIP, vol. 9901, pp. 424–432. Springer, Cham (2016). https://doi.org/10.1007/978-3-319-46723-8_49
9. Dosovitskiy, A., et al.: An image is worth 16×16 words: transformers for image recognition at scale. arXiv preprint arXiv:2010.11929 (2020)
10. Karargyris, A., et al.: Federated benchmarking of medical artificial intelligence with MedPerf. Nat. Mach. Intell. 1–12 (2023)
11. Li, Y., Xie, X., Fu, H., Luo, X., Guo, Y.: A compact transformer for adaptive style transfer. In: 2023 IEEE International Conference on Multimedia and Expo (ICME), pp. 2687–2692. IEEE (2023)
12. Long, J., Shelhamer, E., Darrell, T.: Fully convolutional networks for semantic segmentation. In: Proceedings of the IEEE Conference on Computer Vision and Pattern Recognition, pp. 3431–3440 (2015)
13. Menze, B.H., et al.: The multimodal brain tumor image segmentation benchmark (BraTS). IEEE Trans. Med. Imaging **34**(10), 1993–2024 (2014)
14. Oktay, O., et al.: Attention U-Net: learning where to look for the pancreas. arXiv preprint arXiv:1804.03999 (2018)
15. Ostrom, Q.T., et al.: CBTRUS statistical report: primary brain and central nervous system tumors diagnosed in the united states in 2008–2012. Neuro-Oncology **17**(suppl_4), iv1–iv62 (2015)
16. Pati, S., et al.: The federated tumor segmentation (FETS) challenge. arXiv preprint arXiv:2105.05874 (2021)
17. Reina, G.A., et al.: OpenFL: an open-source framework for federated learning. arXiv preprint arXiv:2105.06413 (2021)
18. Ronneberger, O., Fischer, P., Brox, T.: U-Net: convolutional networks for biomedical image segmentation. In: Navab, N., Hornegger, J., Wells, W., Frangi, A. (eds.) MICCAI 2015. LNIP, vol. 9351, pp. 234–241. Springer, Cham (2015). https://doi.org/10.1007/978-3-319-24574-4_28

19. Schlemper, J., et al.: Attention gated networks: learning to leverage salient regions in medical images. Med. Image Anal. **53**, 197–207 (2019)
20. Su, R., Yu, Q., Xu, D.: STVGBert: a visual-linguistic transformer based framework for spatio-temporal video grounding. In: IEEE International Conference on Computer Vision (ICCV), pp. 1533–1542 (2021)
21. Tang, Z., et al.: Human-centric spatio-temporal video grounding with visual transformers. IEEE Trans. Circuits Syst. Video Technol. (2021)
22. Vaswani, A., et al.: Attention is all you need. Adv. Neural Inf. Process. Syst. (NeurIPS) **30** (2017)
23. Wang, W., Chen, C., Ding, M., Yu, H., Zha, S., Li, J.: TransBTS: multimodal brain tumor segmentation using transformer. In: de Bruijne, M., et al. (eds.) MICCAI 2021. LNIP, vol. 12901, pp. 109–119. Springer, Cham (2021). https://doi.org/10.1007/978-3-030-87193-2_11
24. Wang, X., Girshick, R., Gupta, A., He, K.: Non-local neural networks. In: Proceedings of the IEEE Conference on Computer Vision and Pattern Recognition, pp. 7794–7803 (2018)
25. Xie, X., Li, Y., Huang, H., Fu, H., Wang, W., Guo, Y.: Artistic style discovery with independent components. In: Proceedings of the IEEE/CVF Conference on Computer Vision and Pattern Recognition (CVPR), pp. 19870–19879, June 2022
26. Zhao, L., Cai, D., Sheng, L., Xu, D.: 3DVG-transformer: relation modeling for visual grounding on point clouds. In: IEEE International Conference on Computer Vision (ICCV), pp. 2928–2937 (2021)
27. Zhao, L., Guo, J., Xu, D., Sheng, L.: Transformer3D-Det: improving 3D object detection by vote refinement. IEEE Trans. Circuits Syst. Video Technol. **31**(12), 4735–4746 (2021)
28. Zhou, Z., Rahman Siddiquee, M.M., Tajbakhsh, N., Liang, J.: UNet++: a nested U-Net architecture for medical image segmentation. In: Stoyanov, D., et al. (eds.) DLMIA ML-CDS 2018. LNIP, vol. 11045, pp. 3–11. Springer, Cham (2018). https://doi.org/10.1007/978-3-030-00889-5_1

Evaluating STU-Net for Brain Tumor Segmentation

Ziyan Huang[1,2], Jin Ye[1], Haoyu Wang[1,2], Zhongying Deng[3], Yanzhou Su[1], Tianbin Li[1], Junlong Cheng[1], Jianpin Chen[1], Sizheng Guo[1], Yiqing Shen[1], and Junjun He[1(✉)]

[1] Shanghai AI Laboratory, Shanghai, China
ziyanhuang@sjtu.edu.cn, {yejin,hejunjun}@pjlab.org.cn
[2] Institute of Medical Robotics, Shanghai Jiao Tong University, Shanghai, China
[3] University of Cambridge, Cambridge, UK

Abstract. Brain tumor segmentation is vital in addressing the tumor's high heterogeneity, enhancing accurate diagnosis, guiding effective treatment, and improving prognosis predictions. In recent years, state-of-the-art methods in this domain have primarily evolved from U-Net-based architectures, demonstrating notable advancements in glioma radiographic segmentation. While large-scale models pre-trained on extensive datasets have significantly propelled deep learning progress, most current medical image segmentation models remain small-scale, encompassing only tens of millions of parameters. As the BraTS competition amasses more data and with the advancements of large-scale models in the past year, there emerges a compelling need to investigate the potential benefits of larger network architectures for adult glioma segmentation. In this context, we utilize the Scalable and Transferable U-Net (STU-Net) and its pre-trained variants on the RSNA-ASNR-MICCAI Brain Tumor Segmentation (BraTS) 2023 dataset. Being one of the most extensive medical image segmentation models, STU-Net's sizes range between 14 million to 1.4 billion parameters. Our research seeks to evaluate STU-Net's efficacy and transferability on the BraTS23 dataset, encapsulating diverse MRI scans of brain tumor patients. The code and pre-trained models are available at https://github.com/uni-medical/STU-Net.

Keywords: Segmentation · Pre-training · Large-scale model · Brain tumor

1 Introduction

Brain tumors, particularly glioblastomas, have long been regarded as some of the most aggressive and lethal malignancies in adults. Their inherent heterogeneity in appearance, shape, and histology not only poses significant challenges in diagnosis but also in determining the most effective therapeutic strategies. The global landscape of medical imaging has been progressively shifting towards automated solutions, primarily due to their potential to offer more precise and consistent evaluations. In this context, the accurate segmentation of these tumors from radiographic images becomes paramount for various clinical applications, ranging from early-stage diagnosis to predicting the response to therapy and aiding surgical planning.

The International Brain Tumor Segmentation (BraTS) challenge commenced in 2012 and initially worked with a modest volume of data [2,5,11]. BraTS has since focused on generating a standardized environment for the delineation of adult brain gliomas. By providing standardized datasets, the challenge stimulates advancements in this field, ultimately aiming for improvements in patient care. Over the years, there has been a significant increase in the data volume, expanding to approximately 4,500 cases in the most recent challenge. This substantial expansion includes additional populations (e.g., sub-Saharan Africa patients), tumors (e.g., meningioma), clinical concerns (e.g., missing data), and technical considerations (e.g., augmentations).

The increasing complexity and volume of the dataset in BraTS challenges over the years not only reflects the escalating intricacies in medical imaging but also underscores the need for more sophisticated and larger-scale models for precise analysis. Within the context of the BraTS competition, neural networks, and in particular, the U-Net architecture, have been at the forefront of this transition. They have consistently showcased promising results across numerous BraTS challenges, particularly those methodologies based on the well-regarded nnU-Net [7] framework. Despite these successes, it is noteworthy to mention that the application of more substantial network scales has been relatively rare in the past. The continuous growth of data and complexity in the BraTS challenge necessitates further exploration into larger-scale models, laying the groundwork for the next stages of development in medical imaging.

The Scalable and Transferable U-Net (STU-Net) [6] has emerged as an innovative solution in the medical imaging field. This architecture, built on the nnU-Net framework, offers a new approach to addressing the challenges of scalability and transferability in image segmentation. Unlike conventional models, STU-Net has been designed to adapt to various sizes, with parameter scales ranging from 14 million to an impressive 1.4 billion. This flexibility allows it to fit different computational needs without losing effectiveness. One of the key features of STU-Net is its unique convolutional design and incorporation of residual connections, enabling optimal scaling of model depth and width. Furthermore, STU-Net provides pre-trained models on the current largest supervised medical image dataset, TotalSegmentator [13], facilitating an enhancement in performance across downstream tasks. This thoughtful construction allows it to perform exceptionally well even in complex medical imaging tasks, without excessive computational costs or challenges related to gradient diffusion. The pre-training on the TotalSegmentator dataset acts as a foundational step, harnessing the extensive data to make the network more robust and adaptable to various medical segmentation applications.

In this paper, we rigorously evaluate the performance of the Scalable and Transferable U-Net (STU-Net) in brain tumor segmentation, with a focus on the

BraTS23 dataset. Our exploration encompasses two main inquiries: the effectiveness of utilizing a larger-scale network in enhancing brain tumor segmentation, and the potential advantage of pre-training on a whole-body single modality CT dataset for downstream applications in multi-modal MR brain tumor segmentation. Through a systematic investigation, we aim to shed light on the adaptability and efficiency of STU-Net, providing valuable insights for both the technological advancement in medical imaging and its practical clinical applications.

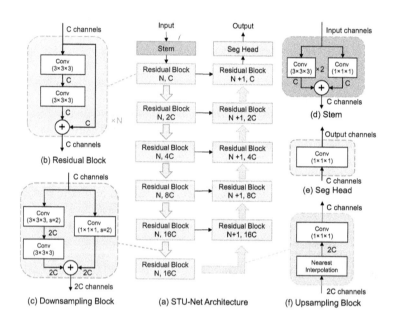

Fig. 1. Illustration of our STU-Net architecture which is built upon the nnU-Net architecture with several modifications to enhance its scalability and transferability. (a) An overview of the STU-Net architecture. The blue arrows denote downsampling while the yellow ones represent upsampling. (b) Residual blocks to achieve a large-scale model. (c) Downsampling in the first residual block of each encoder stage. (d–e) Stem and segmentation head for channel conversion of input and output. (f) Weight-free interpolation for upsampling, which effectively addresses the issue of weight mismatch across different tasks.

2 Method

In our challenge paper, we employ STU-Net, a model that builds upon the nnU-Net framework by introducing enhancements for scalability and transferability. The details of STU-Net are shown in Fig. 1:

Table 1. Our proposed STU-Net with different scales. Depth refers to the number of residual blocks in each resolution stage, and width denotes the channel count in each resolution stage. Parameter calculations are based on a single-channel input and a 105-channel output, which accounts for 104 foreground classes and 1 background class in the TotalSegmentator dataset. FLOPs calculations are based on input patch sizes of $128 \times 128 \times 128$.

Model	depth	width	Params (M)	FLOPs (T)
STU-Net-S	(1,1,1,1,1,1)	(16,32,64,128,256,256)	14.60	0.13
STU-Net-B	(1,1,1,1,1,1)	(32,64,128,256,512,512)	58.26	0.51
STU-Net-L	(2,2,2,2,2,2)	(64,128,256,512,1024,1024)	440.30	3.81
STU-Net-H	(3,3,3,3,3,3)	(96,192,384,768,1536,1536)	1457.33	12.60

2.1 Basic Block Tweaks

STU-Net introduces residual connections in the basic blocks to tackle gradient diffusion, a common challenge in deep networks. Additionally, it innovatively integrates downsampling within the first residual block of each stage, maintaining a neat architecture. These modifications improve optimization and enable effective scaling.

2.2 Upsampling Tweaks

To address weight mismatch issues in transfer learning, STU-Net replaces the default transpose convolution with interpolation and a $1 \times 1 \times 1$ convolution. The use of nearest neighbor interpolation not only offers faster processing but also ensures comparable performance, making it transfer-friendly.

2.3 Scaling Strategy

STU-Net implements a compound scaling strategy that maintains symmetry in the model. This involves simultaneous scaling of encoder and decoder and maintaining the same ratio for depth and width scaling in each resolution stage. Table 1 displays the different scales of STU-Net, with the suffixes 'S, B, L, H' representing 'Small, Base, Large, and Huge,' respectively.

2.4 Large-Scale Supervised Pre-training

For better transferability, STU-Net is pre-trained on the TotalSegmentator dataset. Specific modifications to the training procedure, such as mirror data augmentation and adjusted epoch numbers, enhance the generalization and transfer performance on downstream tasks.

3 Experiment and Results

3.1 Dataset

We participated in Tasks 1 to 5 of BraTS 2023: BraTS-GLI [2–5,11], BraTS-SSA [1], BraTS-PED [9], BraTS-MET [12], and BraTS-MEN [10]. These are all segmentation tasks, and they are consistent in terms of the input modalities and segmentation categories. These scans encompass native (T1), post-contrast T1-weighted (T1Gd), T2-weighted (T2), and T2 Fluid Attenuated Inversion Recovery (T2-FLAIR) volumes. Annotations, approved by experienced neuro-radiologists, include the GD-enhancing tumor (ET - label 3), peritumoral edematous/invaded tissue (ED - label 2), and necrotic tumor core (NCR - label 1). The ground truth data have been pre-processed to a standard resolution (1 mm^3) and skull-stripped. These tasks also have some differences in data sources, tumor types, and data volumes. We carried out our experiments using the provided training data and followed an 8:2 split for training and testing. For supervised pre-training, we use the TotalSegmentator [13] dataset. Next, we will briefly introduce each in turn:

BraTS-GLI. This task is the most traditional BraTS task, aimed at segmenting adult brain gliomas. It provides 1,251 cases as the training set with publicly available annotations, and 219 cases as the validation set.

BraTS-SSA. This task focuses on the segmentation of brain gliomas in patients from sub-Saharan Africa. The dataset includes 60 annotated training samples, 15 unannotated validation samples, and 30 test samples.

BraTS-PED. The task aims to segment pediatric brain gliomas from multimodal MR images (mpMRI). The dataset, released in May 2023, includes data from 3 centers totaling 228 cases, with 99 cases in the publicly annotated training set.

BraTS-MET. The task's objective is to segment brain metastases from multimodal MR images (mpMRI). The dataset, released in June 2023, consists of 328 cases in total, with 238 cases in the annotated training set.

BraTS-MEN. The goal of the task is to segment meningiomas from multimodal MR images (mpMRI). The dataset, released in May 2023, includes data from 6 centers totaling 1,650 cases, with 1,000 cases in the annotated training set.

TotalSegmentator. TotalSegmentator is currently the largest publicly available dataset in the field of 3D medical image segmentation, comprising 1,204 CT images that cover 104 types of anatomical structures throughout the body (Table 2).

Table 2. Quantitative results of different models with and without pre-training on the BraTS-GLI dataset. Performance is measured by DSC (%).

Model	w/ Pretrain	Avg DSC	NCR	ED	ET
nnUNet	×	0.8494	0.8087	0.8687	0.8707
STU-Net-B	×	0.8494	0.8089	0.8689	0.8705
STU-Net-B	√	0.8485	0.8033	0.8679	0.8742
STU-Net-L	×	0.8514	0.8130	0.8706	0.8706
STU-Net-L	√	0.8534	0.8102	0.8711	0.8789
STU-Net-H	×	0.8509	0.8077	0.8716	0.8734
STU-Net-H	√	**0.8536**	**0.8083**	**0.8731**	**0.8794**

3.2 Implementation Details

Our experiments were conducted in an environment running Python 3.8, CentOS 7, Pytorch 1.10, and nnU-Net 1.7.0. We largely adhered to the default data preprocessing, data augmentation, and training procedures provided by nnU-Net. We utilized the SGD optimizer with a Nesterov momentum of 0.99 and a weight decay of 1e−3. The batch size was fixed at 2, and each epoch consisted of 250 iterations. We train models for each task for 1,000 epochs, both with and without pre-training. The pre-trained model undergoes training on TotalSegmentator for 4,000 epochs. The learning rate decay followed the poly learning rate policy: $(1-epoch/1000)^{0.9}$. Data augmentation techniques used during training included additive brightness, gamma, rotation, scaling, mirror, and elastic deformation. The pre-training patch size on the TotalSegmentator dataset was 128 × 128 × 128. Fine-tuning patch sizes on downstream tasks were automatically configured by nnU-Net. We submit our results using MedPerf [8].

3.3 Quantitative Results

In this section, we present the quantitative results of our experiments conducted across five different sub-competitions within the BraTS 2023 Challenge, namely GLI, SSA, PED, MET, and MEN. We specifically compared three variants of the STU-Net model (STU-Net-B, STU-Net-L, STU-Net-H), with and without pre-training on the TotalSegmentator dataset, against the baseline nnUNet model. Our aim was to assess the influence of different model sizes and the impact of pre-training in various tumor segmentation scenarios. The summarized results are provided in the following table (Tables 3 and 4):

From the comprehensive analysis presented in the tables, a deeper understanding of the models' performance can be gleaned. It is particularly noticeable that across various sub-competitions, the influence of pre-training on STU-Net variants is profound, with the STU-Net-H model consistently exhibiting remarkable results. The most significant enhancements are discernible in the NCR and ET sub-regions, reflecting the models' advanced ability to delineate the necrotic

Table 3. Quantitative results of different models with and without pre-training on the BraTS-SSA dataset. Performance is measured by DSC (%).

Model	w/ Pretrain	Avg DSC	NCR	ED	ET
nnUNet	×	0.7952	0.7065	0.8373	0.8417
STU-Net-B	×	0.7923	0.7226	0.8235	0.8308
STU-Net-B	√	0.7931	0.7274	0.8262	0.8258
STU-Net-L	×	0.7841	0.7003	0.8155	0.8364
STU-Net-L	√	**0.8256**	**0.8062**	**0.8528**	**0.8178**
STU-Net-H	×	0.7807	0.7016	0.8105	0.8301
STU-Net-H	√	0.7917	0.7027	0.8386	0.8337

Table 4. Quantitative results of different models with and without pre-training on the BraTS-PED dataset. Performance is measured by DSC (%).

Model	w/ Pretrain	Avg DSC	NCR	ED	ET
nnUNet	×	0.4912	0.8254	0.2479	0.4002
STU-Net-B	×	0.4745	0.8082	0.2098	0.4055
STU-Net-B	√	0.4674	0.8050	0.2216	0.3756
STU-Net-L	×	0.4569	0.7879	0.1994	0.3834
STU-Net-L	√	0.4783	0.8234	0.1988	0.4127
STU-Net-H	×	0.4805	0.8121	0.2237	0.4058
STU-Net-H	√	**0.5062**	**0.8431**	**0.2545**	**0.4209**

components of the tumor and accentuate the intricate details. Intriguingly, the larger-scale STU-Net model, when trained from scratch, especially on subtasks with limited data, exhibited a decline in performance. This phenomenon suggests that the scarcity of data might not be sufficient to support the training of such a large-scale model from scratch, and the limited validation set may lead to less solid verification of the results. However, the incorporation of pre-training compensates for this challenge, allowing the larger model to be effectively trained. This not only highlights the importance of appropriate data volumes for training large models but also emphasizes the role of pre-training in enhancing performance, particularly when the available data is scarce. A detailed analysis of each specific subtask follows (Tables 5 and 6):

- **GLI Dataset Analysis:** The STU-Net-H, augmented with pre-training, achieved an exceptional average DSC of 0.8536, surpassing other configurations. This success not only emphasizes the effectiveness of the STU-Net architecture but also the potency of pre-training, particularly observable in the NCR sub-region, where it reached 0.8083.
- **SSA Dataset Analysis:** Pre-trained STU-Net-L marked the highest average DSC of 0.8256. Its superior performance in the ET sub-region, with a score of

Table 5. Quantitative results of different models with and without pre-training on the BraTS-MET dataset. Performance is measured by DSC (%).

Model	w/ Pretrain	Avg DSC	NCR	ED	ET
nnUNet	×	0.6933	0.6111	0.6962	0.7725
STU-Net-B	×	0.6861	0.5946	0.6937	0.7699
STU-Net-B	√	0.6849	0.5890	0.6901	0.7757
STU-Net-L	×	0.6851	0.5703	0.7060	0.7790
STU-Net-L	√	0.6916	0.5749	0.7257	0.7742
STU-Net-H	×	0.6825	0.5801	0.6972	0.7703
STU-Net-H	√	**0.7072**	**0.6089**	**0.7108**	**0.8020**

Table 6. Quantitative results of different models with and without pre-training on the BraTS-MEN dataset. Performance is measured by DSC (%).

Model	w/ Pretrain	Avg DSC	NCR	ED	ET
nnUNet	×	0.6060	0.3350	0.5578	0.9252
STU-Net-B	×	0.5822	0.3105	0.5420	0.8942
STU-Net-B	√	0.6024	0.3470	0.5441	0.9161
STU-Net-L	×	0.6022	0.3401	0.5555	0.9109
STU-Net-L	√	0.6120	0.3416	0.5655	0.9289
STU-Net-H	×	0.6027	0.3269	0.5670	0.9141
STU-Net-H	√	**0.6268**	**0.3828**	**0.5709**	**0.9266**

0.8178, illuminates its enhanced ability to discern complex tumor structures and delineate them precisely.
- **PED Dataset Analysis:** In the PED dataset, STU-Net-H with pre-training excelled with an average DSC of 0.5062, leading across all sub-regions. Its peak in the NCR at 0.8431 demonstrates the model's capacity to generalize, even in the face of complex segmentation challenges.
- **MET Dataset Analysis:** STU-Net-H, bolstered by pre-training, dominated the MET dataset with an average DSC of 0.7072. Excelling in the ET sub-region with a score of 0.8020, it underscores the adaptability of pre-training across diverse tumor types and stages.
- **MEN Dataset Analysis:** In the MEN dataset, STU-Net-H with pre-training recorded an average DSC of 0.6268, and shone in the ET sub-region with an impressive score of 0.9266. These outcomes validate the model's unswerving robustness and consistency across different datasets and tumor domains.

Despite these consistent positive trends, the analysis reveals some variance in specific results. Since the experiments were executed on a single fold, such variations might be a product of the chosen experimental design. This, coupled with the challenges faced by the larger STU-Net model when trained from scratch with limited data, may lead to minor inconsistencies in specific measurements. However, the broader conclusions, especially concerning the advantageous role of pre-training in enhancing the performance of large models, remain well-grounded and substantial.

Intriguingly, the utilization of pre-training on CT images, although unrelated to brain MRIs, manifested as a valuable addition to the brain tumor segmentation task. This novel finding accentuates the transferability of the learned features across different imaging modalities, thereby strengthening the argument for the universal applicability of large-scale models like STU-Net. The unexpected success of CT pre-training in supporting STU-Net's performance across sub-tasks with varying data volumes illustrates the model's flexibility and adaptive capacity. It also suggests that pre-training with diverse data can infuse the model with a richer understanding of underlying patterns, potentially overcoming limitations due to data scarcity. This discovery further inspires avenues for exploration in cross-modality learning, adding an exciting and promising dimension to current methodologies, and paving the way for more integrative and comprehensive approaches to medical image analysis.

3.4 Test Results

The final test results are included in the Tables 7, 8, 9, 10, and 11.

Table 7. Test results on BraTS-GLI.

Metric	mean	std	25 quantile	median	75 quantile
ET LesionWise Score Dice	0.7990	0.2492	0.7618	0.9146	0.9576
TC LesionWise Score Dice	0.8335	0.2628	0.8623	0.9543	0.9787
WT LesionWise Score Dice	0.8235	0.2253	0.7637	0.9404	0.9703
ET LesionWise Score HD95	39.52	90.06	1.00	1.00	3.61
TC LesionWise Score HD95	35.77	88.85	1.00	1.41	4.69
WT LesionWise Score HD95	44.03	82.54	1.00	2.83	10.95
ET Sensitivity	0.8763	0.2067	0.8821	0.9491	0.9778
TC Sensitivity	0.8901	0.2163	0.9096	0.9687	0.9873
WT Sensitivity	0.9300	0.0857	0.9150	0.9565	0.9808
ET Specificity	0.9998	0.0003	0.9997	0.9999	1.0000
TC Specificity	0.9997	0.0009	0.9998	0.9999	1.0000
WT Specificity	0.9995	0.0008	0.9994	0.9997	0.9999

Table 8. Test results on BraTS-SSA.

Metric	mean	std	25 quantile	median	75 quantile
ET LesionWise Score Dice	0.7839	0.2709	0.8144	0.9109	0.9362
TC LesionWise Score Dice	0.7966	0.2751	0.7956	0.9409	0.9678
WT LesionWise Score Dice	0.7920	0.2716	0.6430	0.9439	0.9699
ET LesionWise Score HD95	52.48	107.35	1.00	2.00	9.15
TC LesionWise Score HD95	53.45	106.94	1.31	2.72	12.48
WT LesionWise Score HD95	61.33	103.40	1.85	4.30	59.23
ET Sensitivity	0.8291	0.2222	0.8260	0.9026	0.9474
TC Sensitivity	0.8292	0.2296	0.7408	0.9115	0.9748
WT Sensitivity	0.9314	0.0569	0.8934	0.9621	0.9733
ET Specificity	0.9997	0.0005	0.9998	0.9999	1.0000
TC Specificity	0.9999	0.0002	0.9998	0.9999	1.0000
WT Specificity	0.9993	0.0005	0.9989	0.9993	0.9998

Table 9. Test results on BraTS-MEN.

Metric	mean	std	25 quantile	median	75 quantile
ET LesionWise Score Dice	0.8698	0.2219	0.8942	0.9686	0.9856
TC LesionWise Score Dice	0.8786	0.2058	0.8994	0.9691	0.9865
WT LesionWise Score Dice	0.8446	0.2258	0.8602	0.9566	0.9807
ET LesionWise Score HD95	33.45	82.04	1.00	1.00	2.66
TC LesionWise Score HD95	29.88	74.99	0.25	1.00	2.34
WT LesionWise Score HD95	41.20	84.28	1.00	1.00	4.12
ET Sensitivity	0.9317	0.1519	0.9358	0.9785	0.9896
TC Sensitivity	0.9320	0.1456	0.9382	0.9788	0.9904
WT Sensitivity	0.9203	0.1565	0.9222	0.9711	0.9879
ET Specificity	0.9999	0.0001	0.9999	1.0000	1.0000
TC Specificity	0.9999	0.0005	0.9999	1.0000	1.0000
WT Specificity	0.9998	0.0003	0.9998	0.9999	1.0000

Table 10. Test results on BraTS-MET.

Metric	mean	std	25 quantile	median	75 quantile
ET LesionWise Score Dice	0.5670	0.2626	0.3957	0.5825	0.8052
TC LesionWise Score Dice	0.6104	0.2780	0.4233	0.5842	0.8798
WT LesionWise Score Dice	0.5742	0.2752	0.4185	0.5747	0.8407
ET LesionWise Score HD95	101.55	107.23	1.37	84.52	187.5
TC LesionWise Score HD95	99.81	105.27	1.21	84.41	187.5
WT LesionWise Score HD95	101.75	110.24	2.69	77.53	188.06
ET Sensitivity	0.6935	0.2784	0.5601	0.8078	0.8950
TC Sensitivity	0.7381	0.2953	0.6314	0.8879	0.9380
WT Sensitivity	0.7282	0.2919	0.7045	0.8551	0.9053
ET Specificity	0.9999	0.0001	0.9999	1.0000	1.0000
TC Specificity	0.9999	0.0001	0.9999	1.0000	1.0000
WT Specificity	0.9997	0.0006	0.9995	0.9999	1.0000

Table 11. Test results on BraTS-PED.

Metric	mean	std	25 quantile	median	75 quantile
ET LesionWise Score Dice	0.5267	0.3399	0.1940	0.5967	0.7984
TC LesionWise Score Dice	0.7924	0.1370	0.7961	0.8256	0.8740
WT LesionWise Score Dice	0.8098	0.1469	0.8150	0.8593	0.8797
ET LesionWise Score HD95	108.93	146.82	1.41	9.59	205.29
TC LesionWise Score HD95	22.02	52.13	3.35	5.83	10.36
WT LesionWise Score HD95	23.56	61.60	3.12	4.95	7.67
ET Sensitivity	0.6349	0.3124	0.4487	0.7150	0.8719
TC Sensitivity	0.7464	0.1092	0.6939	0.7855	0.8198
WT Sensitivity	0.7762	0.0667	0.7523	0.7971	0.8219
ET Specificity	0.9996	0.0007	0.9996	1.0000	1.0000
TC Specificity	0.9997	0.0003	0.9997	0.9999	1.0000
WT Specificity	0.9998	0.0003	0.9997	0.9999	1.0000

4 Conclusion

The findings from this study underscore the significant potential of large-scale models like STU-Net and the transformative power of pre-training in the field of brain tumor segmentation. Utilizing the Brain Tumor Segmentation (BraTS) 2023 dataset, our results demonstrate not only the superior performance of the pre-trained STU-Net model across various tumor sub-regions, including the enhancing tumor (ET), tumor core (TC), and whole tumor (WT), but also the critical role of pre-training in enabling such large models to learn effectively, even with limited data.

The analysis reveals the nuanced impact of different training strategies, showing that while larger models might face challenges when trained from scratch with insufficient data, the application of pre-training, even with unrelated modalities such as CT images, can mitigate these challenges and bolster performance. This affirms the effectiveness of pre-training and large-scale modeling in tackling the intricate challenges of glioma segmentation, adding new dimensions to our understanding of cross-modality learning.

These results contribute valuable insights to the broader research community in the context of medical image segmentation, particularly in the complex realm of brain tumors. The deployment of large-scale models like STU-Net, combined with strategic pre-training, opens a promising avenue for further research and application. It heralds an exciting era of innovative methodologies that could revolutionize brain tumor diagnosis, treatment planning, and perhaps extend to other domains within medical imaging. The findings also stimulate further exploration of the universality and adaptability of large-scale models, paving the way for future advancements in the field.

References

1. Adewole, M., et al.: The brain tumor segmentation (BraTS) challenge 2023: glioma segmentation in Sub-Saharan Africa patient population (BraTS-Africa) (2023)
2. Baid, U., et al.: The RSNA-ASNR-MICCAI BraTS 2021 benchmark on brain tumor segmentation and radiogenomic classification (2021)
3. Bakas, S., et al.: Segmentation labels and radiomic features for the pre-operative scans of the TCGA-GBM collection. Cancer Imaging Arch. (2017)
4. Bakas, S., et al.: Segmentation labels and radiomic features for the pre-operative scans of the TCGA-LGG collection. Cancer Imaging Arch. (2017)
5. Bakas, S., et al.: Advancing the cancer genome atlas glioma MRI collections with expert segmentation labels and radiomic features. Sci. Data **4**(1), 170117 (2017)
6. Huang, Z., et al.: STU-Net: scalable and transferable medical image segmentation models empowered by large-scale supervised pre-training (2023)
7. Isensee, F., Jaeger, P.F., Kohl, S.A.A., Petersen, J., Maier-Hein, K.H.: nnU-Net: a self-configuring method for deep learning-based biomedical image segmentation. Nat. Methods **18**(2), 203–211 (2021)
8. Karargyris, A., et al.: Federated benchmarking of medical artificial intelligence with MedPerf. Nat. Mach. Intell. **5**(7), 799–810 (2023)
9. Kazerooni, A.F., et al.: The brain tumor segmentation (BraTS) challenge 2023: focus on pediatrics (CBTN-CONNECT-DIPGR-ASNR-MICCAI BraTS-PEDs) (2024)
10. LaBella, D., et al.: The ASNR-MICCAI brain tumor segmentation (BraTS) challenge 2023: intracranial meningioma (2023)
11. Menze, B.H., et al.: The multimodal brain tumor image segmentation benchmark (BraTS). IEEE Trans. Med. Imaging **34**(10), 1993–2024 (2015)
12. Moawad, A.W., et al.: The brain tumor segmentation (BraTS-METS) challenge 2023: brain metastasis segmentation on pre-treatment MRI (2023)
13. Wasserthal, J., et al.: TotalSegmentator: robust segmentation of 104 anatomic structures in CT images. Radiol.: Artif. Intell. **5**(5), e230024 (2023)

Automated 3D Tumor Segmentation Using Temporal Cubic PatchGAN (TCuP-GAN)

Kameswara Bharadwaj Mantha[✉], Ramanakumar Sankar, and Lucy Fortson

Department of Physics and Astronomy, University of Minnesota Twin Cities, Minneapolis, MN 55455, USA
manth145@umn.edu

Abstract. Development of robust general purpose 3D segmentation frameworks using the latest deep learning techniques is one of the active topics in various bio-medical domains. In this work, we introduce Temporal Cubic PatchGAN (TCuP-GAN), a volume-to-volume translational model that marries the concepts of a generative feature learning framework with Convolutional Long Short-Term Memory Networks (LSTMs), for the task of 3D segmentation. We demonstrate the capabilities of our TCuP-GAN on the data from four segmentation challenges (Adult Glioma, Meningioma, Pediatric Tumors, and Sub-Saharan Africa subset) featured within the 2023 Brain Tumor Segmentation (BraTS) Challenge and quantify its performance using LesionWise Dice similarity and 95% Hausdorff Distance metrics. We demonstrate the successful learning of our framework to predict robust multi-class segmentation masks across all the challenges. This benchmarking work serves as a stepping stone for future efforts towards applying TCuP-GAN on other multi-class tasks such as multi-organelle segmentation in electron microscopy imaging.

Keywords: 3D Segmentation · Convolutional LSTM · PatchGAN

1 Introduction and Motivation

Brain tumors such as gliomas and meningiomas make up some of the most common and aggressive forms of cancers in both adult and pediatric populations, and are quite challenging to treat [1,2]. Diagnosis and management of these tumors intimately depends on imaging guided techniques, notably using Magnetic Resonance Imaging (MRI) to identify and delineate the extent of the different tumor components. As such, study of these tumors along with development of automated methods for tumor segmentation has been a major epicenter for active research. Simultaneously, automated identification and segmentation of different types of cellular organelles within microscopy imaging of different organ tissues is also an open challenge in the domain of bio-medical research and clinical diagnostic applications.

© The Author(s), under exclusive license to Springer Nature Switzerland AG 2024
U. Baid et al. (Eds.): crossMoDA 2023/BraTS 2023, LNCS 14669, pp. 152–164, 2024.
https://doi.org/10.1007/978-3-031-76163-8_14

Efficiently acquiring annotated labels for such 3D volume data sets and building considerable sample sizes is one of the critical steps towards achieving generalized and robust models. Citizen Science (CS) techniques implemented through platforms such as the Zooniverse [3] have become an established method in tackling these issues [3], demonstrating incredible success in various domains and task types including annotating imaging data for bio-medical research purposes [4]. However, given the ever increasing volume of biomedical datasets (such as from volume electron micrographs or MRI scans), there is a need to accelerate the label gathering step, while still retaining accuracy. One of the promising pathways towards efficient and accelerated procurement of annotations and development of generalized and robust machine models is to use "human-in-the-loop" strategies where the humans provide corrections to the machine proposal. As such, development and testing of general-purpose models using novel deep learning concepts and making them available for use on future data sets as a starting point for citizen science efforts is a critical necessity, especially in the paradigm of big data.

Through this work, we aim to leverage the different individual deep learning concepts such as 3D Convolutional Neural Networks (CNNs), U-Nets (e.g., [5,6]), Generative Adversarial Networks (GANs; [7,8]), and Convolutional Long Short-Term Memory Networks (ConvLSTMs; [9]) towards designing a general purpose 3D volume-to-volume translation framework that can learn robust generalized spatial features and sequential correlations, and make segmentation predictions. Our inspiration stems from drawing parallels between the fact that MRI images are 3-dimensional and its third spatial axis can be considered analogous to temporal dimension of video datasets. As such, we anticipate that using ConvLSTMs can be helpful in learning 3D features corresponding to the targets of interest (e.g., lesions/tumors).

2 Related Works

In the past decade, advancements in deep learning and specifically CNNs [10] have enabled new avenues for automated image segmentation. Several frameworks such as U-Nets [5] and mask-RCNNs [11] have been used for 2D segmentation tasks on not only the general terrestrial datasets [12–14], but also biomedical applications such as the segmentation of nuclei [15], blood vessels [16], lung lesions [17], and brain tumors [18].

The latest techniques such as GANs have been demonstrated as robust image-level feature learners in computer vision tasks [7,19]. Recently, both 2D and 3D CNNs within GAN methodologies have been paired with U-Net [5] style architectures to be successful at several computer vision (e.g., PatchGAN; see [8]) and biomedical segmentation tasks (e.g., [20–22]). Simultaneously, LSTMs [23] have been demonstrated to be robust learners of sequentially related data in text-based corpora, and these concepts have been successfully extended to the image domain with 2D Convolutional LSTMs (2DConvLSTMs; [9]) that can learn spatio-sequential features and respective correlations.

Recently, 2DConvLSTMs have been successfully applied to general segmentation tasks in computer vision, e.g., video semantic segmentation [24,25]. The concepts of 2DConvLSTMs have been successfully paired with the U-Net style architectures for the purpose of image segmentation, with extensive exploration in various bio-medical domain related problems (liver lesions [26], retinal vasculature [27], and cells within microscopy imaging [28]). Furthermore, 2DConvLSTMs have also been paired with the U-Net and GAN concepts (e.g., BLU-GAN; [29]) for biomedical imaging segmentation.

Various architectures used in these studies highlight the different methodological choices by which the concepts of 2DConvLSTMs, GANs, and U-Net frameworks have been married. For example, [28] uses 2DConvLSTM layers within the encoder stage of the U-Net architecture, whereas [27,29,30] apply them during the encoder-decoder skip connection stage of the U-Net. Similarly, [29] incorporated adversarial training concepts with a traditional convolutional discriminator in their 2DConvLSTM-GAN framework, and studies such as [31,32] used 3D CNN based PatchGANs on biomedical domain tasks. As such, in this work we are motivated by the unexplored avenue (to the best of our knowledge) of using 2DConvLSTMs in both the encoder and decoder stages of the U-Net along with a 3D PatchGAN framework for biomedical segmentation tasks.

3 Data

In this work, we demonstrate the development and application of the TCuP-GAN on four BraTS 2023 segmentation challenge datasets. Specifically, we use the Adult Glioma (GLI; [33–35]), Meningioma (MEN; [36]), Pediatric Tumor (PED; [37]), and Sub-Saharan Africa (SSA; [38]) training and validation data made accessible via the Synapse platform. Sample sizes of training (and validation) data provided varied greatly, comprising 1251 (219) GLI cases, 1000 (141) MEN cases, 100 (45) PED cases, and 60 (15) SSA. Furthermore, we additionally split the provided training data by a 90% : 10% ratio into train vs. internal-validation samples across all the challenge data sets.

Each data sample across the different challenges is provided in a NIfTI (.nii) format with imaging across four MRI sequences: T1-weighted, T2-weighted, T1-Contrast Enhanced (T1CE), and T2-FLAIR (Fluid Attenuated Inversion Recovery) with dimensions ($240 \times 240 \times 155$). Additionally, each sample's annotated segmentation map is also provided, where the Necrotic Tumor (NC), Edematous Region (ED), and Enhanced Tumor (ET) are labelled as classes 1, 2, and 3, respectively.

For our model training, we perform on-the-fly data pre-processing for each data sample where we normalize each channel data by its 99th percentile pixel value and concatenate the classes together to create a 4 channel image cube. We then resize them to a size of 256×256 on their x, y axes, making each sample a 4D image cube with dimensions ($155 \times 4 \times 256 \times 256$). Additionally, to introduce stochastic variation in the input and enable robust feature learning, we also add a random Gaussian noise to each input cube with $\mu = 0$ and $\sigma = 0.1$ to only the pixels that do not correspond to the background (i.e., pixels with values always > 0). We perform one-hot encoding of the segmentation map with three classes $(1, 2, 3)$ corresponding to the aforementioned NC, ED, and ET classes. Each of the encoded class masks has pixel values 1 for regions corresponding to that particular class. After applying the same resizing method, our target segmentation map has the dimensionality of $(155 \times 3 \times 256 \times 256)$.

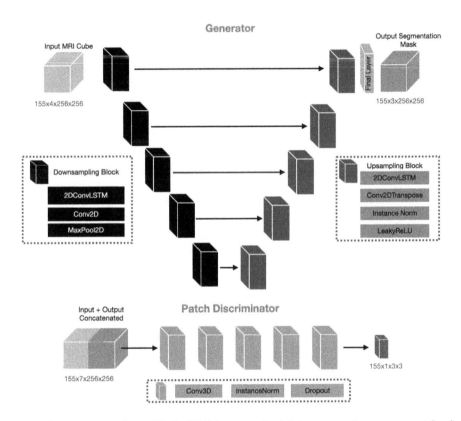

Fig. 1. Architecture of our TCuP-GAN framework with its generative component (top) and discriminator (bottom). Different components of our framework are shown in the legend.

4 Method

4.1 Architecture

Our Temporal Cubic Patch-GAN (TCuP-GAN) is inspired by a generative Image-to-Image translational model (PatchGAN; [8]), which was introduced for performing 2D semantic segmentation of terrestrial datasets. The PatchGAN framework comprises a 2D U-Net generator that predicts an output segmentation mask for a corresponding input image, along with a 2D convolutional patch-wise discriminator that predicts a 2D discriminatory score map for a concatenated image-mask pair input. Additionally, a traditional U-Net framework consists of an encoder portion, which extracts features from the input data and compresses the learnt feature space, and a decoder which uses the compressed representation to generate an output target image. Skip connections are used to transfer the learnt features from the encoder to the decoder, thereby making it easier for the model to learn features specific to the output classes, and stabilize the loss landscape [39].

Our model implementation comprises two components (see Fig. 1) – 1) A U-Net based Generator that accepts an image cube input and produces a corresponding k-class mask for each depth slice in the input image; and 2) A 3D Convolutional patch-wise Discriminator that takes a concatenation of the input image cube and its corresponding ground truth or generated mask and outputs a 3×3 probability matrix per depth slice.

Generator: Our Generator features an extension over the traditional U-Net generator by replacing the 2D Convolutional layers with 2DConvLSTM [9] layers, which are an adaption of the traditional fully connected LSTM layers by making use of 2D Convolution blocks instead of the regular multi-layer perceptrons. These are vital in simultaneously capturing the 2D spatial features and the correlation of these features across the depth axis. The feature vectors (h_t) and the cell state (c) learned by the 2DConvLSTM encodes the spatial features as a function of the third dimension (depth axis for image cubes, or temporal axis for videos), and the cumulative spatial locations of third dimension correlations of these features, respectively.

Following the input, the encoder portion of the generator is designed to extract and bottleneck h_t while preserving the depth axis using 5 down-sampling blocks with incremental number of filters (16, 32, 48, 64, 128). Each block consists of a 2DConvLSTM layer (kernel size 3×3) that outputs h_t and c, followed by a downsampling unit that contains a 2D Convolutional layer (kernel size = 3×3) along with a MaxPooling layer (pool size = 2×2) that act on spatial dimensions of h_t. As such, with an input dimensionality (4, 155, 256, 256), the output of the final block is of dimensions (128, 155, 8, 8).

In the decoder portion of the generator, we expand on the output downsampled h_t feature vector of the encoder with a series of 5 upsampling blocks. Each of these blocks contains a 2DConvLSTM layer (kernel size 3×3), where we skip both the c and h_t vectors across the bottleneck from the encoder side. We concatenate this skipped h_t with the output h_t from the previous decoder block before passing it into the next. In each upsampling block, both the h_t and the spatial dimensions of the feature vector are upsampled using ConvTranspose layers, followed by Instance Normalization, and LeakyReLU activation. Finally, after the 5 upsampling decoder blocks, we have an additional Convolutional layer (kernel size 3×3; stride 1×1) that acts on the spatial dimensions, followed by a final Sigmoid activation layer. Our full generator has 2.3M parameters and its architecture is shown in Fig. 1.

Discriminator: Our discriminator is a 3D CNN patch-wise binary classifier. Following the input layer, it has a series of 4 downsampling blocks with the following filter sizes (16, 32, 64, 128), where each block comprises a 3D Convolutional layer (kernel size $1 \times 3 \times 3$), followed by Instance Normalization, Tanh activation, and Dropout ($= 0.2$) layers. Our fifth and final block performs a 3D Convolution (kernel size $1 \times 3 \times 3$) and has a Sigmoid activated single channel output. Each unit of the output of the discriminator represents a concatenation of 3D patch of the input and output image cubes, and provides the probability that the image + mask patch is real. Figure 1 shows the architecture of the discriminator.

4.2 Training Strategy

In this study, we develop and apply our TCuP-GAN framework on four BraTS 2023 challenge data sets. Here, we describe our general training strategy and hyper-parameters used. Furthermore, as mentioned earlier, some of the challenges come with a relatively small number of training samples (see Sect. 3). As such, we chose to use transfer learning of the model trained on the largest sample size data (GLI) to the others (MEN, PED, SSA).

We train our TCuP-GAN model from scratch on the GLI data set for 30 epochs (with a batch size of 2) by minimizing a scaled, class-weighted Binary Cross-Entropy loss function $BCE' = \gamma \times \mathcal{W} \times BCE$ between the ground truth (GT) and predicted (PD) segmentation mask, where $\mathcal{W} = 1 - \sum_{d,x,y}(GT)/\sum(GT)$. We use $\gamma = 200$ to stabilize the network training at low BCE value regimes. We employ a starting learning rate of $r = 5 \times 10^{-4}$ and $r = 10^{-4}$ for our generator and discriminator, respectively, and decay the learning rates as $r^{0.95}$ every 5 epochs. We find that the GLI model achieved a stable loss at the end of its training with near identical mean BCE' on the internal validation samples. As for the training on the MEN, PED, and SSA challenge data, we initialize the model with GLI-based model weights (at 30th epoch) and further train it for 30 more epochs with a smaller (constant) learning rate of $r = 10^{-4}$ for the generator (and $r = 10^{-4}$ for the discriminator).

In each training step (i.e., for each batch), the input cube is passed through the generator to yield the predicted mask and the BCE' loss is computed between them. Additionally, the concatenated pairs (input, GT) and (input, PD) are passed through the discriminator and two (BCE) losses $\mathcal{L}_\text{real}$ and $\mathcal{L}_\text{fake}$ are computed between the discriminator outputs and corresponding real (unity), fake (zero) matrices, respectively. The total discriminator loss is defined as the average of these aforementioned losses ($\mathcal{L}_\text{disc} = [\mathcal{L}_\text{real} + \mathcal{L}_\text{fake}]/2$). The total generator loss is defined as $\mathcal{L}_\text{gen} = BCE' + \mathcal{L}_\text{fake}$. In Fig. 2, we visually show the generator and discriminator loss computation strategy.

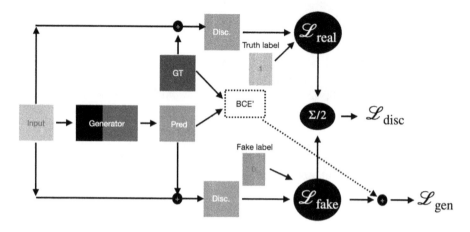

Fig. 2. Illustration of the optimization strategy of our overall generator and discriminator frameworks.

5 Evaluation

Thus far, we described the design and training optimization strategy of the TCuP-GAN model on data from four datasets featured as a part of the BraTS 2023 challenge. In this section, we describe the post-processing of our model's output 3D segmentation masks and quantification of the standard metrics that describe the model performance.

5.1 Model Performance Assessment Metrics

Following the recommendations of the BraTS 2023 challenge evaluation procedures, we quantify the performance of our models using the following core metrics: 'LesionWise' Dice ($\mathcal{D}_{\text{lw}}$) and Hausdorff distances ($\mathcal{H}_{95,lw}$) [40,41], where the average Dice and Hausdorff distance metrics are computed across individual, connected volume regions identified by binary connectivity (referred to as "lesion"), while also penalizing false positive lesion occurrences (with $\mathcal{D}_{\text{lw}} = 0$ and $\mathcal{H}_{95,lw} = 374$). We use the official BraTS 2023 evaluation pipeline[1] to compute these metrics for our internal validation set and present the yielded results after submitting our predicted mask on the provided validation sets. It is worth noting that although the models are trained on the native classes provided by the data sets (NC, ED, and ET), we report the metrics on the "Whole Tumor" (WT = TC + ED), with "Tumor Core" (TC = ET + NT), and "Enhanced Tumor" (ET).

5.2 Post-processing

For each input MRI volume, our trained model outputs a 3D segmentation mask with each voxel denoting the probability of that voxel being a given class (with

---
[1] https://github.com/rachitsaluja/brats_val_2023/.

dimensions $155 \times 3 \times 256 \times 256$), where the second dimension corresponds to the 3 different classes as defined in Sect. 3. Our first step of post-processing involves defining a "background" mask as the $1 - \Sigma_{1,2,3}(\text{PD})$ and concatenating it with PD, yielding a 4-channel mask of dimensions ($155 \times 4 \times 256 \times 256$). Next, we normalize the PD by dividing it with its sum along the class axis and apply the `argmax()` operation to the model output along it, thereby yielding a "combined" segmentation mask where each voxel is labelled one of (0,1,2,3) for background, NC, ED, and ET, respectively.

Next, we further process each combined mask to reject any spurious small-volume regions. This refinement step involves first splitting the combined mask into the BraTS challenge relevant classes – WT, TC, and ET. Next, for each of these three classes, we generate a binary connectivity map (using the *connected-components-3d* library), where connected voxels are uniquely labeled. We then retain those regions that have a mean area (across depth slices) greater than a threshold value ($\mathcal{A}_{\text{thresh}}$) and span at least 5 depth slices. For each model trained on its corresponding BraTS challenge dataset, we run an iterative Monte-Carlo experiment, where we vary the class-wise $\mathcal{A}_{\text{thresh}}$ and chose an optimal value that yielded highest $\mathcal{D}_{\text{lw}}$ on the Internal Validation data. For the GLI, MEN, PED, and SSA models, the chosen class-wise $\mathcal{A}_{\text{thresh}}$ values (WT, TC, ET) are (125, 75, 20), (125, 125, 25), (75, 75, 25), and (75, 100, 5), respectively.

6 Results and Discussion

In this section, we report and discuss the mean and median lesionwise metrics $\mathcal{D}_{\text{lw}}$ and $\mathcal{H}_{95,\text{lw}}$ for the different BraTS challenge datasets (reported in Table 1). Specifically, we report these metrics for both our internal validation set and the team provided validation set.

Generally speaking, we find that our TCuP-GAN framework successfully learns to predict the target multi-class segmentation labels across different datasets. With the reported metrics based on the validation set in context, we note that all the models demonstrated a good performance on the WT class with the mean $\mathcal{D}_{\text{lw}} \sim 0.65$–$0.8$. As for the TC and ET classes, the GLI model showed the highest performance $\mathcal{D}_{\text{lw}} \sim 0.76$, whereas the MEN, PED, and SSA models performed at $\mathcal{D}_{\text{lw}} \sim 0.63$–$0.68$, with the exception of the PED model performing the lowest scores at $\mathcal{D}_{\text{lw}} \sim 0.45$ for the ET class. Additionally, across these three classes and the 4 models, we highlight that the median $\mathcal{D}_{\text{lw}}$ values remain substantially higher (ranging between ~ 0.7–0.9) than the reported means. This can be visually comprehended in Fig. 3, where we show the distributions of $\mathcal{D}_{\text{lw}}$ and $\mathcal{H}_{95,\text{lw}}$ values for the GLI and MEN models applied to the Internal Validation sample. We note that while our model tends to performs very well on a dominant portion of the validation set, a few outlier cases where the models yielded a $\mathcal{D}_{\text{lw}} \sim 0$ or ~ 0.5 impacted the mean $\mathcal{D}_{\text{lw}}$ to be smaller. When our model failed to predict any segmentation regions for a few samples (especially for the TC or ET classes), this resulted in a $\mathcal{D}_{\text{lw}} \sim 0$. Simultaneously, we noticed that the samples that have $0.1 \leq \mathcal{D}_{\text{lw}} \leq 0.5$ are because of the model predicting one to

Table 1. Summary of the LesionWise Dice ($\mathcal{D}_{lw}$) and 95% Hausdorff Distance ($\mathcal{H}_{95\%}$) metrics for the different evaluation datasets across different challenge datasets. The internal validation sample based results are reported in parentheses.

Model Name	Eval. Dataset	Statistic Name	Lesion	Mean	Median
GLI	(Internal) Validation	$\mathcal{D}_{lw}$	WT	0.83 (0.81)	0.9 (0.9)
			TC	0.76 (0.8)	0.9 (0.91)
			ET	0.76 (0.73)	0.84 (0.83)
		$\mathcal{H}_{95,lw}$	WT	29.3 (40.9)	4.1 (4.2)
			TC	43.5 (34.3)	3.3 (2.2)
			ET	35.6 (43.3)	2.0 (1.7)
MEN	(Internal) Validation	$\mathcal{D}_{lw}$	WT	0.67 (0.72)	0.85 (0.88)
			TC	0.68 (0.73)	0.85 (0.88)
			ET	0.68 (0.73)	0.85 (0.88)
		$\mathcal{H}_{95,lw}$	WT	86.8 (66.7)	3.69 (3.0)
			TC	82.2 (65.5)	3.16 (2.2)
			ET	81.8 (65.0)	2.23 (2.0)
PED	(Internal) Validation	$\mathcal{D}_{lw}$	WT	0.74 (0.70)	0.84 (0.87)
			TC	0.66 (0.64)	0.75 (0.76)
			ET	0.45 (0.86)	0.36 (0.80)
		$\mathcal{H}_{95,lw}$	WT	48.8 (77.6)	6.1 (8.0)
			TC	58.7 (89.2)	9.2 (8.0)
			ET	152.9 (1.6)	14.9 (1.4)
SSA	(Internal) Validation	$\mathcal{D}_{lw}$	WT	0.67 (0.63)	0.73 (0.75)
			TC	0.64 (0.44)	0.83 (0.48)
			ET	0.63 (0.42)	0.78 (0.47)
		$\mathcal{H}_{95,lw}$	WT	76 (96.6)	6.92 (24.5)
			TC	74.7 (161.3)	6.1 (102.6)
			ET	72 (159.5)	4.0 (101.6)

two large false-positive (FP) region(s) that incrementally (and asymptotically) down-weight the $\mathcal{D}_{lw}$ (as FP regions are assigned a $\mathcal{D}_{lw} = 0$). For example, in a case where our model predicts a true positive with $\mathcal{D}_{lw} \sim 0.9$ and a false positive, then the averaged $\mathcal{D}_{lw}$ reported is ~ 0.45.

The class-wise performance trends of $\mathcal{D}_{lw}$ (and $\mathcal{H}_{95,lw}$) across different models also mostly follow the same behavior when assessing the internal validation based values, albeit with a worthwhile note that they tend to be sometimes higher when compared to the validation set based results. However, it is to be also noted that the median metric values between the internal validation and validation sets seem to be much more in close agreement with each other than the mean values. This indicates a higher incidence of FPs in the validation set when compared to our internal validation data, however, we are cognizant that such differences are to be expected as our internal validation set is one random realization of the entire sample. Finally, we also highlight that all of our assessments and interpretations based on $\mathcal{D}_{\text{lw}}$ also resonate with $\mathcal{H}_{95,\text{lw}}$ values in a self-consistent way.

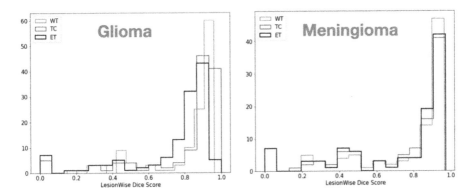

Fig. 3. Distributions of the lesionwise dice ($\mathcal{D}_{\text{lw}}$ based on the GLI and MEN models applied to the internal validation set.

7 Conclusions

In this work, we introduced a 3D volume-to-volume translation model – Temporal Cubic PatchGAN (TCuP-GAN), which leverages the conceptual frameworks of U-Nets, 2DConvLSTMs, and GANs (especially PatchGAN) for the purpose of automated 3D segmentation of brain tumors. We demonstrated the successful application and performance of our framework on four datasets within the BraTS 2023 segmentation challenge aimed at segmenting Gliomas, Meningiomas, and Pediatric tumors. This benchmarking analysis lays critical groundwork for future applications of TCuP-GAN on different biomedical segmentation tasks (e.g., multi-organelle segmentation in microscopy imaging) and interfacing with citizen science platforms such as Zooniverse as a general-purpose segmentation model for project teams to use in a human-in-the-loop strategy.

Acknowledgments. This work was partially supported by the National Science Foundation under grants OAC 1835530 and IIS 2006894. The authors also acknowledge the Minnesota Supercomputing Institute (MSI) at the University of Minnesota for providing resources that contributed to the research results reported within this paper. URL: http://www.msi.umn.edu.

References

1. Dolecek, T.A., Propp, J.M., Stroup, N.E., Kruchko, C.: CBTRUS statistical report: primary brain and central nervous system tumors diagnosed in the united states in 2005–2009. Neuro-Oncology **14**(suppl_5), v1–v49 (2012)
2. Kotecha, R.S., et al.: Meningiomas in children and adolescents: a meta-analysis of individual patient data. Lancet Oncol. **12**(13), 1229–1239 (2011)
3. Trouille, L., Lintott, C.J., Fortson, L.F.: Citizen science frontiers: efficiency, engagement, and serendipitous discovery with human–machine systems. Proc. Natl. Acad. Sci. **116**(6), 1902–1909 (2019). https://doi.org/10.1073/pnas.1807190116. https://www.pnas.org/content/116/6/1902
4. Spiers, H., et al.: Deep learning for automatic segmentation of the nuclear envelope in electron microscopy data, trained with volunteer segmentations. Traffic **22**(7), 240–253 (2021). https://doi.org/10.1111/tra.12789. https://onlinelibrary.wiley.com/doi/abs/10.1111/tra.12789
5. Ronneberger, O., Fischer, P., Brox, T.: U-Net: convolutional networks for biomedical image segmentation. In: Navab, N., Hornegger, J., Wells, W., Frangi, A. (eds.) MICCAI 2015. LNCS, vol. 9351, pp. 234–241. Springer, Cham (2015). https://doi.org/10.1007/978-3-319-24574-4_28
6. Falk, T., et al.: U-Net: deep learning for cell counting, detection, and morphometry. Nat. Methods **16**(1), 67–70 (2019)
7. Goodfellow, I., et al.: Generative adversarial nets. Adv. Neural Inf. Process. Syst. **27** (2014)
8. Isola, P., Zhu, J.Y., Zhou, T., Efros, A.A.: Image-to-image translation with conditional adversarial networks. In: Proceedings of the IEEE Conference on Computer Vision and Pattern Recognition, pp. 1125–1134 (2017)
9. Shi, X., Chen, Z., Wang, H., Yeung, D.Y., Wong, W.K., Woo, W.C.: Convolutional LSTM network: a machine learning approach for precipitation nowcasting. Adv. Neural Inf. Process. Syst. **28** (2015)
10. LeCun, Y., Bengio, Y., Hinton, G.: Deep learning. Nature **521**(7553), 436–444 (2015)
11. He, K., Gkioxari, G., Dollár, P., Girshick, R.: Mask R-CNN. In: Proceedings of the IEEE International Conference on Computer Vision, pp. 2961–2969 (2017)
12. Puri, D.: COCO dataset stuff segmentation challenge. In: 2019 5th International Conference on Computing, Communication, Control and Automation (ICCUBEA), pp. 1–5. IEEE (2019)
13. Freudenberg, M., Nölke, N., Agostini, A., Urban, K., Wörgötter, F., Kleinn, C.: Large scale palm tree detection in high resolution satellite images using U-Net. Remote Sens. **11**(3), 312 (2019)
14. Laxman, K., Dubey, S.R., Kalyan, B., Kojjarapu, S.R.V.: Efficient high-resolution image-to-image translation using multi-scale gradient U-Net. In: Raman, B., Murala, S., Chowdhury, A., Dhall, A., Goyal, P. (eds.) CVIP 2021. CCIS, vol. 1567, pp. 33–44. Springer, Cham (2021). https://doi.org/10.1007/978-3-031-11346-8_4
15. Vuola, A.O., Akram, S.U., Kannala, J.: Mask-RCNN and U-Net ensembled for nuclei segmentation. In: 2019 IEEE 16th International Symposium on Biomedical Imaging (ISBI 2019), pp. 208–212. IEEE (2019)
16. Xiancheng, W., et al.: Retina blood vessel segmentation using a U-Net based convolutional neural network. In: Procedia Computer Science: International Conference on Data Science (ICDS 2018), pp. 8–9 (2018)

17. Shaziya, H., Shyamala, K., Zaheer, R.: Automatic lung segmentation on thoracic CT scans using U-Net convolutional network. In: 2018 International Conference on Communication and Signal Processing (ICCSP), pp. 0643–0647. IEEE (2018)
18. Dong, H., Yang, G., Liu, F., Mo, Y., Guo, Y.: Automatic brain tumor detection and segmentation using U-Net based fully convolutional networks. In: Valdés Hernández, M., González-Castro, V. (eds.) MIUA 2017. CCIS, vol. 723, pp. 506–517. Springer, Cham (2017). https://doi.org/10.1007/978-3-319-60964-5_44
19. Goodfellow, I., et al.: Generative adversarial networks. Commun. ACM **63**(11), 139–144 (2020)
20. Dong, X., et al.: Automatic multiorgan segmentation in thorax CT images using U-Net-GAN. Med. Phys. **46**(5), 2157–2168 (2019)
21. Nema, S., Dudhane, A., Murala, S., Naidu, S.: RescueNet: an unpaired GAN for brain tumor segmentation. Biomed. Sig. Process. Control **55**, 101641 (2020)
22. Choi, J., Kim, T., Kim, C.: Self-ensembling with GAN-based data augmentation for domain adaptation in semantic segmentation. In: Proceedings of the IEEE/CVF International Conference on Computer Vision, pp. 6830–6840 (2019)
23. Hochreiter, S., Schmidhuber, J.: Long short-term memory. Neural Comput. **9**(8), 1735–1780 (1997)
24. Zhou, L., Yuan, H., Ge, C.: ConvLSTM-based neural network for video semantic segmentation. In: 2021 International Conference on Visual Communications and Image Processing (VCIP), pp. 1–5. IEEE (2021)
25. Qiu, Z., Yao, T., Mei, T.: Learning deep spatio-temporal dependence for semantic video segmentation. IEEE Trans. Multimed. **20**(4), 939–949 (2017)
26. Li, J., et al.: Study on strategy of CT image sequence segmentation for liver and tumor based on U-Net and Bi-ConvLSTM. Expert Syst. Appl. **180**, 115008 (2021)
27. Yi, Y., Guo, C., Hu, Y., Zhou, W., Wang, W.: BCR-UNet: bi-directional convLSTM residual u-net for retinal blood vessel segmentation. Front. Public Health **10**, 1056226 (2022)
28. Arbelle, A., Cohen, S., Raviv, T.R.: Dual-task convLSTM-UNet for instance segmentation of weakly annotated microscopy videos. IEEE Trans. Med. Imaging **41**(8), 1948–1960 (2022)
29. Lin, L., Wu, J., Cheng, P., Wang, K., Tang, X.: BLU-GAN: bi-directional convLSTM U-Net with generative adversarial training for retinal vessel segmentation. In: Gao, W., et al. (eds.) FICC 2020. CCIS, vol. 1385, pp. 3–13. Springer, Singapore (2021). https://doi.org/10.1007/978-981-16-1160-5_1
30. Rani, B., Ratna, V.R., Srinivasan, V.P., Thenmalar, S., Kanimozhi, R.: Disease prediction based retinal segmentation using bi-directional convLSTM U-Net. J. Ambient Intell. Humaniz. Comput. 1–10 (2021)
31. Yang, C.J., et al.: Generative adversarial network (GAN) for automatic reconstruction of the 3D spine structure by using simulated bi-planar X-ray images. Diagnostics **12**(5), 1121 (2022)
32. Abramian, D., Eklund, A.: Generating FMRI volumes from T1-weighted volumes using 3D cycleGAN. arXiv preprint arXiv:1907.08533 (2019)
33. Baid, U., et al.: The RSNA-ASNR-MICCAI BraTS 2021 benchmark on brain tumor segmentation and radiogenomic classification. arXiv preprint arXiv:2107.02314 (2021)
34. Menze, B.H., et al.: The multimodal brain tumor image segmentation benchmark (BraTS). IEEE Trans. Med. Imaging **34**(10), 1993–2024 (2014)
35. Lloyd, C.T., Sorichetta, A., Tatem, A.J.: High resolution global gridded data for use in population studies. Sci. Data **4**(1), 1–17 (2017)

36. LaBella, D., et al.: The ASNR-MICCAI brain tumor segmentation (BraTS) challenge 2023: intracranial meningioma (2023)
37. Kazerooni, A.F., et al.: The brain tumor segmentation (BraTS) challenge 2023: focus on pediatrics (CBTN-CONNECT-DIPGR-ASNR-MICCAI BraTS-PEDs). arXiv preprint arXiv:2305.17033 (2023)
38. Adewole, M., et al.: The brain tumor segmentation (BraTS) challenge 2023: glioma segmentation in Sub-Saharan Africa patient population (BraTS-Africa). arXiv preprint arXiv:2305.19369 (2023)
39. Wang, L., Shen, B., Zhao, N., Zhang, Z.: Is the skip connection provable to reform the neural network loss landscape? In: IJCAI (2020)
40. Bakas, S., et al.: Advancing the cancer genome atlas glioma MRI collections with expert segmentation labels and radiomic features. Sci. Data **4**(1), 1–13 (2017)
41. Bakas, S., et al.: Segmentation labels and radiomic features for the pre-operative scans of the TCGA-LGG collection. Cancer Imaging Arch. **286** (2017)

An Optimization Framework for Processing and Transfer Learning for the Brain Tumor Segmentation

Tianyi Ren[✉], Ethan Honey, Harshitha Rebala, Abhishek Sharma, Agamdeep Chopra, and Mehmet Kurt

University of Washington, Seattle, WA 98105, USA
tr1@uw.edu

Abstract. Tumor segmentation from multi-modal brain MRI images is a challenging task due to the limited samples, high variance in shapes and uneven distribution of tumor morphology. The performance of automated medical image segmentation has been significant improvement by the recent advances in deep learning. However, the model predictions have not yet reached the desired level for clinical use in terms of accuracy and generalizability. In order to address the distinct problems presented in Challenges 1, 2, and 3 of BraTS 2023, we have constructed an optimization framework based on a 3D U-Net model for brain tumor segmentation. This framework incorporates a range of techniques, including various pre-processing and post-processing techniques, and transfer learning. On the validation datasets, this multi-modality brain tumor segmentation framework achieves an average lesion-wise Dice score of 0.79, 0.72, 0.74 on Challenges 1, 2, 3 respectively.

Keywords: Brain Tumor Segmentation · U-Net · Deep Learning · Diffusion · Transfer Learning · Magnetic Resonance Imaging

1 Introduction

Brain tumors are a deadly type of cancer that have long-term impacts on a patient's health [2]. Treatments of surgery, radiation therapy, and drug therapy are pursued depending on the type and condition of the patient's brain tumor [5]. These insights into the brain tumor are often obtained through Magnetic Resonance Imaging (MRI) scans, which require experienced radiologists to manually segment tumor sub-regions [5]. This is a long process that is unscalable to the needs of all patients. Thus, the recent growth of deep learning technologies holds promise to provide a reliable and automated solution to segmentation to save time and help medical professionals with this process [14].

The BraTS Challenge encourages advancement in the field of tumor segmentation of brain MRI images by providing challenges geared toward specific brain

---

T. Ren, E. Honey and H. Rebala—These authors contributed equally to this work.

tumors. Challenge 1 focuses on adult glioblastoma, which is one of the most common tumors. Over the past 20 years, there has been little to no change in the average patient prognosis of 14 months [5,6,15]. This highlights the need of faster yet accurate tumor segmentation for clinical treatments and experiments.

Challenge 2 is centered on glioblastoma in Sub-Saharan Africa, where cases and mortality rates are still rising [2]. These MRI scans are often lower in resolution and contrast and thus require tailored segmentation models to bridge this gap [2]. The use of an automatic and accurate segmentation would improve healthcare access to more patients in Sub-Saharan Africa since most of the current tumor segmentation analysis is limited to high-resource urban areas.

The focus of Challenge 3 is intracranial meningioma. Since imaging is one of the most common ways to diagnose meningioma, automated segmentation would be pivotal in assisting surgical and radiotherapy planning by approximating tumor volume and sub-regions [13].

For all challenges, each model is evaluated by computing the Dice similarity coefficient and Hausdorff distance (95%) (HD95) between each region of interest in the ground truth and the corresponding prediction. In previous years, these metrics were calculated over the whole brain volume; however, this year they are computed lesion-wise, giving equal weight to each tumor lesion regardless of its size. There are also extra penalties for false negative (FN) and false positive (FP) predictions. Consequently, we investigated new pre- and post-processing techniques alongside a range of loss functions to maximize our performance in the new lesion-wise metrics, particularly to minimize the number of FP predictions.

Various deep learning architectures, including classical convolutional neural networks, widely used U-Net [7], recently popular vision transformers [8] and swin transformer [10], have been applied in automating brain tumor segmentation and classification tasks. The state-of-the-art models in brain tumor segmentation are based on the encoder-decoder architectures such as U-Net [11] and its variants. For instance, Luu et al. [14] modified the nnU-Net model by adding an axial attention in the decoder. Futrega et al. [9] optimized the U-Net model by adding foreground voxels to the input data, increasing the encoder depth and convolutional filters. Siddiquee et al. [16] applied adaptive ensembling to minimize redundancy under perturbations.

Consequently, we propose deep learning framework for automatic brain tumor segmentation. This frameworkaims to solve various problems in multiple tasks such as model prediction using of U-Net, image pre-processing techniques given a certain criteria, post-processing of the model prediction, and transfer learning training strategies for low-quality images.

2 Methods

We employed the same overall pipeline for Challenges 1 and 3, which we will outline in Subsects. 2.1–2.6.

2.1 Data and Pre-Processing

The BraTS mpMRI scans for each patient comprise of a native T1, post-contrast T1-weighted, T2-weighted, and T2 Fluid Attenuated Inversion Recovery (T2-FLAIR) volumes. The dataset was preprocessed by applying DICOM to NIfTI file conversions, and coregistration to the same SRI24 anatomical template. The preprocessing techniques of resampling to a uniform isotropic resolution (1mm3) and skull-stripping to maintain anonymity were also done [2,5,13]. In addition to the standardized preprocessing applied to all BraTS mpMRI scans by the BraTS Challenge organizers, our team experimented with further processing techniques to improve the quality and comparability of the dataset.

Z-Score Normalization. The Z-score normalization technique was used to address the varying intensity distributions across the dataset as seen in [14]. Z-score normalization can be computed by calculating the mean and standard deviation of voxels and then transforming the value of the voxel by first subtracting the mean and dividing it by the standard deviation. This technique standardizes the intensity values of each voxel and allows for better direct comparisons between the different patient data by removing outliers.

Rescaling Voxel Intensities. Segmentation relies on the ability to identify important features and structures, so we aimed to improve the visibility of such features by rescaling voxel intensities. The voxel intensity percentiles were calculated and we defined the 2nd and 98th percentiles to be the range of voxel intensity to be stretched to cover the entire intensity range. This technique increases the contrast and provides more insight into the subtle features in the data.

Histogram Contrast Matching. Histogram contrast matching helps in better aligning the intensity distributions between the image contrasts. This technique transforms the source data's voxel values in a manner that ensures that the new histogram matches a reference data sample.

2.2 Model Architecture

We used the optimized U-Net [9] as our baseline model for challenge 1 and 3 which can be seen in Fig. 1a. We used Challenge 1's model, froze its decoder layers as seen in Fig. 1a and then continued training on Challenge 2 dataset for transfer learning.

2.3 Loss Functions

The selection of loss functions plays an important role in guiding accurate segmentation results, so we explored various loss functions to determine the most effective ones.

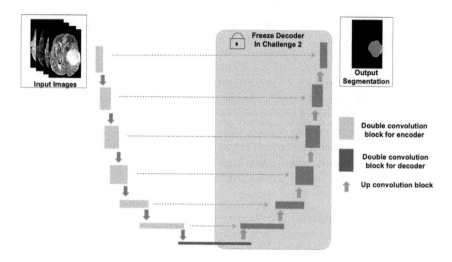

Fig. 1. (a) Baseline U-Net model [9]

We first investigated the Mean Squared Error (MSE) loss to enhance the model's accuracy. MSE provides the average squared difference between the predicted and ground truth voxels and therefore is useful in attaining accuracy at the voxel-level by heavily penalizing large deviations. Next, we explored Cross-Entropy (CE) loss, which measures the dissimilarity between predicted and ground truth labels [12] and penalizes false negatives and false positives. Another contender was Dice loss (Dice) since it acts as a strong indicator of similarity by calculating the overlap between the predicted and ground truth regions [12]. This made it a natural fit for handling class imbalance and enhancing the model's ability to accurately segment the regions of interest. We also considered Focal loss (Focal) to enhance the model's focus on segmenting difficult regions. Focal loss focuses learning by assigning a higher weight to challenging data [12]. In order to reinforce correct boundary deformation and overcome intensity dependence, we introduced an Edge loss (Edge) component, as described in [1]. Edges were obtained by computing and normalizing the magnitude of the extracted intensity gradients. The Edge loss was calculated by comparing the edges of the predicted image to the target image edges using MSE.

2.4 Training Details

The ground truth segmentations provided by the BraTS organizers are in the following format: each voxel in the volume has one of the following labels: 1 for necrotic tumor core (NCR), 2 for peritumoral edematous/invaded tissue (ED), 3 for enhancing tumor (ET) and 0 for background voxels (no tumor). However, the evaluation is performed with partially overlapping regions. These consist of enhancing tumor; tumor core (TC), the union of ET and NCR; and whole tumor (WT), the union of ET, NCR and ED. Thus, from the ground truth labels we produce three channels that correspond to the partially overlapping regions ET, TC and WT. We compute the loss between these channels and our model output, so that the model output for a given voxel is a set of probabilities that the voxel lies in each of these overlapping regions. For our loss functions described above, we compute the loss between the ground truth and model output for each channel separately and then average them.

We used the Adam optimizer with no weight decay and learning rate equal to 6e-5. Additionally, we implemented exponential decay of the learning rate. We divided the official training dataset into a 90:10 split, holding 10% of the dataset for validation rather than training. After every epoch, we iterate through this validation hold, calculating the Dice and HD95 score between our prediction and the ground truth for the regions of ET, TC, and WT and then averaging these scores. We then average this over each subject in the validation hold and save the model checkpoints with the highest such score.

2.5 Inference

As mentioned, we construct the training of our model such that it outputs a probability for each voxel being in each of the overlapping regions ET, TC and WT. However, the final output of our model must associate to each voxel a single label that is either 1 (NCR), 2 (ED), 3 (ET) or 0 (no tumor). Thus, we implement a thresholding strategy as in [9] to convert the probabilities for overlapping regions to actual predictions for the disjoint labels.

Firstly, consider the WT probability for a given voxel. If it is not large enough (less than 0.45), we do not consider the voxel to be in the tumor and set its label to 0 (no tumor), otherwise, we consider the voxel in the tumor. Next, consider the TC probability for the voxel. If it is not large enough (less than 0.4), we do not consider the voxel to be in TC and set its label to 2 (ED), otherwise, we consider the voxel to be in TC. Finally, consider the ET probability for the voxel. If it is not large enough (less than 0.45), we do not consider the voxel to be in ET and set its label to 1 (NCR), otherwise, we consider the voxel as ET and set its label to 3.

2.6 Post-processing

To prepare our final predictions, we perform the following strategy. We identify all connected components of ET voxels and remove any that have a volume less than or equal to 50 voxels, by relabelling the prediction labels to 0 for these voxels. (We call this removing 'dust'.) Then we examine the TC voxels (ET + NCR) and check if any of the ET voxels that we removed created any holes[1] in this region; if so, we change these voxels to be NCR (label 1). Next we remove any dust that still exists in the TC voxels, before examining the WT voxels (ET + NCR + ED) and filling any holes created by the removal of TC dust by

---

[1] By holes, we mean a connected component of background voxels that is fully enclosed by the corresponding tumor region voxels.

changing these voxels to be ED (label 2). Finally, we remove any dust that still exists in the WT voxels.

2.7 Transfer Learning for Challenge 2

We applied the same pre- and post-processing techniques for the Challenge 2 data as we used for Challenges 1 and 3, but opted for a different training approach. One major hurdle for Challenge 2 was the limited training dataset of 60 patients which made training a full-scale, accurate model difficult. Therefore, we decided to implement transfer learning [3] which uses a pre-trained model that already understands the important features of the task and then freezes or adds new layers to adapt the model to a new yet similar task. In our case, we utilized our model from Challenge 1 (also focused on glioma) and continued training on Challenge 2 data while experimenting with different frozen layers. Different strategies has been investigated such as freezing the encoder, decoder, and no layers. We also froze the middle layers, which included convolutional layers 5 to 7 in the encoder and layers 6 to 4 in the decoder.

Freezing in this context of transfer learning refers to the designated layer's weights and biases being prevented from updating during training. Instead, the layers retain the values and thus the learned features from the pre-trained model. In the context of Challenge 2, we considered freezing to be the optimal solution to prevent overfitting to the small dataset and maintain feature retention from Challenge 1's model, which was trained on higher-resolution data. For our final model, we froze the decoder, as illustrated by the grey box as seen in Fig. 1a.

3 Results

3.1 Pre-processing

To determine the most effective pre-processing technique, we tested Z-score normalization, rescaling voxel intensities, and histogram contrast matching. We ran an experiment by randomly selecting a subset of 100 glioblastoma patients and applying different pre-processing techniques before training. The data was processed in the following manners for each trial: (1) no additional pre-processing (2) Z-score normalization, (3) Z-score & rescaling, and (4) Z-Score & rescaling & histogram-matching. The model was then validated on a random sample of 30 glioblastoma patients, and we recorded the overall average Dice score for the ED, ET and NCR across all patients. The model's features were kept consistent throughout these experiments and the pre-processing experiment results can be found in Table 1. As a result, we rescale the voxel intensity after Z-Score normalization as the preprocessing protocol for all the 3 challenges.

3.2 Loss Functions

Different loss functions were also been investigated, including MSE, CE, Focal, Dice Loss, and a previously developed loss function Edge loss [1]. We examined

Table 1. Average Dice across tumor sub-regions for different pre-processing techniques

Preprocessing Techniques	Dice
No Additional Preprocessing	0.7539
Z-score normalization	0.7432
Z-Score & Rescaling	**0.8153**
Z-Score & Rescaling & Histogram-matching	0.8017

three distinct combinations for our loss functions: (1) MSE, CE, and Edge. We obtained their respective weights of 0.25, 0.0044 and 0.00015 through hyperparameter optimization using Optuna [4]. (2) Dice, Focal, and Edge. The weights were set to sensible values of 1, 1, and 0.05, respectively. (3) Similar to combination 2, Dice, Focal, and Edge were included in the compound loss. However, the weight edge loss is set to 0.005. The weights of Dice and Focal are still 1.

The weight of Dice and Focal losses were set to 1, as they were on a similar scale, and the weights edge loss was set to 0.05 or 0.005, based on the relative scale of the output of the Edge loss function in comparison to Dice and Focal losses. Models were trained on the entire Challenge 1 dataset with these different loss function combinations and evaluated during the validation phase. The results can be seen in Table 2.

Table 2. Lesion-wise Dice and HD95 scores for Challenge 1 Loss Function Combinations

Loss functions	Dice			HD95		
	ET	TC	WT	ET	TC	WT
MSE + CE + Edge	**0.7696**	**0.7980**	0.8024	**22.40**	**28.59**	46.06
Dice + Focal + 0.05*Edge	0.7413	0.7796	**0.8296**	39.26	34.59	**32.30**
Dice + Focal + 0.005*Edge	0.7523	0.7742	0.8257	30.61	30.69	35.72

Analyzing the results, combination 1 performed the best on ET and TC as per the Dice and HD95 evaluation metrics from the validation phase. However, it was important to note its HD95 score for WT was significantly larger compared to the other experiments. Combination 3's Dice scores were on par with combination 2 and its average HD95 score was lower. Therefore, combination 1 and 3 became our top contenders and we further tested on Challenge 3, meningioma. This was done similarly to the previous experiment by training with the different loss function combinations on the same datasets. The results in Table 3 show that using a compound loss function including Dice loss, Focal loss, and Edge loss gives us better results in Dice socre and HD95 score which is consistent with challenge 1.

Table 3. Lesion-wise Dice and HD95 scores for Challenge 3 Loss Function Combinations

Loss functions	Dice			HD95		
	ET	TC	WT	ET	TC	WT
MSE + CE + Edge	0.7494	0.7136	0.7240	49.52	65.31	59.39
Dice + Focal + 0.005*Edge	**0.7602**	**0.7565**	**0.7322**	**43.90**	**44.26**	**55.99**

3.3 Post-processing

Our models' results were predicting numerous small connected components that were being classified as false positives (FPs) under the new lesion-wise evaluation metrics and decreasing our scores. We experimented with post-processing strategies to address this.

Our main idea was to find any small connected components (of any overlapping region) and reset their labels to 0, referred to as removing 'dust' by connected-components-3d [17], a Python package employed in the official evaluation code that we also utilized in our pipeline. We removed any components of 50 voxels or fewer, mirroring how the official evaluation code ignored ground truth lesions of this size. We also experimented with replacing the dust with the modal label of its neighboring voxels, which took a lot more computation time for very little gain.

The removal of dust from ET and TC created small holes in the predictions of TC and WT respectively. To resolve this, any holes that were created in TC were relabeled as NCR, and holes in WT as ED. This adjustment saw a very marginal increase in performance but definitely seemed more robust. The comparison of our final post-processing technique with no post-processing is shown in Table 4.

Table 4. Lesion-wise Dice and HD95 scores with and without post-processing

Post-processing strategy	Dice			HD95		
	ET	TC	WT	ET	TC	WT
No post-processing	0.6337	0.7024	0.5722	84.31	57.57	138.30
Removing dust and filling holes	**0.7130**	**0.7672**	**0.8090**	**43.91**	**26.76**	**40.40**

3.4 Transfer Learning for Challenge 2

Finally, we conducted an experiment on the transfer learning approach to determine which model if pre-trained on challenge 1 data can help improve segmentation performance for challenge 2. We use two baselines in this experiments: 1) baseline 1: model trained on challenge 2 data only (challenge 2 model), 2) baseline 2: model trained on challenge 1 data only (challenge 1 model). We also investigated which layers in the model contribute to improvements in performance. Thus, we selected our pre-trained challenge 1 model trained with the loss functions of Dice, Focal, and Edge Loss, and continued training the model on challenge 2's dataset using the same loss functions and weights, but with specific layers frozen. The results evaluated during the validation phase show that freezing the decoder gives us the best results (Table 5).

Table 5. Lesion-wise scores for challenge 2 Freezing Layers Experiment

Experiments	Dice				HD95			
	ET	TC	WT	mean	ET	TC	WT	mean
Challenge 2 model	0.6524	0.6925	0.5972	0.6474	81.96	70.49	120.81	91.09
Challenge 1 model	0.7188	0.7424	0.6433	0.7015	**52.35**	**48.16**	101.58	**67.36**
Freeze encoder layers	0.6745	0.7143	0.5810	0.6566	80.40	69.80	142.55	97.58
Freeze middle layers	**0.7392**	**0.7533**	0.6484	0.7136	57.27	55.10	114.41	75.59
Freeze decoder layers	0.7200	0.7358	**0.7039**	**0.7199**	59.21	60.21	**86.48**	68.63
Freeze nothing	0.7159	0.7214	0.6764	0.7046	68.72	67.43	103.55	79.90

4 Discussion

The introduction of lesion-wise evaluation criteria pushed us to rethink our approach to automatic brain tumor segmentation. We systematically implemented and compared different strategies at different stages of the model training. For pre-processing, we wanted to ensure that our model has improved visibility into the four image modalities to identify the tumor sub-regions correctly. Our experiments with pre-processing techniques revealed that the best Dice score was achieved by applying both Z-score normalization and rescaling voxel intensities as seen in Table 1. As a result, we decided to move forward with these two techniques for all the challenges. For model training, we investigated several combinations of loss functions. We first ran an experiment on challenge 1 as seen in Table 2 and then tested our top two combinations on challenge 3. Examining the challenge 3 results from Table 3, The results shows that a compound loss function includes Dice, Focal, and Edge loss combination with the respective weights of 1, 1, 0.05. obtained the best scores across all evaluation metrics. When computing the loss between the three output channels of our model and three corresponding channels of ground truth segmentations, there were two options for how to prepare the ground truth channels. They could be the disjoint labels NCR, ED, and ET, which is the format in which they are provided, or the partially overlapping regions WT, TC, and ET. We experimented with both options and observed marginal differences in the results. As a result, we picked the overlapped regions for training Since the official BraTS evaluation metrics are on the overlapping regions.

Also, we performed a rudimentary hyperparameter search using Optuna(A hyperparameter optimization framework) [4] to find the thresholds for converting model output probabilities to actual predictions, so that each voxel had exactly one label assigned to it. The results show that any thresholds below 0.9 worked reasonably well, since the model's output probabilities were usually around 0.9 for voxels that it believed to be in the tumor region of interest. Thus, we chose thresholds based on [9].

As mentioned before, decrease in performance was observed if the model was evaluated using the new lesion-wise metrics when compared to the 'legacy' scores of BraTS challenges from previous years. This is because the extra penalties that false positive (FP) components receive. We investigated several approaches to overcome this problem, The best solution we found was in post-processing, as we see from Table 4, our final post-processing strategy improved overall performance in both Dice and HD95 scores in each of the partially overlapping regions. However, this post-processing strategy did decrease scores for certain subjects by removing small components in our prediction that did match up with the ground truth.

To understand why the so-called 'dust' was being predicted by our models in the first place, we further analyzed the ground truth data (for challenge 1). We found that the ground truth segmentations themselves contain a large amount of dust, which is likely why the model was learning to predict this. However, as mentioned, the official evaluation code ignored any lesions that are 50 voxels or fewer from its calculations. Thus, we tried applying the dust-removal strategy as a pre-processing technique on the training data, to remove such lesions from the ground truth. For each region, we identify lesions using the same strategy as the official evaluation code (by considering separate connected components whose dilations overlap with each other as one lesion).

We implemented this for the training of our final model for Challenge 1, however, this still predicted a lot of FP components that we had to remove in post-processing. This is likely due to identifying lesions in the same way as the official evaluation code, which combines separate connected components into one lesion if they are still close enough to each other. Thus, the underlying ground truth still contained connected components of 50 voxels or fewer, so our model still learned to predict these structures.

Furthermore for Challenge 2, we investigated transfer learning approach to overcome the problem of small training data associated with the challenge. Freezing layers of Challenge 1's model, and continuing training on Challenge 2's dataset shows good results as seen in Table 5.

We compared the results from freezing different layers against the performance of 2 baseline models: model trained on challenge 2 data only, and model trained on challenge 1 data only. Surprising, model trained on Challenge 1 data only performed better on challenge 2 than the one trained challenge 2 data. Indicating the inadequacy of challenge 2 data, and the need to enhance challenge 2 dataset both in quantity and quality.

Overall we found that finetuning the model pretrained on challenge 1 data, lead to some improvements over the model trained only on challenge 1 data. Freezing the encoder led to decrease in performance over the challenge 1 model baseline, in terms of both Dice and HD95 scores. Freezing no layers and freezing the middle layers improved the Dice scores but HD95 saw a dip in performance. Freezing the decoder improved Dice scores across all tumor sub-regions and comparable HD95 scores (especially for WT). Looking ahead, we will be further experimenting with other frozen layer configurations, notably those focused on the decoder.

The strategies we implemented show improvements in tumor segmentation, however, there is still a lot of room for improvement regarding better lesion-wise performance.

We note that the state-of-the-art models, at least in adult glioma patients, achieve Dice scores close to 0.90 or above, and we recognize that many more techniques can be implemented to push performance even higher, such as data augmentation, deep supervision, dropout, addition of extra input channels and complex loss functions that drive more focused learning. Further investigation will be done using such techniques to further optimize deep learning models in the realm of automatic brain tumor segmentation.

5 Conclusion

Overall, our final models achieved fair performance in the BraTS 2023 validation phase, with the following lesion-wise Dice scores averaged across all three regions of interest: 0.79 in Challenge 1; 0.72 in Challenge 2; and 0.74 in Challenge 3. We were able to thoroughly test and implement optimizing strategies for data pre-processing, prediction post-processing and transfer learning via the fine-tuning of models trained on one challenge to another challenge.

References

1. Abderezaei, J., Pionteck, A., Chopra, A., Kurt, M.: 3D Inception-Based Trans-Morph: Pre-and Post-operative Multi-contrast MRI Registration in Brain Tumors. arXiv preprint arXiv:2212.04579 (2022)
2. Adewole, M., et al.: The brain tumor segmentation (brats) challenge 2023: Glioma segmentation in sub-saharan africa patient population (brats-africa) (2023)
3. Ahuja, S., Panigrahi, B., Gandhi, T.: Transfer learning based brain tumor detection and segmentation using superpixel technique. In: 2020 International Conference on Contemporary Computing and Applications (IC3A), pp. 244–249 (2020). https://doi.org/10.1109/IC3A48958.2020.233306
4. Akiba, T., Sano, S., Yanase, T., Ohta, T., Koyama, M.: Optuna: a next-generation hyperparameter optimization framework. In: Proceedings of the 25th ACM SIGKDD International Conference on Knowledge Discovery and Data Mining (2019)
5. Baid, U., et al.: The RSNA-ASNR-MICCAI brats 2021 benchmark on brain tumor segmentation and radiogenomic classification. arXiv preprint arXiv:2107.02314 (2021)

6. Bakas, S., et al.: Advancing the cancer genome atlas glioma MRI collections with expert segmentation labels and radiomic features. Sci. Data **4** (2017). https://doi.org/10.1038/sdata.2017.117
7. Çiçek, Ö., Abdulkadir, A., Lienkamp, S.S., Brox, T., Ronneberger, O.: 3D U-Net: learning dense volumetric segmentation from sparse annotation. In: Ourselin, S., Joskowicz, L., Sabuncu, M.R., Unal, G., Wells, W. (eds.) MICCAI 2016. LNCS, vol. 9901, pp. 424–432. Springer, Cham (2016). https://doi.org/10.1007/978-3-319-46723-8_49
8. Dosovitskiy, A., et al.: An image is worth 16x16 words: transformers for image recognition at scale. arXiv preprint arXiv:2010.11929 (2020)
9. Futrega, M., Milesi, A., Marcinkiewicz, M., Ribalta, P.: Optimized U-net for brain tumor segmentation. In: International MICCAI Brainlesion Workshop, pp. 15–29. Springer, Cham (2021)
10. Hatamizadeh, A., Nath, V., Tang, Y., Yang, D., Roth, H.R., Xu, D.: Swin UNETR: swin transformers for semantic segmentation of brain tumors in MRI images. In: International MICCAI Brainlesion Workshop, pp. 272–284. Springer, Cham (2021)
11. Isensee, F., Jaeger, P.F., Kohl, S.A., Petersen, J., Maier-Hein, K.H.: nnU-Net: a self-configuring method for deep learning-based biomedical image segmentation. Nat. Methods **18**(2), 203–211 (2021)
12. Jadon, S.: A survey of loss functions for semantic segmentation. In: 2020 IEEE Conference on Computational Intelligence in Bioinformatics and Computational Biology (CIBCB), pp. 1–7. IEEE (2020)
13. LaBella, D., et al.: The ASNR-MICCAI brain tumor segmentation (brats) challenge 2023: Intracranial meningioma (2023)
14. Luu, H., Park, S.H.: Extending nn-UNet for Brain Tumor Segmentation, pp. 173–186 (2022)
15. Menze, B.H., et al.: The multimodal brain tumor image segmentation benchmark (brats). IEEE Trans. Med. Imaging **34**(10), 1993–2024 (2015). https://doi.org/10.1109/TMI.2014.2377694
16. Siddiquee, M.M.R., Myronenko, A.: Redundancy reduction in semantic segmentation of 3D brain tumor MRIs. arXiv preprint arXiv:2111.00742 (2021)
17. Silversmith, W.: CC3D: connected components on multilabel 3D & 2D images (2021). https://zenodo.org/record/5535251

All Sizes Matter: Improving Volumetric Brain Segmentation on Small Lesions

Ayhan Can Erdur[1,2(✉)], Daniel Scholz[2,3], Josef A. Buchner[1],
Stephanie E. Combs[1,4,5], Daniel Rueckert[2,6], and Jan C. Peeken[1,4,5]

[1] Department of Radiation Oncology, TUM School of Medicine and Health, Klinikum rechts der Isar, Technical University of Munich, Munich, Germany
can.erdur@tum.de
[2] Chair for AI in Healthcare and Medicine, Technical University of Munich (TUM) and TUM University Hospital, Munich, Germany
[3] Department of Neuroradiology, TUM School of Medicine and Health, Klinikum rechts der Isar, Technical University of Munich, Munich, Germany
[4] Deutsches Konsortium für ur Translationale Krebsforschung (DKTK), Partner Site Munich, Munich, Germany
[5] Institute of Radiation Medicine (IRM), Helmholtz Zentrum Munich, Munich, Germany
[6] Department of Computing, Imperial College London, London, UK

Abstract. Brain metastases (BMs) are the most frequently occurring brain tumors. The treatment of patients having multiple BMs with stereotactic radiosurgery necessitates accurate localization of the metastases. Neural networks can assist in this time-consuming and costly task that is typically performed by human experts. Particularly challenging is the detection of small lesions since they are often underrepresented in existing approaches. Yet, lesion detection is equally important for all sizes. In this work, we develop an ensemble of neural networks explicitly focused on detecting and segmenting small BMs. To accomplish this task, we trained several neural networks focusing on individual aspects of the BM segmentation problem: We use blob loss that specifically addresses the imbalance of lesion instances in terms of size and texture and is, therefore, not biased towards larger lesions. In addition, a model using a subtraction sequence between the T1 and T1 contrast-enhanced sequence focuses on low-contrast lesions. Furthermore, we train additional models only on small lesions. Our experiments demonstrate the utility of the additional blob loss and the subtraction sequence. However, including the specialized small lesion models in the ensemble deteriorates segmentation results. We also find domain-knowledge-inspired postprocessing steps to drastically increase our performance in most experiments. Our approach enables us to submit a challenge entry to the ASNR-MICCAI BraTS Brain Metastasis Challenge 2023.

Keywords: Metastasis segmentation · Small lesion detection · Brain MRI · Blob loss

---

A. C. Erdur, D. Scholz and J. A. Buchner—Contributed equally.

© The Author(s), under exclusive license to Springer Nature Switzerland AG 2024
U. Baid et al. (Eds.): crossMoDA 2023/BraTS 2023, LNCS 14669, pp. 177–189, 2024.
https://doi.org/10.1007/978-3-031-76163-8_16

Brain metastases (BMs) occur approximately ten times more frequently than primary malignant brain tumors [24]. In addition, nearly 10% of patients with malignant tumors in the United States are expected to develop brain metastases [8]. While surgical resection is recommended for particularly large BMs, stereotactic radiosurgery (STS) is a possible treatment for patients with multiple BMs [31]. To minimize radiation exposure to healthy tissue, precise delineation of the target lesion in magnetic resonance imaging (MRI) is required for STS. Brain lesion delineation is a time-consuming task in clinical practice and also prone to interrater variability, i.e., deviations between annotators, especially for small BMs [10,30].

Various machine learning algorithms [22,27] opened the possibility of automatic segmentation of such lesions. The potential of such approaches for automatic segmentation of primary brain tumors has been shown in previous brain tumor segmentation (BraTS) Challenges [2,18]: The neural network-based segmentations are not only faster but also independent of the rater. Moreover, recent research suggests that experts consistently score automatically created segmentations by neural networks higher than human-curated reference labels [14].

While only a small fraction of glioma patients suffer from multicentric lesions [17], nearly 50% of patients with BMs are affected by multiple metastases [7,9]. This has a direct impact on measuring segmentation performance as well as on ranking contributions to segmentation challenges: To evaluate large and small lesions equally, segmentation performance must be measured per lesion rather than cumulatively for all lesions combined.

The goal of this work is to develop an algorithm based on neural networks for the segmentation of the non-enhancing tumor core, enhancing tumor, and surrounding non-enhancing Fluid Attenuated Inversion Recovery (FLAIR) hyperintensity of BMs as a contribution to the ASNR-MICCAI BraTS Brain Metastasis Challenge [12,21]. We aim to improve the small lesion segmentation performance by employing data augmentations, loss functions, and domain-knowledge-based postprocessing.

1 Methods

This section outlines the three key components of our challenge submission: first, the provided dataset and our preprocessing pipeline; second, our baseline model and training configurations; and finally, our proposed pre- and post-training improvements to the baseline.

1.1 Data

Datasets. The provided data in this project consists of two parts: 238 patients provided directly by the BraTS challenge organizers [21] as well as 488 additional patients from the listed external datasets included in the challenge [23,28].

In total, four MRI sequences are supplied per patient as the following: pre-contrast T1-weighted sequence (t1w), post-contrast T1-weighted sequence (t1c), T2-weighted sequence (t2w), and T2-weighted FLAIR sequence.

A segmentation map of three labels (enhancing tumor (ET), non-enhancing tumor core (NETC), and surrounding non-enhancing FLAIR hyperintensity (SNFH)) is also provided along MRI sequences to be the reference in training.

Preprocessing. All sequences were supplied as co-registered, skull-stripped sequences with an isotropic resolution of 1 mm in SRI24 space [26] with dimensions of 240 × 240 × 155 voxels. We further normalize the orientation to (Left, Right), (Posterior, Anterior), (Inferior, Superior), ensure 1mm isotropic resolution, and scale intensities of each MRI sequence individually to [0, 1] based on percentiles. Best percentiles are determined visually by experts (*cf.* Fig. 1).

To ensure gapless segmentations, we create 3-channel targets for our networks by merging the labels as whole tumor (WT), combination of ET, NETC, and SNFH, tumor core (TC), combination of ET and NETC, and enhancing tumor (ET).

Data Augmentations. Based on prior research in brain metastasis segmentation on a multi-center dataset of MRI images [3], we determine a fixed set of data augmentations that are shared among all experiments. The augmentations and the corresponding parameters are shown in Table 1.

Table 1. Data augmentations and their corresponding parameters used during training.

Augmentation	Probability	Parameters	
Random Flip	0.5	**Axis**	
		0	
Random Affine	0.5		
Random Gaussian Noise	0.5	**Mean**	**Std**
		0.0	0.1
Random Spatial Crops	1	**Crop size**	n_{crops}
		[192,192,32]	2

1.2 Training

Base Model: SegResNetVAE. For our experiments, we use the SegResNet-VAE [22] model, which is a 3D adaptation of the U-Net architecture [27] with modified residual blocks and a branch for image reconstruction using a variational autoencoder principle. The additional branch functions as an auxiliary regularization on the learning task. The model is visualized in Fig. 2.

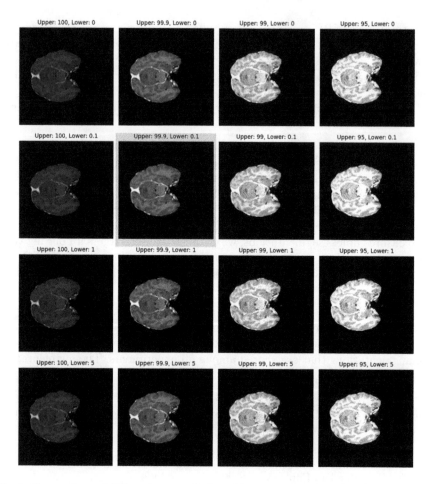

Fig. 1. Comparison of different percentile-based intensity rescaling thresholds to obtain the best percentiles. We choose the 0.1th and the 99.9th as the lower and upper percentiles, respectively, (highlighted in yellow) to strike a balance between avoiding outliers and losing contrast. (Color figure online)

Loss Functions. In segmentation tasks, it is common practice to use the Dice loss [19] or a weighted sum of the pixel-wise cross-entropy and the Dice loss (DiceCE) for training. An equally weighted sum of the pixel-wise cross-entropy and the Dice loss is used as a loss function for our training runs.

Training Configurations. We first train a baseline model with default settings and incrementally add extra methods to the training or inference to improve the final segmentation performance. Our baseline consists of the SegResNetVAE model with the DiceCE loss function. For the input, all four of the available MRI sequences are concatenated to form a multi-channel image.

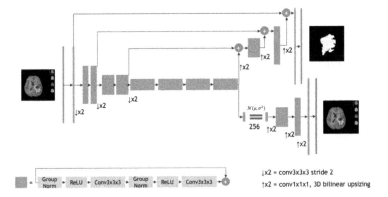

Fig. 2. SegResNetVAE architecture with segmentation decoder at the top and variational autoencoder (VAE) branch for image reconstruction on the bottom. We replace the RELU activations in each residual block with Mish [20] functions. The input is a four-channel image of concatenated MRI sequences, and the output segmentation map has three channels representing WT, TC, and ET labels, respectively.

As the default training settings for all models, we set the maximum number of epochs to 200 epochs and use AdamW optimizer with a weight decay parameter of $1e-5$. The batch size is selected as 5, and the learning rate is $1e-4$.

As shown in Table 1, the images are cropped into smaller patches during training with two crops per patient, increasing the effective batch size from 5 to 10. In the testing stage, we use the *sliding window inference* method with an overlap of 0.75 to obtain the segmentations matching the original input size. We use MONAI [5] library as the basis for the model implementations, loss functions, data preprocessing, and augmentation tools in our pipeline.

We created a training, validation, and test split consisting of 80%, 10%, and 10% portions, respectively, and used the same splits throughout all experiments for model tuning and comparison.

1.3 Improvements

In this section, we present steps taken to improve the segmentations overall and with special focus on small lesions compared to our baseline.

Blob Loss. Kofler *et al.* [15] have shown that the Dice loss is biased toward larger lesions and performs poorly with an unbalanced set of instances, i.e., differences in size, texture, and morphology. They have proposed a loss function, *blob loss*, that addresses the imbalance by treating each lesion individually. The blob loss functions as a wrapper around any segmentation loss to mask out all lesions but one, calculate the loss value per lesion, and compute the final loss by averaging the lesion losses of a patient. With this method, they improve overall and instance-wise detection and segmentation performance in multi-lesion cases.

Following the suggestions of Kofler *et al.* [15], we always formulate the blob loss as an auxiliary term to DiceCE loss. Throughout the paper, we refer to a weighted summation of the losses as the blob loss. This consists of a global DiceCE term and a lesion-focused blob loss term:

$$\mathcal{L}_{\text{final}} = 2 \cdot \mathcal{L}_{\text{DiceCE}} + \mathcal{L}_{\text{blob}}\left[\text{Dice}\right], \tag{1}$$

with $\mathcal{L}_{\text{blob}}\left[\text{Dice}\right]$ depicting the vanilla Dice loss wrapped in blob loss as the lesion-wise evaluator.

To detect small lesions in BM patients and to achieve better instance-wise performance, we choose to use blob loss in our experiments. We also provide a comparison with DiceCE loss under the same settings.

Subtraction Sequence. Other works have included a subtraction sequence between t1w and t1c for BM segmentation [29], creating an image with highlighted contrast-enhancing lesions and almost zeroed out remaining tissue. We adopt this domain knowledge and use the subtraction sequence $||t1c - t1w||^2$ as an additional channel in our input combination.

We keep the network architecture identical across experiments by swapping t2w with the subtraction sequence. The t2w sequence contributes minimally to the results, such that identical or better performance can be achieved without it [4].

Small Lesions Model. Smaller lesions are generally overlooked by the original Dice loss formulation since larger errors in larger lesions contribute more to the score. To overcome this shortcoming, we propose additional measures to improve the detection of small lesions. By following a similar strategy to the protected group models approach by Puyol *et al.* [25], we train a separate model for small lesions. To this end, we mask out all lesions that are larger than a certain threshold τ. Since some of the samples end up with no remaining lesions, we filter these patients from the dataset for this specific training. In our experiments, we set the lesion size thresholds to $\tau = 1000$ voxels.

Test Time Augmentations. Buchner *et al.* [3] improve metastasis segmentation on MR images employing a set of test time augmentations. Following their work, we apply additive Gaussian noise sampled from $\mathcal{N}(0, 0.001)$ and randomly flips along the sagittal and coronal planes. We repeat these test time augmentations four times and calculate the output as the average of all iterations.

Ensembling. Previous research shows that combining the predictions of multiple networks increases the segmentation performance and robustness [11]. Therefore, we combine the predictions of our baseline, blob-loss and subtraction sequence models into an ensemble for our final submission. As presented in the following results chapter, the models trained only on the small lesions are excluded. We compare a mean ensembling approach, i.e., averaging over the outputs, with the *SIMPLE* [16] algorithm implemented in the BraTS Toolkit [13], which is an iterative majority-voting approach.

Postprocessing. To aggregate the 3-channel outputs of our neural networks into a final segmentation map, we perform the inverse of input label merging, which is described in the preprocessing section. Then, individual blobs of the respective labels are detected using a connected components analysis utilizing the Python library connected-components-3d [1]. To remove small lesions, which can be a result of the inversed label merging, we employ a postprocessing step based on the following rules:

- WT: Blobs smaller than 25 voxels get removed.
- NETC: Blobs smaller than 20 voxels are added to the ET label.
- SNFH: Blobs smaller than 20 voxels get removed.
- ET: Blobs smaller than 10 voxels get removed.

An example of the resulting changes can be seen in Fig. 3.

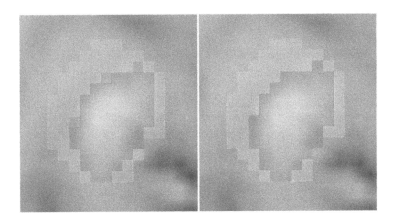

Fig. 3. Comparison of an segmentation before (left) and after (right) postprocessing. Since the NETC (in green) is created by subtracting the ET (in red) from the TC, some border voxels may get labeled NETC. These get removed and labeled to ET by our postprocessing. (Color figure online)

1.4 Metrics

To determine the performance of our models, we use the evaluation script provided by the challenge organizers [6,21]. We report the cumulative Dice Similarity Coefficient (cDSC) across all lesions as well as the DSC per lesion (lDSC) for the ET, TC, and WT. The 95th percentile of the Hausdorff Distance is also reported cumulatively (cHD95) and per lesion (lHD95). For a more granular analysis of our experiments, we also measure false positives (FPs), i.e., additional detections, and false negatives (FNs), i.e., missed detections, averaged per patient. Unless otherwise specified, we report the mean metric across all three labels.

2 Results

2.1 Final Results

We report our results in Table 2 on a hold-out test set from the provided challenge training data. We find that both the additional blob loss and the subtraction sequence yield substantial improvement over the baseline. Our contributions primarily cause a reduction in FP lesion detections, leading to better segmentations. However, test time augmentations only reduce the number of FPs per patient at the expense of more FNs. The DSC and the Hausdorff distance remain constant. Combining the baseline model with the models that additionally utilize the blob loss and the subtraction sequence by using the iterative SIMPLE ensemble method, we improve the performance compared to the individual models and the mean ensemble.

Table 2. Results on our hold-out test set after postprocessing comparing our submission model to the baseline.

Model	lDSC (↑)	cDSC (↑)	lHD95 (↓)	cHD95 (↓)	FP (↓)	FN (↓)
Baseline	0.43	0.69	267	32	0.75	0.63
+ Blob Loss [15]	0.46	0.70	**249**	**23**	0.69	0.63
+ Sub. Seq. [29]	0.47	0.72	**249**	24	0.50	0.69
+ TTA [3]	0.47	0.71	250	24	**0.41**	0.72
SIMPLE Ensemble [16]	**0.49**	**0.74**	254	**23**	0.57	**0.45**

Preliminary Challenge Results. We report our preliminary results on the validation set obtained from the official challenge evaluation platform. Our final model ensemble achieves a 0.47 average lDSC (0.45 ET, 0.50 TC, 0.47 WT) and a 158 average lHD95 (163 ET, 158 TC, 152 WT).

Challenge Performance. Disclosed later on by the organizers, our submission has reached average scores of 0.4047 lDSC (0.3918 ET, 0.4269 TC, 0.3963 WT) and 175 lHD95 (174 ET, 174 TC, 176 WT) on the official test cohort of the ASNR-MICCAI BraTS Brain Metastasis Challenge 2023.

2.2 Complementary Analysis of Our Proposed Methods

We provide complementary analysis, justifying our choice of improvements leading to our main results.

Postprocessing Based on Domain Knowledge. By incorporating domain knowledge into our model predictions via postprocessing, we achieve better lesion-wise volumetric segmentation performance (*cf.* Table 3). Furthermore, we are able to reduce the number of FPs at the expense of more FNs.

Table 3. Comparing model performance with and without domain specific postprocessing (PP). Our postprocessing improves primarily lesion-wise metrics compared to the unprocessed results. We observe a drastic reduction in false positives indicated by the mean FP lesions per patient, while the FNs increase.

Model	lDSC (↑)		cDSC (↑)		lHD95 (↓)		cHD95 (↓)		FP (↓)		FN (↓)	
		+ PP		+ PP		+ PP		+ PP		+ PP		+ PP
Baseline	0.38	**0.43**	0.69	0.69	286	**267**	28	32	2.00	**0.75**	**0.48**	0.63
+ Blob Loss [15]	0.35	**0.46**	0.70	0.70	281	**249**	28	**23**	2.46	**0.69**	**0.49**	0.63
+ Sub. Seq. [29]	0.38	**0.47**	0.72	0.72	270	**249**	27	**24**	1.94	**0.50**	**0.52**	0.69
+ TTA [3]	0.41	**0.47**	**0.72**	0.71	257	**250**	25	**24**	1.49	**0.41**	**0.55**	0.72
Mean Ensemble	0.41	**0.47**	**0.73**	0.72	269	**261**	**24**	30	1.56	**0.59**	**0.35**	0.51
SIMPLE [16]	0.43	**0.49**	0.74	0.74	261	**254**	23	23	1.40	**0.57**	**0.34**	0.45

Ensembling Methods. We evaluate different algorithms to combine the predictions of our best models into an ensemble. Namely, we compare a mean ensemble to the *SIMPLE* method implemented by BraTS Toolkit [13]. We show that the latter method performs better in both lesion wise and cumulative DSC (*cf.* Table 4).

Table 4. Comparing the mean ensemble with the more sophisticated SIMPLE ensembling method [13].

Ensemble	lDSC (↑)	cDSC (↑)	lHD95 (↓)	cHD95 (↓)	FP (↓)	FN (↓)
Mean	0.47	0.72	261	30	0.59	0.51
SIMPLE [16]	**0.49**	**0.74**	**254**	**23**	**0.57**	**0.45**

Small Lesion Networks. We report segmentation results for the networks only trained on up to 1000 voxel-sized lesions on only these test images that contain lesions smaller than 1000 voxels (*cf.* Table 5). The model performs worse with respect to general DSC and HD95 compared to the all-lesions-model. To evaluate the impact of incorporating a small-lesion-model into our existing ensemble, we test the performance of an ensemble of our all-lesion-models models with the small-lesion-model.

In order to combine the small-lesion-model with the former ensemble and to obtain final predictions, a second ensembling step is introduced. Namely, we apply the voxel-wise maximum operation between the outputs of the small-lesion-model and the all-lesion-models. This ensemble did not improve the volumetric segmentation performance compared to the ensemble without the small lesion models while being computationally more expensive. Consequently, we exclude the small lesion model from our final models for the challenge submission.

Table 5. Segmentation performance of models trained solely on small lesions. We report individual model performance and as an ensemble with our best models.

Model	lDSC (↑)	cDSC (↑)	lHD95 (↓)	cHD95 (↓)	FP (↓)	FN (↓)
Small Lesions ($\tau = 1000$)	0.27	0.27	334	67	0.80	1.52
SIMPLE Ensemble [16]	**0.49**	0.74	254	**23**	**0.57**	0.45
+ Small Lesions	0.48	0.74	**239**	24	0.84	**0.37**

3 Discussion

In this work, we developed an algorithm for automatically detecting and segmenting BMs. We added dedicated components to a baseline segmentation model focusing on the detection and segmentation of small lesions. Compared to a baseline model, we improved our lDSC by 14%. Most of the improvement can be attributed to using blob loss, adding a subtraction sequence, and the model ensembling.

The introduction of blob loss improved both the lDSC and the cDSC, with the former being more affected. This is likely due to a better segmentation quality of mainly small lesions, while the segmentation quality of larger lesions did not change significantly.

Using domain-specific postprocessing with fixed thresholds, we reduced the number of false positives by up to 75%. For this work, we choose a threshold that balances specificity and sensitivity. In contrast, in many clinical applications, the risk of missing BMs outweighs the additional manual effort of removing FPs, and the threshold should be adjusted accordingly. Ultimately, our competition entry aims to inspire the research community to improve the detection of small lesions in the future.

References

1. Silversmith, W., Kemnitz, N.: seung-lab/connected-components-3d. seung-lab (2020). https://github.com/seung-lab/connected-components-3d
2. Baid, U., et al.: The RSNA-ASNR-MICCAI brats 2021 benchmark on brain tumor segmentation and radiogenomic classification (2021). https://arxiv.org/abs/2107.02314v2
3. Buchner, J.A., et al.: Development and external validation of an MRI-based neural network for brain metastasis segmentation in the aurora multicenter study. Radiother. Oncol. **178**, 109425 (2023)
4. Buchner, J.A., et al.: Identifying core MRI sequences for reliable automatic brain metastasis segmentation. medRxiv, vol. 16, 2023.05.02.23289342 (2023). https://doi.org/10.1101/2023.05.02.23289342. https://www.medrxiv.org/content/10.1101/2023.05.02.23289342v2. https://www.medrxiv.org/content/10.1101/2023.05.02.23289342v2.abstract
5. Cardoso, M.J., et al.: MONAI: an open-source framework for deep learning in healthcare (2022). https://doi.org/10.48550/arXiv.2211.02701
6. Chung, V.: Brats 2023 lesion-wise performance metrics evaluation (2023). https://github.com/rachitsaluja/brats_val_2023
7. Delattre, J.Y., Krol, G., Thaler, H.T., Posner, J.B.: Distribution of brain metastases. Arch. Neurol. **45**, 741–744 (1988). https://doi.org/10.1001/ARCHNEUR.1988.00520310047016. https://jamanetwork.com/journals/jamaneurology/fullarticle/587837
8. Eichler, A.F., Chung, E., Kodack, D.P., Loeffler, J.S., Fukumura, D., Jain, R.K.: The biology of brain metastases–translation to new therapies. Nat. Rev. Clin. Oncol. **8**, 344–356 (2011). https://doi.org/10.1038/nrclinonc.2011.58. https://www.nature.com/articles/nrclinonc.2011.58
9. Fabi, A., et al.: Brain metastases from solid tumors: disease outcome according to type of treatment and therapeutic resources of the treating center. J. Exp. Clin. Cancer Res. **30**, 1–7 (2011). https://doi.org/10.1186/1756-9966-30-10/TABLES/5. https://jeccr.biomedcentral.com/articles/10.1186/1756-9966-30-10
10. Growcott, S., Dembrey, T., Patel, R., Eaton, D., Cameron, A.: Inter-observer variability in target volume delineations of benign and metastatic brain tumours for stereotactic radiosurgery: results of a national quality assurance programme. Clin. Oncol. (Royal College of Radiologists (Great Britain)) **32**, 13–25 (2020). https://doi.org/10.1016/J.CLON.2019.06.015. https://pubmed.ncbi.nlm.nih.gov/31301960/
11. Kamnitsas, K., et al.: Ensembles of multiple models and architectures for robust brain tumour segmentation. In: Crimi, A., Bakas, S., Kuijf, H., Menze, B., Reyes, M. (eds.) BrainLes 2017. LNCS, vol. 10670, pp. 450–462. Springer, Cham (2018). https://doi.org/10.1007/978-3-319-75238-9_38
12. Karargyris, A., et al.: Federated benchmarking of medical artificial intelligence with medperf. Nat. Mach. Intell. **5**, 799–810 (2023). https://doi.org/10.1038/s42256-023-00652-2. https://www.nature.com/articles/s42256-023-00652-2
13. Kofler, F., et al.: Brats toolkit: translating brats brain tumor segmentation algorithms into clinical and scientific practice. Front. Neurosci. 125 (2020)
14. Kofler, F., et al.: Are we using appropriate segmentation metrics? Identifying correlates of human expert perception for CNN training beyond rolling the dice coefficient. Mach. Learn. Biomed. Imaging **2**, 27–71 (2021). https://doi.org/10.59275/j.melba.2023-dg1f. https://arxiv.org/abs/2103.06205v4

15. Kofler, F., et al.: Blob loss: instance imbalance aware loss functions for semantic segmentation. In: International Conference on Information Processing in Medical Imaging, pp. 755–767. Springer, Cham (2023)
16. Langerak, T.R., Heide, U.A.V.D., Kotte, A.N., Viergever, M.A., Vulpen, M.V., Pluim, J.P.: Label fusion in atlas-based segmentation using a selective and iterative method for performance level estimation (simple). IEEE Trans. Med. Imaging **29**, 2000–2008 (2010). https://doi.org/10.1109/TMI.2010.2057442. https://pubmed.ncbi.nlm.nih.gov/20667809/
17. Lasocki, A., Gaillard, F., Tacey, M., Drummond, K., Stuckey, S.: Multifocal and multicentric glioblastoma: improved characterisation with flair imaging and prognostic implications. J. Clin. Neurosci. Off. J. Neurosurg. Soc. Australas. **31**, 92–98 (2016). https://doi.org/10.1016/J.JOCN.2016.02.022. https://pubmed.ncbi.nlm.nih.gov/27343042/
18. Menze, B.H., et al.: The multimodal brain tumor image segmentation benchmark (brats). IEEE Trans. Med. Imaging **34**, 1993–2024 (2015). https://doi.org/10.1109/TMI.2014.2377694
19. Milletari, F., Navab, N., Ahmadi, S.A.: V-net: fully convolutional neural networks for volumetric medical image segmentation. In: 2016 Fourth International Conference on 3D Vision (3DV), pp. 565–571. IEEE (2016)
20. Misra, D.: Mish: a self regularized non-monotonic activation function. arXiv preprint arXiv:1908.08681 (2019)
21. Moawad, A.W., et al.: The brain tumor segmentation (brats-mets) challenge 2023: brain metastasis segmentation on pre-treatment MRI (2023). https://arxiv.org/abs/2306.00838v1
22. Myronenko, A.: 3D MRI brain tumor segmentation using autoencoder regularization. In: Crimi, A., Bakas, S., Kuijf, H., Keyvan, F., Reyes, M., van Walsum, T. (eds.) BrainLes 2018. LNCS, vol. 11384, pp. 311–320. Springer, Cham (2019). https://doi.org/10.1007/978-3-030-11726-9_28
23. Oermann, M.L.E.: Nyumets_brain v1.0 (2022). https://nyumets.org/2022/03/29/nyumets-brain-v1/
24. Ostrom, Q.T., Wright, C.H., Barnholtz-Sloan, J.S.: Brain metastases: epidemiology. In: Handbook of Clinical Neurology, vol. 149, pp. 27–42 (2018). https://doi.org/10.1016/B978-0-12-811161-1.00002-5
25. Puyol-Antón, E., et al.: Fairness in cardiac MR image analysis: an investigation of bias due to data imbalance in deep learning based segmentation. In: de Bruijne, M., et al. (eds.) MICCAI 2021. LNCS, vol. 12903, pp. 413–423. Springer, Cham (2021). https://doi.org/10.1007/978-3-030-87199-4_39
26. Rohlfing, T., Zahr, N.M., Sullivan, E.V., Pfefferbaum, A.: The SRI24 multichannel atlas of normal adult human brain structure. Hum. Brain Mapp. **31**, 798–819 (2010). https://doi.org/10.1002/HBM.20906
27. Ronneberger, O., Fischer, P., Brox, T.: U-Net: convolutional networks for biomedical image segmentation. In: Navab, N., Hornegger, J., Wells, W.M., Frangi, A.F. (eds.) MICCAI 2015. LNCS, vol. 9351, pp. 234–241. Springer, Cham (2015). https://doi.org/10.1007/978-3-319-24574-4_28
28. Rudie, J.D., et al.: The university of California San Francisco, brain metastases stereotactic radiosurgery (UCSF-BMSR) MRI dataset (2023). https://arxiv.org/abs/2304.07248v2
29. Rudie, J.D., et al.: Three-dimensional u-net convolutional neural network for detection and segmentation of intracranial metastases. Radiol. Artif. Intell. **3**(3), e200204 (2021)

30. Sandström, H., Jokura, H., Chung, C., Toma-Dasu, I.: Multi-institutional study of the variability in target delineation for six targets commonly treated with radiosurgery. Acta Oncologica **57**, 1515–1520 (2018). https://doi.org/10.1080/0284186X.2018.1473636/SUPPL_FILE/IONC_A_1473636_SM2616.ZIP. https://www.tandfonline.com/doi/abs/10.1080/0284186X.2018.1473636
31. Vogelbaum, M.A., et al.: Treatment for brain metastases: asco-sno-astro guideline. J. Clin. Oncol. **40**, 492–516 (2022). https://doi.org/10.1200/JCO.21.02314

3D-TransUNet for Brain Metastases Segmentation in the BraTS2023 Challenge

Siwei Yang[1], Xianhang Li[1], Jieru Mei[2], Jieneng Chen[2], Cihang Xie[1], and Yuyin Zhou[1](✉)

[1] University of California, Santa Cruz, USA
yzhou284@ucsc.edu
[2] The Johns Hopkins University, Baltimore, USA

Abstract. Segmenting brain tumors is complex due to their diverse appearances and scales. Brain metastases, the most common type of brain tumor, are a frequent complication of cancer. Therefore, an effective segmentation model for brain metastases must adeptly capture local intricacies to delineate small tumor regions while also integrating global context to understand broader scan features. The TransUNet model, which combines Transformer self-attention with U-Net's localized information, emerges as a promising solution for this task. In this report, we address brain metastases segmentation by training the 3D-TransUNet [6] model on the Brain Tumor Segmentation (BraTS-METS) 2023 challenge dataset. Specifically, we explored two architectural configurations: the **Encoder-only 3D-TransUNet**, employing Transformers solely in the encoder, and the **Decoder-only 3D-TransUNet**, utilizing Transformers exclusively in the decoder. For Encoder-only 3D-TransUNet, we note that Masked-Autoencoder pre-training is required for a better initialization of the Transformer Encoder and thus accelerates the training process.

We identify that the Decoder-only 3D-TransUNet model should offer enhanced efficacy in the segmentation of brain metastases, as indicated by our 5-fold cross-validation on the training set (The code and models are available at https://github.com/Beckschen/3D-TransUNet). However, our use of the Encoder-only 3D-TransUNet model already yield notable results, with an average lesion-wise Dice score of 59.8% on the test set, securing second place in the BraTS-METS 2023 challenge.

Keywords: Brain Tumor Segmentation · Transformer

1 Introduction

Tumors, with their subtle intensity variations compared to surrounding tissues, often pose difficulties, as evidenced by inconsistencies in even expert-driven manual annotations [1,8,9,13,24]. Additionally, the wide variance in tumor appearances and dimensions across patients challenges the efficacy of traditional shape and location models [15,19]. Brain metastases, which are brain tumors that originate from primary cancers elsewhere in the body, represent the most prevalent malignant tumors in the central nervous system. With an annual incidence of 24 per 100,000 individuals [3,11,17], brain metastases outnumber the occurrence of all primary brain cancers combined.

In terms of segmentation methods, Convolutional Neural Networks (CNNs), especially Fully Convolutional Networks (FCNs) [14], have established their prominence. Among various architectures, the u-shaped architecture, popularly known as U-Net [20], stands out for its symmetrical encoder-decoder framework and skip-connections, excelling at preserving image intricacies. However, these methods often struggle with modeling long-range dependencies due to convolution's inherent locality. To address this, researchers have turned to Transformers, which rely solely on attention mechanisms, showcasing success in capturing global contexts [22]. An example is TransUNet [5], a hybrid CNN-Transformer model, seamlessly blending localized convolution's efficiency with global attention's comprehension. Anchored in the encoder-decoder paradigm, this innovation leverages and elevates both paradigms, promising a new frontier in segmentation precision.

This report aims to validate the performance of 3D-TransUNet [6] on the segmentation of brain metastases in the BraTS 2023 challenge. 3D-TransUNet has two opted self-attention modules: 1) A *Transformer encoder*, which tokenizes image patches extracted from CNN feature maps to capture extensive global contexts using transformer blocks, and 2) A *Transformer decoder*, which innovatively redefines the process of medical image segmentation by treating it as a mask classification task and dynamically refining organ queries through cross-attention with multi-scale CNN decoding features. Specifically, we experiment with two architectures: **Encoder-only** (CNN encoder + Transformer encoder + CNN decoder) and **Decoder-only** (CNN encoder + Transformer decoder + CNN decoder). Notably, Masked-Autoencoder (MAE) Pre-training can be used to accelerate the training of the Encoder-only model. To introduce stronger supervision, we employ deep supervision across all levels of our decoder. Our model yielded average lesion-wise Dice scores of 59.6% and 59.8%, respectively, on the validation set and test set of BraTS-METS 2023 datasets.

2 Method

In this work, we adopt 3D-TransUNet [6] to segment brain metastases. This model leverages the advantages of integrating transformers within the encoder and decoder of the U-Net architecture, as shown in Fig. 1. We first studied the encoder to verify if transformer blocks can extract representative features. We also explore combining the U-Net pixel decoder with a Transformer decoder for prediction. The U-Net pixel decoder upsamples the low-resolution features generated by the image encoder. Simultaneously, the Transformer decoder enhances these features through a cross-attention mechanism, effectively refining the final prediction.

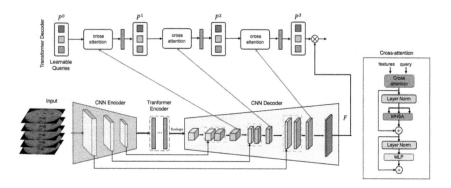

Fig. 1. Overview of our adaptation of 3D-TransUNet [6] for BraTS-METS 2023 [2].

2.1 Transformer as Encoder

Image Sequentialization. An input feature map $\mathbf{x}$ are first tokenized and reshaped into a sequence of 3D patches, noted as $\{\mathbf{x}_i^p \in \mathbb{R}^{P^3 \cdot C} | i = 1, .., N\}$. The size of each 3D patch is $P \times P \times P$, and the total patch number is $N = \frac{DHW}{P^3}$.

Patch Embedding. 3D patches $\mathbf{x}^p$ are linearly projected into a d_{enc}-dimensional embedding space. Learnable positional embeddings are added to retain spatial information. The final embeddings are formulated as follows:

$$\mathbf{z}_0 = [\mathbf{x}_1^p \mathbf{E}; \mathbf{x}_2^p \mathbf{E}; \cdots; \mathbf{x}_N^p \mathbf{E}] + \mathbf{E}^{pos}, \tag{1}$$

where $\mathbf{E} \in \mathbb{R}^{(P^2C) \times d}$ and $\mathbf{E}^{pos} \in \mathbb{R}^{N \times d}$ denotes the linear projection and position embedding accordingly.

The Transformer encoder consists of L_{enc} layers of Multi-head Self-Attention (MSA) Eq. (2) and Multi-Layer Perceptron (MLP) blocks Eq. (3). Therefore, the final output $\mathbf{z}_\ell$ of the ℓ-th layer is

$$\mathbf{z}'_\ell = \text{MSA}(\text{LN}(\mathbf{z}_{\ell-1})) + \mathbf{z}_{\ell-1}, \tag{2}$$
$$\mathbf{z}_\ell = \text{MLP}(\text{LN}(\mathbf{z}'_\ell)) + \mathbf{z}'_\ell, \tag{3}$$

where $\text{LN}(\cdot)$ is layer normalization operator and $\mathbf{z}_\ell$ is the encoded image representation.

2.2 Transformer as Decoder

The segmentation task can be reformulated into a binary mask classification problem inspired by the set prediction mechanism proposed in DETR [4]. As shown in Fig. 1, we train the CNN decoder and the Transformer decoder simultaneously, allowing for the refinement of organ queries and feature maps. Specifically, in the t-th layer of the Transformer decoder, the refined organ queries are denoted by $\mathbf{P}^t \in \mathbb{R}^{N \times d_{dec}}$. Alongside, an intermediate feature from the U-Net is transformed into a d_{dec}-dimensional feature, represented by $\mathcal{F}$. The number of upsampling blocks in the CNN decoder aligns with the Transformer decoder layers, so multi-scale CNN features are effectively projected into the feature space $\mathcal{F} \in \mathbb{R}^{(D_t H_t W_t) \times d_{dec}}$, where D_t, H_t, and W_t define the spatial dimensions of the feature map at the t-th upsampling block. Transitioning from the t-th to the $t+1$-th layer, the organ queries $\mathbf{P}^t$ are updated through the cross-attention mechanism as described by the following formula:

$$\mathbf{P}^{t+1} = \mathbf{P}^t + \text{Softmax}\left((\mathbf{P}^t \mathbf{w}_q)(\mathcal{F}^t \mathbf{w}_k)^\top\right) \mathcal{F}^t \mathbf{w}_v, \qquad (4)$$

where $\mathbf{w}_q \in \mathbb{R}^{d_{dec} \times d_q}$, $\mathbf{w}_k \in \mathbb{R}^{d_{dec} \times d_k}$, and $\mathbf{w}_v \in \mathbb{R}^{d_{dec} \times d_v}$ are the weight matrices that linearly project the t-th query features, keys, and values for the subsequent layer. This process is repeated, with a residual connection updating $\mathbf{P}$ after each layer, in line with the previous method [7]. The final prediction, $\mathbf{Z}^T$, is derived through Eq. 5, which details the process of converting $\mathbf{P}^T$ into the binarized segmentation map. It involves a dot product with U-Net's last block feature, $\mathbf{F}$, resulting in $\mathbf{Z}^T$.

$$\mathbf{Z}^T = g(\mathbf{P} \times \mathbf{F}^\top), \qquad (5)$$

where $g(\cdot)$ is sigmoid activation followed by a hard thresholding operation with a threshold set at 0.5, such to decode region-wise binary brain tumor masks.

Note that unlike [6], we do not use masked attention here due to the observed training instability.

2.3 3D-TransUNet Variants

Two 3D-TransUNet variants, *i.e.*, Encoder-only and Decoder-only, are involved in the experiment. Encoder-only 3D-TransUNet is used as the main architecture for all of our submissions since Decoder-only 3D-TransUNet requires longer training compared to the Encoder-only 3D-TransUNet. This is mainly due to its use of high-resolution features in the Transformer decoder. Additionally, the Hungarian matching process used to match binary masks to ground truth in the Decoder-only model is slower compared to directly computing cross-entropy and Dice loss.

Encoder-Only. The Transformer encoder along with the CNN encoder compose a CNN-Transformer hybrid encoder in this variant. Feature maps are first extracted by CNN then patchified and tokenized before being fed to the Transformer encoder. A standard U-Net is used as the decoder without the Transformer decoder.

Decoder-Only. This variant uses a conventional CNN encoder only for the encoding phase while both CNN and Transformer are used as the decoder. Before being processed by the Transformer decoder, they are augmented with learnable positional embeddings following Eq. (1).

2.4 Training Details

Masked-Autoencoder (MAE) Pre-training. For our **Encoder-only 3D-TransUNet**, we first pre-train the transformer encoder in an MAE style [12]. Specifically, We initially tokenized 3D input using a 2D patch embedding layer along the z-axis, then flattened it into a 1D sequence. We randomly mask out 75% of the tokens and then utilize just one lightweight decoder block to predict the masked tokens. Following [12], we calculate the reconstruction loss $L_{\text{recon}} = \frac{1}{N}\sum_{i=1}^{N}(x_i - \hat{x}_{i,\text{masked}})^2$, where L_{recon} is the mean square error, x_i are the original pixel values, $\hat{x}_{i,\text{masked}}$ denotes the predicted pixel values for the masked tokens, and N represents the total count of masked tokens. Following [12], we adopt pixel normalization on each patch. Specifically, we compute the mean and standard deviation of all pixels in a patch and use them to normalize this patch. After pre-training, we discard the patch embedding layer and decoder block and solely initialize all transformer encoder blocks with the pre-trained weights. We observe that utilizing a pre-trained encoder significantly speedup model convergence. For instance, with MAE pre-training, the model attains an average Dice score across five folds of 58.2% with only 300 epochs of training, whereas a model trained from scratch needs 600 epochs to achieve comparable performance.

Training Loss. Unless indicated otherwise, we mainly follow the training details of 3D-TransUNet [6]. In addressing the challenge posed by setting the number of coarse candidates N considerably greater than the class count K, it becomes inevitable that predictions for each class will exhibit false positives. To mitigate this, we employ a post-processing step to refine the coarse candidates, drawing on a matching process between predicted and ground truth segmentation masks. Taking cues from prior work [4,23], we utilize the Hungarian matching approach to establish the correspondence between predictions and ground-truth segments. The resulting matching loss is formulated as follows:

$$\mathcal{L} = \lambda_0(\mathcal{L}_{ce} + \mathcal{L}_{dice}) + \lambda_1 \mathcal{L}_{cls}, \tag{6}$$

Here, the pixel-wise losses $\mathcal{L}_{ce}$ and $\mathcal{L}_{dice}$ denote the binary cross-entropy and dice loss [16] respectively, while $\mathcal{L}_{cls}$ represents the classification loss computed using the cross-entropy for each candidate region. The hyper-parameters λ_0 and λ_1 serve to strike a balance between per-pixel segmentation and mask classification loss.

Deep Supervision. To introduce stronger supervision, every intermediate level of the 3D-TransUNet decoder produces a prediction map on which the loss function is applied during training.

3 Experiments and Results

3.1 Experimental Setting

Implementation Details. All experiments are conducted with a single NVIDIA A5000. Batch size and base learning rate are set as 2 and 2e−3 accordingly. The learning rate follows polynomial decay with a power factor of 0.9. Augmentation including random rotation, scaling, flipping, white Gaussian noise, Gaussian blurring, color jittering, low-resolution simulation, Gamma transformation. Our main experiments in Table 2 are conducted using Encoder-only 3D-TransUNet. The architecture combines a 3D nn-UNet with a pre-trained 12-layer Vision Transformer (ViT) as the Transformer encoder, utilizing Masked Autoencoder (MAE) weights. The latent dimension d is set at 768. For decoder-only, the number of layers is 3. And d_{dec} is set to 192. For training loss 6, λ_0 and λ_1 are set as 0.7 and 0.3. During the testing phase, we train our model on the entire training set for 600 epochs and submit the predictions on the validation set. During the testing phase, we applied 10-fold cross-validation, where we trained an individual model for every fold for 1,000 epochs.

MAE Pretraining Settings. The input has a shape of $128 \times 128 \times 128$ after random cropping. We train all data on 8 GPUs distributedly for our MAE training, with a batch size of 2 on each GPU. We train the model in 4800 epochs, including a warm-up period of 40 epochs. The base learning rate is set to 1.5e−4, accompanied by a weight decay 0.05. AdamW optimizer is used by default.

Datasets. We report results on BraTS-MET 2023 [17] which is pivotal for crafting sophisticated algorithms to detect and segment brain metastases, aiming for easy clinical integration. This dataset encompasses a collection of untreated brain metastases mpMRI scans, sourced from multiple institutions and conducted under regular clinical protocols. It should be noted that we didn't use other officially allowed datasets, *e.g.*, NYUMets [18], UCSF-BMSR [21], BrainMetsShare [10] as these datasets don't share the same mpMRI modalities and annotation format as the BraTS-MET 2023.

It should be noted that we only use BraTS-METS 2023 for training as these datasets share the mpMRI modalities and annotation format.

Evaluation Metrics. In assessing the accuracy of a medical image segmentation model, various metrics offer insights into different aspects of performance:

1. **Lesion-wise Dice Score**: Dice score represents the similarity between two binary segmentations. It is given by:

$$\text{Dice}(\mathbf{A}, \mathbf{B}) = \frac{2|\mathbf{A} \cap \mathbf{B}|}{|\mathbf{A}| + |\mathbf{B}|} \qquad (7)$$

where $\mathbf{A}$ and $\mathbf{B}$ denote the binary segmentations.
In this challenge, dice scores localized to individual lesions are adopted for lesion-specific evaluation. The Lesion-wise Dice for a designated lesion is:

$$\text{Dice}_{\text{lesion-wise}}(\mathbf{A}_i, \mathbf{B}_i) = \frac{2|\mathbf{A}_i \cap \mathbf{B}_i|}{|\mathbf{A}_i| + |\mathbf{B}_i|} \qquad (8)$$

This formula assesses the overlap between the ith ground-truth lesion $\mathbf{B}_i$ and all the lesions that overlap with it $\mathbf{A}_i$.

Table 1. Ablation Performance of 3D-TransUNet on the training set of BraTS-METS 2023 [17] under 5-fold cross-validation.

Method	Lesion-wise Dice (↑)				HD95 (↓)			
	ET	TC	WT	Avg.	ET	TC	WT	Avg.
Encoder-only 3D-TransUNet [6]	54.79%	58.96%	56.05%	56.60%	108.9	107.6	109.5	108.7
Decoder-only 3D-TransUNet [6]	56.80%	61.12%	60.09%	59.34%	99.4	95.9	93.97	96.4

Table 2. Performance of Encoder-only 3D-TransUNet on the validation and test set of BraTS-METS 2023 [17].

Dataset Split	Lesion-wise Dice (↑)				HD95 (↓)			
	ET	TC	WT	Avg.	ET	TC	WT	Avg.
Validation	59.2%	63.4%	56.5%	59.6%	94.8	94.8	110.9	100.1
Test	57.4%	62.0%	59.9%	59.8%	103.0	99.8	99.6	100.8

2. **Hausdorff Distance (95%)**: A metric quantifying the maximum of minimum distances between two binary images at the 95-th percentile to mitigate outlier effects. Mathematically:

$$H(A, B) = \max \left\{ \sup_{a \in A} \inf_{b \in B} d(a, b), \sup_{b \in B} \inf_{a \in A} d(a, b) \right\} \quad (9)$$

Model Ensemble and Test-Time Augmentation. During testing phase, five models are randomly chosen from ten models trained on each fold for ensemble. Predictions from these five models were averaged to ensemble predictions. To further boost the model's performance with test-time augmentation, predictions from augmented views with flipping and rotation (90°, 180°, 270°) are averaged to produce the final predictions.

3.2 Encoder-Only v.s. Decoder-Only

In order to compare the effectiveness between the Encoder-only model and the Decoder-only model, we apply 5-fold cross-validation on the entire 238 training cases and report the average Dice and HD95 for all testing cases. The 5 models from the 5 folds of BraTS-METS 2023 training set are trained for 200 epochs. In Table 1, we report the comparison between Encoder-only 3D-TransUNet and Decoder-only 3D-TransUNet on BraTS-METS 2023's training set with 5-fold cross-validation are presented in Table 1. Compared to our internal validation results with the baseline nnUNet, which yielded average Dice scores of 54.90%, 58.67%, and 55.75% for segmenting ET, TC, and WT, respectively, resulting in an overall average Dice score of 56.44%, it becomes evident that while the Encoder-only model offers only marginal improvement in segmentation, the Decoder-only model demonstrates a substantial increase in Dice

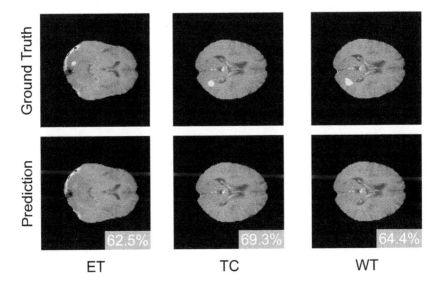

Fig. 2. Visual comparison between ground-truths and predictions from Encoder-only 3D-TransUNet on BraTS-METS 2023. The lesion-wise Dice score of each category on this patient is also listed (best viewed in color).

score by 2.9%. It is important to note that MAE pretraining was not applied to the Encoder-only model in this evaluation. However, with MAE pretraining, the advantages of the Encoder-only model are expected to be more pronounced, albeit still inferior to the Decoder-only model.

3.3 Main Results

Since the Decoder-only 3D-TransUNet requires longer training, due to the time and computation limit, we were only able to submit results from the Encoder-only 3D-TransUNet during the validation phase and testing phase, where the official evaluation results are presented in Table 2. Specifically, we achieve average lesion-wise Dice scores of 59.6% and 59.8% on the validation and test set, securing the second place in the BraTS 2023 challenge. We also display a qualitative example to further demonstrate our method's effectiveness, as shown in Fig. 2.

4 Conclusion

Brain tumors, especially brain metastases, present challenges in segmentation due to their diverse appearances and sizes. The TransUNet model, combining Transformer self-attention and U-Net's features, shows promise for this task. We trained the 3D-TransUNet model on the BraTS-METS 2023 dataset for brain metastases segmentation, exploring Encoder-only and Decoder-only configurations. Pre-training the Encoder-only model with Masked-Autoencoder improves initialization, facilitating faster training. Although the Decoder-only model is expected to perform better, the Encoder-only model achieved notable results in a shorter timeframe, securing second place in the BraTS-METS 2023 challenge with a 59.8% average lesion-wise Dice score on the test set.

References

1. Adewole, M., et al.: The brain tumor segmentation (brats) challenge 2023: Glioma segmentation in sub-saharan africa patient population (brats-africa) (2023)
2. Adewole, M., et al.: The brain tumor segmentation (brats) challenge 2023: Glioma segmentation in sub-saharan africa patient population (brats-africa). arXiv preprint arXiv:2305.19369 (2023)
3. Boire, A., Brastianos, P.K., Garzia, L., Valiente, M.: Brain metastasis. Nat. Rev. Cancer **20**(1), 4–11 (2020)
4. Carion, N., Massa, F., Synnaeve, G., Usunier, N., Kirillov, A., Zagoruyko, S.: End-to-end object detection with transformers. In: Vedaldi, A., Bischof, H., Brox, T., Frahm, J.-M. (eds.) ECCV 2020. LNCS, vol. 12346, pp. 213–229. Springer, Cham (2020). https://doi.org/10.1007/978-3-030-58452-8_13
5. Chen, J., et al.: Transunet: transformers make strong encoders for medical image segmentation. arXiv preprint arXiv:2102.04306 (2021)
6. Chen, J., et al.: 3D transunet: advancing medical image segmentation through vision transformers. arXiv preprint arXiv:2310.07781 (2023)
7. Cheng, B., Misra, I., Schwing, A.G., Kirillov, A., Girdhar, R.: Masked-attention mask transformer for universal image segmentation. In: Proceedings of the IEEE/CVF Conference on Computer Vision and Pattern Recognition, pp. 1290–1299 (2022)
8. Fathi Kazerooni, A., et al.: Automated tumor segmentation and brain tissue extraction from multiparametric MRI of pediatric brain tumors: a multi-institutional study. Neuro-Oncol. Adv. **5**(1), vdad027 (2023)
9. Greenwald, N.F., et al.: Whole-cell segmentation of tissue images with human-level performance using large-scale data annotation and deep learning. Nat. Biotechnol. **40**(4), 555–565 (2022)
10. Grøvik, E., Yi, D., Iv, M., Tong, E., Rubin, D., Zaharchuk, G.: Deep learning enables automatic detection and segmentation of brain metastases on multisequence MRI. J. Magn. Reson. Imaging **51**(1), 175–182 (2020)
11. Habbous, S., et al.: Incidence and real-world burden of brain metastases from solid tumors and hematologic malignancies in Ontario: a population-based study. Neuro-Oncol. Adv. **3**(1), vdaa178 (2021)
12. He, K., Chen, X., Xie, S., Li, Y., Dollár, P., Girshick, R.: Masked autoencoders are scalable vision learners. In: Proceedings of the IEEE/CVF Conference on Computer Vision and Pattern Recognition, pp. 16000–16009 (2022)
13. Kazerooni, A.F., et al.: The brain tumor segmentation (brats) challenge 2023: focus on pediatrics (cbtn-connect-dipgr-asnr-miccai brats-peds) (2024)
14. Long, J., Shelhamer, E., Darrell, T.: Fully convolutional networks for semantic segmentation. In: Proceedings of the IEEE Conference on Computer Vision and Pattern Recognition, pp. 3431–3440 (2015)
15. Ma, J., He, Y., Li, F., Han, L., You, C., Wang, B.: Segment anything in medical images. Nat. Commun. **15**(1), 654 (2024)

16. Milletari, F., Navab, N., Ahmadi, S.A.: V-net: fully convolutional neural networks for volumetric medical image segmentation. In: 3DV (2016)
17. Moawad, A.W., et al.: The brain tumor segmentation (brats-mets) challenge 2023: brain metastasis segmentation on pre-treatment MRI. arXiv preprint arXiv:2306.00838 (2023)
18. Oermann, E., et al.: Longitudinal deep neural networks for assessing metastatic brain cancer on a massive open benchmark (2023)
19. Renard, F., Guedria, S., Palma, N.D., Vuillerme, N.: Variability and reproducibility in deep learning for medical image segmentation. Sci. Rep. **10**(1), 13724 (2020)
20. Ronneberger, O., Fischer, P., Brox, T.: U-Net: convolutional networks for biomedical image segmentation. In: Navab, N., Hornegger, J., Wells, W.M., Frangi, A.F. (eds.) MICCAI 2015. LNCS, vol. 9351, pp. 234–241. Springer, Cham (2015). https://doi.org/10.1007/978-3-319-24574-4_28
21. Rudie, J.D., et al.: The university of California San Francisco, brain metastases stereotactic radiosurgery (UCSF-BMSR) MRI dataset. arXiv preprint arXiv:2304.07248 (2023)
22. Vaswani, A., et al.: Attention is all you need. In: Advances in Neural Information Processing Systems, pp. 5998–6008 (2017)
23. Wang, H., Zhu, Y., Adam, H., Yuille, A., Chen, L.C.: Max-deeplab: end-to-end panoptic segmentation with mask transformers. In: Proceedings of the IEEE/CVF Conference on Computer Vision and Pattern Recognition, pp. 5463–5474 (2021)
24. Wang, S., et al.: Annotation-efficient deep learning for automatic medical image segmentation. Nat. Commun. **12**(1), 5915 (2021)

Towards SAMBA: Segment Anything Model for Brain Tumor Segmentation in Sub-Saharan African Populations

Mohannad Barakat[1,2], Noha Magdy[1,2(✉)], Jjuuko George William[3], Ethel Phiri[4], Raymond Confidence[5,6], Dong Zhang[7], and Udunna C. Anazodo[5,6,8,9,10]

[1] Engineering and Applied Sciences, Nile University, Giza, Egypt
n.magdy@nu.edu.eg
[2] Computer Science, Friedrich-Alexander-Universität, Erlangen, Germany
mohannad.barakat@fau.de
[3] Makerere University, Kampala, Uganda
[4] Malawi University of Science and Technology, Mikolongwe, Malawi
[5] Medical Artificial Intelligence Laboratory (MAI Lab), Lagos, Nigeria
[6] Lawson Health Research Institute, London, Canada
[7] Electrical and Computer Engineering, University of British Columbia, Vancouver, Canada
[8] Montreal Neurological Institute, McGill University, Montréal, Canada
[9] Medicine, University of Cape Town, Cape Town, South Africa
[10] Clinical and Radiation Oncology, University of Cape Town, Cape Town, South Africa

Abstract. Gliomas, the most prevalent primary brain tumors, require precise segmentation for diagnosis and treatment planning. However, this task poses significant challenges, particularly in the African population, where limited access to high-quality imaging data hampers algorithm performance. In this study, we propose a new approach combining the Segment Anything Model (SAM) and a voting network for multi-modal glioma segmentation. By fine-tuning SAM with bounding box-guided prompts (SAMBA), we adapt the model to the complexities of African datasets. Our ensemble strategy, utilizing multiple modalities and views, produces a robust consensus segmentation, addressing the intratumoral heterogeneity. This study was conducted on the Brain Tumor Segmentation (BraTS) Africa (BraTS-Africa) dataset, which provides a valuable resource for addressing challenges specific to resource-limited settings and facilitating the development of effective and more generalizable segmentation algorithms. To illustrate our approach's potential, our experiments on the BraTS-Africa dataset yielded compelling results, with SAMBA attaining a Dice coefficient of 86.6% for binary segmentation and 60.4% for multi-class segmentation. Although the low quality of the scans currently presents difficulties, SAMBA has the potential to facilitate more generalizable segmentations for real world clinical problems with future applications to other types of brain lesions.

Keywords: SAM · BraTS · voting network · prompt encoder · Glioma · MRI · Africa

---

M. Barakat and N. Magdy—Equal contribution.

1 Introduction

Brain tumors represent a significant global health challenge, affecting millions of lives each year [1]. Among these tumors, gliomas being the most prevalent primary brain tumor is characterized by their heterogeneous and infiltrative nature, making diagnosis and treatment challenging [1]. The complexity of gliomas stems from their morphological and biological variations, leading to intricate sub-regions with distinct characteristics. Precise segmentation of these sub-regions, such as the active tumor core, peritumoral edema, and enhancing tumor regions, is crucial for understanding the tumor's behavior and guiding personalized treatment strategies [2]. However, achieving precise glioma segmentation remains a challenging task [3], particularly in resource-limited settings where access to high quality advanced brain imaging tools and skilled personnel to manually analyze high volume of imaging data, remain scarce [4]. Specifically, for Sub-Saharan African populations, accurate segmentation is critical because of the usual delayed disease presentation and the high propensity for comorbidities such as infectious disease. This leads to misdiagnosis and worse outcomes [5, 6]. Thus, this study aims to provide an adaptive and robust methodology that can improve the accuracy of glioma segmentation in low-resourced settings and pave the way for advancements in neuro-oncology research.

In recent years, various approaches have been explored for the segmentation of brain tumor data [8], each aiming to achieve improved performance. These include learning frameworks for automatic detection of tumor boundaries, such as DeepSeg [9], nnU-Net [10], and DeepSCAN [11] based on convolutional neural networks, as well as approaches such as Swin UNETR [12] based on vision transformers. Another promising method, trained on multiple U-net-like neural networks with deep supervision and stochastic weight averaging, produces segmented brain tumor subregions by assembling models from different training pipelines [13]. More recently, the Segment Anything Model (SAM) [14] was introduced as a pioneering image segmentation solution, known for its exceptional ability to generate high-quality object masks. Whether prompted by points or boxes, SAM effortlessly produces accurate masks for diverse objects within images [14]. Trained on a vast dataset of 11 million images and 1.1 billion masks, SAM's revolutionary zero-shot capabilities set it apart from conventional methods, making it indispensable for various segmentation tasks. [14]. The adoption of SAM in the medical field has shown potential, particularly when fine-tuned [15, 16]. By fine-tuning SAM [14], we adapt the model to focus on the region of interest within the brain, making it better equipped to handle the complexities of African datasets. This targeted fine-tuning process enables SAM to extract relevant features from the limited and potentially noisy imaging data, enhancing the accuracy of glioma segmentation. The integration of multiple imaging modalities, including FLAIR, T1-weighted, T2-weighted, and T1-weighted contrast enhanced, is vital for gaining a comprehensive understanding of the glioma's characteristics. To this end, we utilize a voting network ensemble strategy, which combines individual segmentations from SAM generated using different modalities and image views. This ensemble approach aims to mitigate the uncertainties and artifacts present in individual modalities, ultimately providing a more robust consensus segmentation.

Since 2012, the Brain Tumor Segmentation (BraTS) Challenge has offered open MRI training data, annotations, and model evaluation metrics, catalyzing machine learning (ML) progress in glioma diagnosis [4]. Uncertainty persists about whether advanced ML methods developed from BraTS data can be applied in Sub-Saharan clinical settings given their unique challenges including the limited number of annotated cases for model training and validation, the lower resolution of acquired MRI, and fewer access to high powered computational resources. Here, we leveraged the recently introduced BraTS-Africa dataset [6] to explore the potential of fine-tuning SAM to improve the accuracy of glioma segmentation and provide a viable solution to overcome these unique challenges.

2 Methodology

2.1 The Dataset

The dataset comprised of 60 (45 training, 15 validation) pre-operative adult glioma cases from the MICCAI-CAMERA-Lacuna Fund BraTS-Africa 2023 Challenge data [6] and 250 (200 training, 50 validation) adult glioma cases from the BraTS 2021 Challenge data [6, 7]. Each case included routine multi-parametric MRI T1-weighted, (T1-w), T2-weighted (T2-w), T2-FLAIR (FLAIR), and T1-post-contrast enhanced (T1CE) scans, meticulously annotated by experienced neuroradiologists for training, validation, and testing (Fig. 1) [6, 7]. The annotated sub-regions are the "Enhancing tumor" (ET), "Non-enhancing tumor core" (NETC), and "Surrounding non-enhancing FLAIR hyper-intensity" (SNFH). The ET are areas with increased T1 signal on postcontrast images, while the NETC comprises of the non-enhancing tumor core regions, including necrosis and cystic changes, and the SNFH refers to FLAIR signal abnormality surrounding the tumor but not part of the tumor core [6].

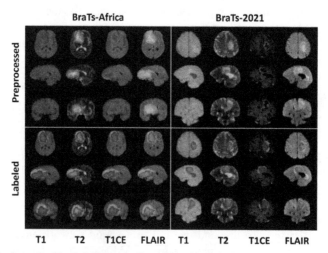

Fig. 1. Clinical standard brain MRI typically acquired in Sub-Saharan African Populations illustrated in a glioma patient (left) shows the conventional lower image resolution compared to the BraTS 2021 data (right). Adapted from [6]

2.2 The SAM Model

The Segment Anything Model (SAM) incorporates a promptable design that facilitates interactive specification of the target area for image segmentation. SAM's design includes an image encoder, a prompt encoder, and a lightweight decoder for generating segmentation masks (Fig. 2). Drawing inspiration from chat-based Large Language Models, SAM allows users to provide prompts to guide the segmentation process effectively [13].

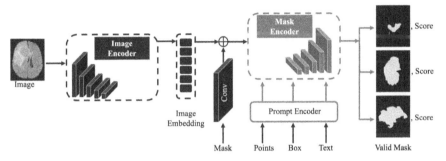

Fig. 2. SAM model architecture

SAM supports three distinct types of prompts:

1. Point Prompt: Users select a point in the image to define the target area.
2. Bounding Box Prompt: Users draw a bounding box around the object to be segmented.
3. Rough Mask Prompt: Users manually draw a basic mask outlining the target object.

Experiments were conducted in this research with various prompts to guide SAM for glioma segmentation. However, implementing the "points" prompt, lead to significant variations in the generated masks with minor pixel changes, due to its high sensitivity (see Eq. 1). To clarify, selecting a positive point within the tumor as a prompt, and subsequently choosing another point within the tumor with a slight pixel shift, may result in the generation of two entirely disparate masks which makes point prompt very sensitive to slight changes in the input points. Similarly, using the "bounding box" prompt around the entire brain image proved ineffective, as SAM struggled to discern the tumor area amidst the extensive brain region. As a result, we decided to focus on the "bounding box" prompt around the tumor area, as it had shown promising initial results even before fine-tuning when using manually created bounding boxes. Table 1 summarizes the prompts experimentation.

$$Assume\ prompt\ p_1 = (x, y)\ with\ mask\ m_1$$
$$prompt\ p_2 = (x + 1, y)\ with\ mask\ m_2$$

$$A\ non\text{-}sensitive\ prompt\ means\ that\ IoU(m_1, m_2) \approx 1 \quad (1)$$

To obtain the desired bounding box during inference, we fine-tuned a YOLO v8 localizer [17] for 150 epochs by providing the 2D MRI data of the ground truth tumor

Table 1. Advantages and disadvantages for different modes of SAM.

Prompt	Explanation	Dis/Advantage	Status
Point	Point(s) inside the lesion	- Easy to compute - SAM is not stable with this prompt	Needs investigation
Box	Bounding box around lesion	- Easy to compute - SAM is stable with this prompt	**This paper**
Mask	Initial binary mask covering part of or the whole lesion	- Hard to get	Future work
Text	Input text describing the type of lesion to segment	- Allows SAM to segment all lesion - Hardest to train	Future work

labels as bounding box prompts. The bounding boxes were extracted from the BraTS-2021 and BraTS-Africa labels using the phyton implementation of the Open Source Computer Vision Library (Open CV; http://opencv.org). The YOLO localizer, based on the You Only Look Once algorithm [17], excels in real-time object detection by simultaneously predicting bounding boxes and class probabilities. By using these localized bounding boxes as prompts, SAM's segmentation was targeted, leading to improved and robust glioma segmentations.

2.3 SAMBA: Finetuning SAM

This study proposes two distinct approaches for fine-tuning SAM using the bounding box prompt mode to address the task of accurate glioma segmentation (SAMBA). In both approaches, a localizer is employed to generate bounding boxes encompassing the glioma regions, providing spatial information to guide SAM's segmentation. In the first approach, SAM's image and prompt encoders remain frozen, while the decoder is specifically fine-tuned for binary segmentation of gliomas without specifying the three classes. Subsequently, a compact voting network is introduced to amalgamate the binary segmentation outputs from SAM across various modalities and image views, yielding a final three-class glioma segmentation that effectively captures intra-tumoral heterogeneity. Figure 3A shows the SAMBA architecture for this approach. The second approach also involves freezing the encoders and fine-tuning the decoder, but this time, it is tailored to directly output the three designated segmentation classes. Optionally, a voting network is integrated to further enhance the results by leveraging the encoder's output to capture finer details not entirely captured by SAM. Figure 3B shows the architecture of SAM multi class finetuning (SAMBA-mc).

In the binary segmentation approach (SAMBA), SAM was trained for 15 epochs on BraTS-Africa and BraTS-2021 datasets, whereas in the multi-class segmentation approach (SAMBA-mc), SAM was trained for 50 epochs on BraTS-Africa data in both approaches the model was trained to minimize the Dice loss. The shorter training duration

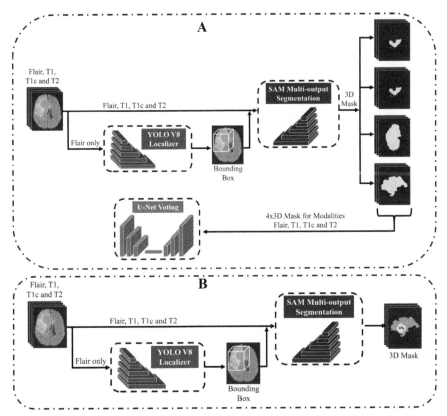

Fig. 3. The architecture for SAM decoder fine-tuning for binary segmentation (SAMBA) (3A) and for multi-class segmentation (SAMBA-mc) (3B)

for binary segmentation was sufficient to achieve satisfactory results, as it involved a simpler task of distinguishing the presence or absence of the tumor. On the other hand, the multi-class segmentation task required a more extended training period to accurately classify the tumor into three distinct classes: edema, enhancing tumor, and non-enhancing tumor. The different training epochs were tailored to the complexity and requirements of each segmentation task, optimizing the performance of SAM in both scenarios. Due to the nature of the SAM model as a type of foundation model that does not generally require a large volume of data to achieve its tasks we opted to train the model without any data augmentation. The BraTS-Africa and BraTS-2021 datasets were trained separately with five finetuned SAM models on BraTS-Africa and two finetuned models on BraTS 2021.

2.4 The Voting Network

The voting network used in our study is a 3D U-Net [18] with approximately 200,000 parameters minimizing the Dice loss. The network takes as input the output of SAM for the different MRI modalities and it serves two primary purposes: Firstly, it addresses

SAM's limitations in capturing fine details by refining the segmentation results. Secondly, it performs a crucial voting process by aggregating the binary segmentation outputs from SAM across different modalities (T1-w, T2-w, FLAIR, T1CE). By combining the segmented outputs through voting, the voting network produces the final three-class segmentation. The incorporation of the voting network significantly enhances the robustness and accuracy of the glioma segmentation, addressing both SAM's limitations and the complexities posed by multi-modal data.

The code used in this study is available at: https://github.com/CAMERAMRI/SPARK2023/tree/main/SPARK_SAMBA.

3 Results

We observed that the fine-tuning of SAM's decoder for binary segmentation (SAMBA) resulted in a Dice coefficient of 63.3%, which represented a decrease compared to the 72.2% achieved on higher-quality images from the BraTS 2021 dataset when trained using a bounding box around the whole brain. However, when SAM was fine-tuned using the manually created bounding box around the tumor region, the Dice coefficient improved to 84.6% on the BraTS-Africa data and 89.4% on the better-quality data from BraTS 2021 (Fig. 4).

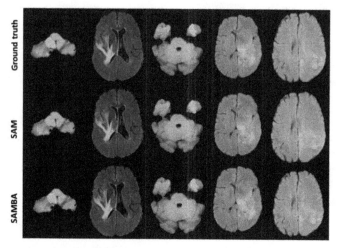

Fig. 4. An example of SAM results illustrating improvement before and after fine-tuning for binary segmentation in BraTS-Africa. The results also show the limitation of SAM on capturing fine details.

Notably, SAM without fine-tuning achieved a Dice coefficient of 73.6% when using a bounding box around the tumor on the BraTS 2021 dataset. This highlights the efficacy of SAM's promptable design, as it performed well even without specific fine-tuning on the high-quality dataset, further demonstrating its potential for accurate glioma segmentation. Figure 6 shows the improvement of SAM before and after fine-tuning.

Table 2. Dice scores for finetuned SAM (SAMBA) model on the BraTS-Africa data and BraTS 2021 data for binary and multi-class segmentations.

Experiment	BraTS-Africa (Dice)	BraTS 2021 (Dice)
Binary, full brain bounding box	63.3%	72.2%
Binary, tumor bounding box	84.6%	89.4%
Binary, tumor bounding box with YOLO	33.7%	-
Multi class tumor bounding box	60.4% (mean over ET, TC, WT)	-
Multi class tumor bounding with YOLO	12.8% (ET), 16.8% (TC), 50.9% (WT)	-

For the multi-class segmentation task, SAM was trained on the African data, and its Dice coefficient reached the value of 60.4%. Integrating YOLO into the pipeline decreased the Dice coefficient value, impacting segmentation results. SAM performed well initially using manually generated bounding boxes, but when tested with YOLO-generated bounding boxes, the Dice coefficient decreased. Enhancing YOLO's performance could improve the overall Dice coefficient, highlighting the need to refine the interaction between YOLO and SAM for better segmentation results. Table 2 summarize SAM results. These findings suggest that fine-tuning SAM using the localized bounding box around the tumor region improved the segmentation results, particularly in the African dataset, which is characterized by lower image quality. The results demonstrate the potential of SAM's adaptability to different data qualities and its ability to produce accurate segmentations with appropriate guidance.

The YOLO v8 localization network achieved a high Dice score of 96.7% in correctly differentiating between images with bounding boxes (i.e., slices containing tumors) and background images (i.e., slices without tumors). For the bounding boxes generated by the model, the box loss was 1.24, indicating accurate localization, with an average box confidence of 87%. Some examples of the results shown in Fig. 5. These improved results demonstrate the effectiveness of the YOLO v8 localizer in accurately detecting and localizing tumor regions within the brain images, providing valuable bounding boxes to guide the glioma segmentation process in our research. With the constraint imposed by YOLO, the overall Dice coefficient reached approximately 43%, showcasing the voting network's valuable contribution to mitigating the impact of this limitation.

4 Discussion

This study demonstrated the effectiveness of SAM in glioma segmentation, particularly when guided by bounding boxes around the tumor region. Fine-tuning SAM (SAMBA) with localized bounding boxes significantly improved segmentation results, achieving Dice coefficients of 84.6% on the BraTS-Africa dataset and 89% on the higher-quality BraTS 2021 dataset. Notably, SAM performed well even without fine-tuning, achieving a

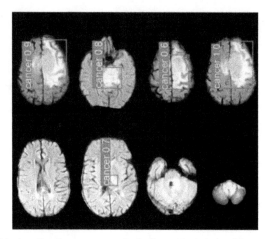

Fig. 5. Example of the localization output results indicated by box confidence score for the BRATS Africa dataset. The box outlined in red and the confidence of the model on detecting the class "cancer" are overlaid on the figured where the tumor was identified. (Color figure online)

Dice coefficient of 73% on BraTS 2021 dataset when a bounding box was placed around the tumor. SAM demonstrated the ability to achieve high Dice coefficient when fine-tuning on limited data (only 45 cases), an important finding for low-resourced settings where training and validation datasets are often scarce.

Using SAM with multi-class segmentation does not yield improved results. This may be due to the difference between the purpose of the multi-class segmentation in SAM and SAMBA. In SAM each layer represented a sub-object to the inferior layer. While this remains the same for SAMBA, SAMBA has multiple outputs where it should only have one or two outputs not three. Fine tuning SAM with a fixed prompt around the brain didn't yield good Dice score. However, this was for fine tuning the decoder only. Fine tuning the encoder and decoder together might give better results and will be investigated in future work. The incorporation of a lightweight U-Net voting network further enhanced segmentation results, addressing SAM's limitations in capturing fine details. The voting network effectively combined binary segmentation outputs from different modalities and views, producing robust three-class glioma segmentations. Moreover, the utilization of the YOLO v8 localization network for accurate tumor detection proved instrumental in providing reliable bounding boxes to guide SAM's segmentation process. This approach proved particularly valuable for datasets with lower image quality, such as the African dataset, where access to high quality imaging data is limited. Although YOLO v8 made SAMBA possible by providing prompts, it clearly degraded the overall loss by introducing some false positives and false negatives.

Overall, our findings demonstrate the potential clinical impact of SAM for brain tumor imaging and treatment planning, especially in regions with limited imaging resources. The adaptability and versatility of SAM make it a valuable tool for accurate and efficient lesion segmentation, paving the way for extension of SAMBA to brain metastasis and other types of brain lesions to further improved diagnostic and treatment decisions.

5 Future Work

For future work, we propose to explore fine-tuning the entire SAM, including both the encoder and decoder, using the LoRA fine-tuning technique [19]. Given the substantial size of the encoder, LoRA fine-tuning offers a more efficient approach to update the model's parameters while preserving its learned knowledge. We anticipate that fine-tuning the full SAM will yield significantly improved segmentation results compared to the current approach. Additionally, we plan to develop a specialized version of SAM tailored specifically for brain tumor segmentation, capable of generalizing beyond gliomas to other brain tumor types. Examples of these brain tumor types could include meningiomas, metastatic tumors, pituitary adenomas, and others. By incorporating diverse tumor types in the training data, the fine-tuned SAM encoder will be able to learn the distinct characteristics and variations across these tumor types, ultimately leading to highly accurate segmentations for each specific tumor type.

Acknowledgment. The authors would like to thank the all the faculty and instructors of the Sprint AI Training for African Medical Imaging Knowledge Translation (SPARK) Academy 2023 summer school on deep learning in medical imaging for providing insightful background knowledge that informed the research presented here. The authors thank Linshan Liu for administrative assistance in supporting SPARK and acknowledge the computational infrastructure support from the Digital Research Alliance of Canada (The Alliance) and the knowledge translation support from the McGill University Doctoral Internship Program through student exchange program for the SPARK Academy. The authors are grateful to McMedHacks for providing foundational information on python programming for medical image analysis as part of the 2023 SPARK Academy program. This research was funded by the Lacuna Fund for Health and Equity (PI: Udunna Anazodo, grant number 0508-S-001) and National Science and Engineering Research Council of Canada (NSERC) Discovery Launch Supplement (PI: Udunna Anazodo, grant number DGECR-2022-00136).

References

1. Aldape, K., Brindle, K.M., Chesler, L., Chopra, R., et al.: Challenges to curing primary brain tumours. Nat. Rev. Clin. Oncol. **16**(8), 509–520 (2019)
2. Anazodo, U.C., Ng, J.J., Ehiogu, B., Obungoloch, J., Fatade, A., et al.: A framework for advancing sustainable magnetic resonance imaging access in Africa. NMR Biomed. **36**(3), e4846 (2023)
3. Zhang, D., Confidence, R., Anazodo, U.: Stroke lesion segmentation from low quality and few-shot mris via similarity-weighted self-ensembling framework. In: Wang, L., Dou, Q., Fletcher, P.T., Speidel, S., Li, S. (eds.) Medical Image Computing and Computer Assisted Intervention – MICCAI 2022. MICCAI 2022. Lecture Notes in Computer Science, vol. 13435. Springer, Cham (2022)
4. Cahall, D.E., et al.: Inception Modules Enhance Brain Tumor Segmentation (2019). https://doi.org/10.3389/FNCOM.2019.00044
5. Kanmounye, U.S., Karekezi, C., Nyalundja, A.D., Awad, A.K., et al.: Adult brain tumors in Sub-Saharan Africa: a scoping review. Neuro Oncol. **24**(10), 1799–1806 (2022)
6. Adewole, M., Rudie, J.D., Gbadamosi, A., et al.: The Brain Tumor Segmentation (BraTS) Challenge 2023: Glioma Segmentation in Sub-Saharan Africa Patient Population (BraTS-Africa). arXiv preprint arXiv:2305.19369 (2023)

7. Baid, U., Ghodasara, S., Mohan, S., Bilello, M., Calabrese, E., et al.: The RSNA-ASNR-MICCAI- BraTS 2021 benchmark on brain tumor segmentation and radiogenomic classification. arXiv preprint arXiv:2107.02314 (2021)
8. Menze, B.H., Jakab, A., Bauer, S., Kalpathy-Cramer, J., et al.: The multimodal brain tumor image segmentation benchmark (BRATS). IEEE Trans. Med. Imaging **34**(10), 1993–2024 (2014)
9. Zeineldin, R.A., Karar, M.E., Burgert, O., Mathis-Ullrich, F.: Multimodal CNN networks for brain tumor segmentation in MRI: a BraTS 2022 challenge solution. arXiv preprint arXiv: 2212.09310 (2022)
10. Isensee, F., Jäger, P.F., Full, P.M., Vollmuth, P., Maier-Hein, K.H.: nnU-Net for brain tumor segmentation. In: Brainlesion: Glioma, Multiple Sclerosis, Stroke and Traumatic Brain Injuries: 6th International Workshop, BrainLes 2020, Held in Conjunction with MICCAI 2020, Lima, Peru, October 4, 2020, Revised Selected Papers, Part II 6 2021, pp. 118–132. Springer, Cham (2020)
11. Gong, Q., et al.: DeepScan: Exploiting deep learning for malicious account detection in location-based social networks. IEEE Commun. Mag. **56**(11), 21–27 (2018)
12. Hatamizadeh, A., Nath, V., Tang, Y., Yang, D., Roth, H.R., Xu, D.: Swin unetr: swin transformers for semantic segmentation of brain tumors in MRI images. In: International MICCAI Brain- lesion Workshop 2021 Sep 27, pp. 272–284. Springer, Cham (2021)
13. Henry, T., et al.: Brain tumor segmentation with self-ensembled, deeply-supervised 3D U-net neural networks: a BraTS 2020 challenge solution. In: Brainlesion: Glioma, Multiple Sclerosis, Stroke and Traumatic Brain Injuries: 6th International Workshop, BrainLes 2020, Held in Conjunction with MICCAI 2020, Lima, Peru, October 4, 2020, Revised Selected Papers, Part I 6 2021, pp. 327–339. Springer, Cham (2020)
14. Kirillov, A., Mintun, E., Ravi, N., Mao, H., Rolland, C., et al.: Segment anything. arXiv preprint arXiv:2304.02643 (2023)
15. Ma, J., Wang, B.: Segment anything in medical images. arXiv preprint arXiv:2304.12306 (2023)
16. Liu, Y., Zhang, J., She, Z., Kheradmand, A., Armand, M.: SAMM (segment any medical model): A 3D Slicer integration to SAM. arXiv preprint arXiv:2304.05622 (2023)
17. Terven, J., Cordova-Esparza, D.: A comprehensive review of YOLO: From YOLOv1 to YOLOv8 and beyond. arXiv preprint arXiv:2304.00501 (2023)
18. Ronneberger, O., Fischer, P., Brox, T.: U-net: convolutional networks for biomedical image segmentation. In: Medical Image Computing and Computer-Assisted Intervention–MICCAI 2015: 18th International Conference, Munich, Germany, October 5–9, 2015, Proceedings, Part III 18 2015, pp. 234–241. Springer, Cham (2015)
19. Hu, E.J., et al.: Lora: low-rank adaptation of large language models. arXiv preprint arXiv: 2106.09685 (2021)

Automated Ensemble Method for Pediatric Brain Tumor Segmentation

Shashidhar Reddy Javaji[1], Advait Gosai[1], Sovesh Mohapatra[1,2], and Gottfried Schlaug[2,3,4](✉)

[1] Manning College of Information and Computer Sciences, University of Massachusetts Amherst, Amherst, MA 01002, USA
[2] Institute for Applied Life Sciences, University of Massachusetts Amherst, Amherst, MA 01003, USA
gschlaug@umass.edu
[3] Department of Biomedical Engineering, University of Massachusetts Amherst, Amherst, MA 01002, USA
[4] Department of Neurology, Baystate Medical Center, and UMass Chan Medical School - Baystate Campus, Springfield, MA 01199, USA

Abstract. Brain tumors remain a critical global health challenge, necessitating advancements in diagnostic techniques and treatment methodologies. A tumor or its recurrence often needs to be identified in imaging studies and differentiated from normal brain tissue. In response to the growing need for age-specific segmentation models, particularly for pediatric patients, this study explores the deployment of deep learning techniques using magnetic resonance imaging (MRI) modalities. By introducing a novel ensemble approach using ONet and modified versions of UNet, coupled with innovative loss functions, this study achieves a precise segmentation model for the BraTS-PEDs 2023 Challenge. Data augmentation, including both single and composite transformations, ensures model robustness and accuracy across different scanning protocols. The ensemble strategy, integrating the ONet and UNet models, shows greater effectiveness in capturing specific features and modeling diverse aspects of the MRI images which result in lesion wise Dice scores of 0.52, 0.72 and 0.78 on unseen validation data and scores of 0.55, 0.70, 0.79 on final testing data for the "enhancing tumor", "tumor core" and "whole tumor" labels respectively. Visual comparisons further confirm the superiority of the ensemble method in accurate tumor region coverage. The results indicate that this advanced ensemble approach, building upon the unique strengths of individual models, offers promising prospects for enhanced diagnostic accuracy and effective treatment planning and monitoring for brain tumors in pediatric brains.

Keywords: UNet · ONet · Hybrid Loss · Majority Ensemble

S. R. Javaji, A. Gosai and S. Mohapatra—Contributed equally.

© The Author(s), under exclusive license to Springer Nature Switzerland AG 2024
U. Baid et al. (Eds.): crossMoDA 2023/BraTS 2023, LNCS 14669, pp. 211–220, 2024.
https://doi.org/10.1007/978-3-031-76163-8_19

1 Introduction

Brain tumor has been a major global health challenge, impacting not only adults but also children and adolescents [1]. In 2022, the United States alone reported an estimated 40,594 individuals, from infancy to 19 years of age, diagnosed with primary brain or other central nervous system (CNS) tumors. Among these, pilocytic astrocytoma was the predominant histopathologic group, accounting for 8,264 cases. Given that survival rates following a diagnosis are particularly low among infants, there is a huge need to develop age-specific segmentation models [2]. These models could enable precise and automated detection of tumor regions within pediatric brains, thereby facilitating more efficient and fast diagnosis and treatment.

With the increasing use of deep learning techniques in conjunction with different modalities of MRI, different models, especially the U-shaped architectures, have demonstrated precise and accurate performance across various medical image segmentation tasks [3–5]. Various models have been employed for whole brain segmentation, yet certain architectural designs have been observed to perform better in segmenting specific regions within the brain [6]. This phenomenon can be attributed to the intricate relationship between the complexities inherent in both the architecture and the brain's structure. Just as different modalities provide complementary information about anomalous regions in the brain, different architectures may be more adept at handling particular areas of the brain [7].

In this paper, we are focused on using the CBTN-CONNECT-DIPGr-ASNR-MICCAI BraTS-PEDs 2023 Challenge data which constitutes four different modalities (native T1, post-contrast T1-weighted (T1Gd), T2-weighted (T2), and T2 Fluid Attenuated Inversion Recovery (T2-FLAIR)) [8]. We introduce a novel ensemble approach using ONet and various modified versions of UNet along with modified loss functions which yielded a more precise segmentation for the pediatric tumors.

2 Methodology

2.1 Data Augmentation

Due to the inherent variability and noise that can occur during acquisition using different scanners, the integration of various physics-inspired augmentation techniques is essential. By populating the training data with these techniques, the model becomes robust and accurate across diverse scanning protocols [9].

In this study, we used two different approaches of augmentation: single and composite transformation. For the single transformation, we used techniques like flip, affine transformation, elastic deformation, noise, rescale Intensity, and random bias field. Additionally, in composite transformation, a combination of some or all of the aforementioned techniques was applied to further enrich the dataset [10–13].

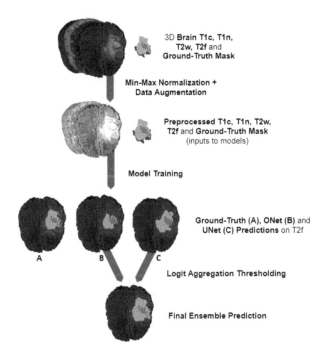

Fig. 1. Comprehensive workflow visualizing the end-to-end process with model training and ensemble approaches.

2.2 Model Architectures

UNet3D Family. In this work, we implemented eight unique variations using two fundamental base architectures, each paired with different loss functions (further explained in Sect. 2.3) and tailored hyperparameters. Figure 2 illustrates the architecture for one of the variants of the UNet3D configurations.

The UNet variations are as follows (Fig. 1):

- **3D UNet**: This is the standard configuration utilizing an input channel size of 4, output class size of 3, and a channel size of 32.
- **3D UNet GELU**: A variant of the standard 3D UNet where the ReLU activation function is substituted with GELU (Gaussian Error Linear Unit) to potentially improve non-linear learning capabilities.
- **3D UNet SingleConv**: This version modifies the typical double convolution process in each upscaling and downscaling step, replacing it with a single convolution, which might affect the model's ability to capture complex features.
- **3D UNet Attention**: Incorporates an attention mechanism into the 3D UNet structure, aiming to enhance the model's focus on relevant features for improved segmentation.
- **3D UNet Dropout**: Introduces dropout layers into the 3D UNet architecture to prevent overfitting and promote generalization.

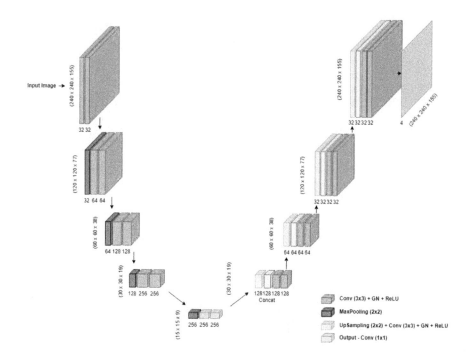

Fig. 2. Core UNet3D Architecture.

ONet3D Family. We also explore variations within the ONet3D family, which differs from the UNet3D by concatenating the encoder-decoder sections before the output convolution layer:

- **3D ONet SingleConv Kernel_1**: Utilizes a single convolution with a kernel size of 1 in the ONet3D architecture.
- **3D ONet SingleConv Kernel_5**: Adopts a single convolution with a kernel size of 5, offering a broader receptive field compared to Kernel_1.
- **3D ONet DoubleConv Kernel_1**: Features double convolution operations with a kernel size of 1, potentially enhancing the model's ability to extract fine-grained features.

2.3 Loss Functions

In our segmentation framework, we explored different loss functions to optimize the model performance. Specifically, we employed two distinct loss combinations: Binary Cross-Entropy (BCE) [14] plus Dice Loss, and Generalized Dice Loss [15] plus BCE. The choice of these loss functions is motivated by their abilities to tackle the class imbalance problem often encountered in medical image segmentation.

Binary Cross-Entropy Combined with Dice Loss. The Binary Cross-Entropy (BCE) loss is commonly used for binary classification tasks and computes the cross-entropy between the true labels and predicted probabilities. To enhance the model's sensitivity to the region of interest, we combined BCE with Dice Loss. The Dice Loss computes the overlap between the predicted segmentation and the ground truth, providing a spatially aware metric that is sensitive to the shape of the segmented structures.

The BCE loss is defined as:

$$BCE(y, \hat{y}) = -\frac{1}{N} \sum_{i=1}^{N} (y_i \log(\hat{y}_i) + (1 - y_i) \log(1 - \hat{y}_i)) \quad (1)$$

and the Dice Loss is defined as:

$$Dice(y, \hat{y}) = 1 - \frac{2 \sum_{i=1}^{N} y_i \hat{y}_i + \varepsilon}{\sum_{i=1}^{N} y_i + \sum_{i=1}^{N} \hat{y}_i + \varepsilon} \quad (2)$$

where ε is a small constant to avoid division by zero. The combined loss function is:

$$Loss(y, \hat{y}) = \alpha \cdot BCE(y, \hat{y}) + \beta \cdot Dice(y, \hat{y}) \quad (3)$$

where α and β are weights that balance the contribution of each term.

Generalized Dice Loss Combined with BCE. Recognizing the limitations of standard Dice Loss in handling cases with varying object sizes, we also experimented with Generalized Dice Loss (GDL). GDL extends the traditional Dice Loss by incorporating class-wise weights, thus accommodating the imbalanced class distribution. This loss function is especially well-suited to medical image segmentation where certain classes or labels may be underrepresented.

The GDL is defined as:

$$GDL(y, \hat{y}) = 1 - \frac{2 \sum_{c=1}^{C} w_c \sum_{i=1}^{N} y_{ci} \hat{y}_{ci} + \varepsilon}{\sum_{c=1}^{C} w_c (\sum_{i=1}^{N} y_{ci} + \sum_{i=1}^{N} \hat{y}_{ci}) + \varepsilon} \quad (4)$$

where C is the number of classes, w_c is the weight for class c, defined as:

$$w_c = \frac{1}{(\sum_{i=1}^{N} y_{ci})^2} \quad (5)$$

Here, ε is again a small constant to avoid division by zero.

2.4 Ensemble Strategy

The ensemble strategy integrates the predictive capabilities of ONet and UNet models, capitalizing on their complementary strengths. Initial predictions from the models are combined through a summation of logits, followed by thresholding. A majority vote across the models for each voxel finalizes the ensemble prediction, aiming to capture specific features and model diverse aspects of the MRI images.

2.5 Post Processing

Post-processing techniques are applied to the combined predictions to refine segmentation quality:

- Size Filtering Based on Voxel Volumes: This technique removes small isolated regions, eliminating noise.
- Morphological Reconstruction: A more advanced method for interpolation of voxels violating constraints and smoothing boundaries for all labels.

3 Results

3.1 Evaluation Metrics

The BraTS challenge evaluates submitted models using two primary metrics: the lesion-wise (LW) Dice score and the 95th percentile lesion-wise Hausdorff distance (HD95). These metrics are used to assess segmentations across three distinct tumor sub-regions: the whole tumor (WT), tumor core (TC), and enhancing tumor (ET).

The Lesion-wise Dice Score and 95th Percentile Lesion-wise Hausdorff Distance (HD95) are key metrics for evaluating segmentation models in medical imaging. The Dice score, ranging from 0 (no overlap) to 1 (perfect overlap), measures the accuracy of predicted segmentations against the true segmentations on a lesion-by-lesion basis, penalizing False Positives and False Negatives by assigning a 0 score. The HD95 metric quantifies the maximum deviation between predicted and actual segmentations for each lesion, with False Positives and False Negatives receiving a fixed penalty value of 374. Mean scores for both metrics are calculated across case IDs. These evaluations offer a detailed insight into the model's segmentation performance, highlighting areas for potential enhancement.

3.2 Quantitative Performance

Table 1. Comparison of evaluation metrics for Enhancing Tumor on validation data

Models	LW Dice ↑	Dice ↑	LW HD95 ↓	HD95 ↓
UNet3D	0.43	0.44	168.68	114.03
ONet3D	0.52	0.48	131.28	121.74
Ensemble (BCE, Dice)	0.38	0.38	186.73	141.84
Ensemble (BCE, GD)	**0.52**	**0.49**	**127.11**	**105.46**

In our assessment of various models, we submitted the results to the synapse portal for testing the results on the validation. The findings revealed that the

Table 2. Comparison of evaluation metrics for Tumor Core on validation data

Models	LW Dice ↑	Dice ↑	LW HD95 ↓	HD95 ↓
UNet3D	0.70	0.75	44.68	12.19
ONet3D	0.71	0.74	33.26	19.82
Ensemble (BCE, Dice)	0.64	0.73	60.00	17.68
Ensemble (BCE, GD)	**0.72**	**0.74**	**23.84**	**11.48**

Table 3. Comparison of evaluation metrics for Whole Tumor on validation data

Models	LW Dice ↑	Dice ↑	LW HD95 ↓	HD95 ↓
UNet3D	0.75	0.82	45.51	11.85
ONet3D	0.76	0.80	32.88	19.31
Ensemble (BCE, Dice)	0.70	0.82	61.74	15.97
Ensemble (BCE, GD)	**0.78**	**0.82**	**25.88**	**10.89**

ensemble training approach demonstrates better effectiveness in comparison to the single model training approach, across almost all of the validation cases (Tables 2 and 3).

Furthermore, an individual evaluation of predictions indicated that the single-model training approach of the ONet3D model matches the ensemble training approach for lesion-wise dice as outlined in Table 1. This indicates that there can be an ensemble model which might be robust and be generalizable for a larger dataset. However for specific types of segmentation and evaluation metrics, the approaches might differ (Table 4).

Table 4. Evaluation metrics for sub-regions on **Final Test Data**

Sub-region	LW Dice ↑	Dice ↑	LW HD95 ↓	HD95 ↓
ET	**0.55**	65.23	**0.55**	**0.99**
TC	**0.71**	31.61	**0.61**	**0.99**
WT	**0.79**	22.36	**0.70**	**0.99**

In the evaluation of our brain tumor segmentation model on the BraTS test set, the results demonstrate varying degrees of performance across different tumor sub-regions, indicating the model's proficiency in distinguishing between tumor core (TC), enhancing tumor (ET), and whole tumor (WT) regions. Specifically, the model achieved Dice scores of 0.5519, 0.7054, and 0.7938 for ET, TC, and WT, respectively, suggesting a higher accuracy in segmenting the whole tumor region compared to the more challenging enhancing tumor and tumor core regions. Similarly, the Hausdorff distance (95th percentile) metrics, which assess the model's precision in outlining tumor boundaries, show values of 65.23, 31.61, and 22.36 for ET, TC, and WT, respectively, indicating the model's increased boundary precision in WT segmentation. The sensitivity scores-0.5544 for ET, 0.6096 for TC, and 0.7010 for WT-further highlight the model's ability to correctly identify tumor pixels, with WT regions being most accurately detected. In contrast, the specificity scores, which are consistently high across all regions (0.9997 for ET, 0.9998 for TC, and 0.9999 for WT), underscore the model's effectiveness in correctly classifying non-tumor pixels. These results collectively underscore the model's robustness in brain tumor segmentation, with notable strengths in whole tumor delineation and high specificity across tumor sub-regions. In the end it's evident from the validation and test results that the model generalizes well.

3.3 Visual Comparison

Figure 3 illustrates a side-by-side comparison of prediction results derived from two separate methodologies for modeling: individual model training and the ensemble approach.

The comparison reveals a noticeable difference between the two approaches. The predictions stemming from the single model training method, as evidenced by UNet3D and ONet3D, demonstrate to capture less core tumor region and region affected by the tumor (enhancing tumor). This limitation is contrasted by the predictions generated through the ensemble training method.

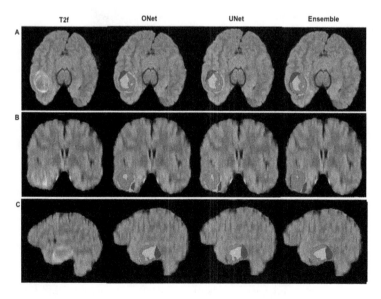

Fig. 3. A, B, and C depict three slice planes (sagittal, coronal, axial) from the same CaseID, showcasing predictions generated by three different models-UNet3D, ONet3D, and the ensemble model respectively.

The ensemble approach adds the strengths of multiple individual models, potentially leading to more accurate and robust predictions. In the context of the figure, it becomes evident that employing the ensemble method results in more effective coverage of tumor regions. This might suggest that the ensemble training not only compensates for the limitations observed in the single model training but possibly enhances the overall predictive capability.

4 Discussion and Conclusion

The integration of ONet and UNet models through an ensemble technique, together with the novel proposed post-processing strategy, creates an advanced approach to medical image segmentation. This method builds upon the unique strengths of both ONet and UNet models, combining them in an interdependent manner that leverages their individual capabilities. By doing so, the approach not only amplifies the robustness of the segmentation but also adds a level of precision that might be unattainable with a single-model training strategy. The clinical significance of this methodology lies in its potential to offer enhanced diagnostic accuracy and effective treatment planning.

References

1. Mackay, A., et al.: Integrated molecular meta-analysis of 1,000 pediatric high-grade and diffuse intrinsic pontine glioma. Cancer Cell **32**(5), 520-537.e5 (2017)
2. Ostrom, Q.T., et al.: CBTRUS statistical report: pediatric brain tumor foundation childhood and adolescent primary brain and other central nervous system tumors diagnosed in the united states in 2014-2018. Neuro-oncology **24**(Suppl. 3), iii1–iii38 (2022). https://doi.org/10.1093/neuonc/noac161
3. Ronneberger, O., Fischer, P., Brox, T.: U-Net: convolutional networks for biomedical image segmentation. In: Navab, N., Hornegger, J., Wells, W.M., Frangi, A.F. (eds.) MICCAI 2015. LNCS, vol. 9351, pp. 234–241. Springer, Cham (2015). https://doi.org/10.1007/978-3-319-24574-4_28
4. Hatamizadeh, A., et al.: Swin UNETR: swin transformers for semantic segmentation of brain tumors in MRI images. In: Brandlesion: Glioma, Multiple Sclerosis, Stroke and Traumatic Brain Injuries, pp. 272–284. Springer, Cham (2022)
5. Heiliger, L., et al.: AutoPET Challenge: Combining nn-Unet with Swin UNETR Augmented by Maximum Intensity Projection Classifier. arXiv [eess.IV] (2022)
6. Mohapatra, S., et al.: Meta-Analysis of Transfer Learning for Segmentation of Brain Lesions. arXiv [eess.IV] (2023)
7. Ranjbarzadeh, R., et al.: Brain tumor segmentation based on deep learning and an attention mechanism using MRI multi-modalities brain images. Sci. Rep. **11**(1), 10930 (2021)
8. Kazerooni, A.F., et al.: The Brain Tumor Segmentation (BraTS) Challenge 2023: Focus on Pediatrics (CBTN-CONNECT-DIPGR-ASNR-MICCAI BraTS-PEDs). arXiv (2023)
9. Alsaif, H., et al.: A novel data augmentation-based brain tumor detection using convolutional neural network. Appl. Sci. **12**(8), 3773 (2022). https://doi.org/10.3390/app12083773

10. Nalepa, J., et al.: Data augmentation for brain-tumor segmentation: a review. Front. Comput. Neurosci. **13**, 83 (2019). https://doi.org/10.3389/fncom.2019.00083
11. Castro, E., Cardoso, J.S., Pereira, J.C.: Elastic deformations for data augmentation in breast cancer mass detection. In: 2018 IEEE EMBS International Conference on Biomedical & Health Informatics (BHI), Las Vegas, NV, USA, pp. 230–234 (2018). https://doi.org/10.1109/BHI.2018.8333411
12. Abdalla, P.A., Mohammed, B.A., Saeed, A.M.: The impact of image augmentation techniques of MRI patients in deep transfer learning networks for brain tumor detection. J. Electr. Syst. Inf. Technol. **10**, 51 (2023). https://doi.org/10.1186/s43067-023-00119-9
13. Kalaivani, S., Asha, N., Gayathri, A.: Geometric transformations-based medical image augmentation. In: Solanki, A., Naved, M. (eds.) GANs for Data Augmentation in Healthcare. Springer, Cham (2023). https://doi.org/10.1007/978-3-031-43205-7_8
14. Cox, D.R.: The regression analysis of binary sequences. J. Roy. Stat. Soc. Ser. B (Methodol.) **20**(2), 215–242 (1958). http://www.jstor.org/stable/2983890. Accessed 13 Mar 2024
15. Sudre, C.H., Li, W., Vercauteren, T., Ourselin, S., Jorge Cardoso, M.: Generalised dice overlap as a deep learning loss function for highly unbalanced segmentations. In: Cardoso, M.J., et al. (eds.) DLMIA/ML-CDS -2017. LNCS, vol. 10553, pp. 240–248. Springer, Cham (2017). https://doi.org/10.1007/978-3-319-67558-9_28

Model Ensemble for Brain Tumor Segmentation in Magnetic Resonance Imaging

Daniel Capellán-Martín[1,2], Zhifan Jiang[1], Abhijeet Parida[1], Xinyang Liu[1], Van Lam[1], Hareem Nisar[1], Austin Tapp[1], Sarah Elsharkawi[1,3], María J. Ledesma-Carbayo[2], Syed Muhammad Anwar[1,4], and Marius George Linguraru[1,4(✉)]

[1] Sheikh Zayed Institute for Pediatric Surgical Innovation, Children's National Hospital, Washington, DC 20010, USA
mlingura@childrensnational.org
[2] Biomedical Image Technologies, ETSI Telecomunicación, Universidad Politécnica de Madrid, Madrid 28040, Spain and CIBER-BBN, ISCIII, Madrid, Spain
[3] Princeton University, Princeton, NJ 08544, USA
[4] School of Medicine and Health Sciences, George Washington University, Washington, DC 20052, USA

Abstract. Segmenting brain tumors in multi-parametric magnetic resonance imaging enables performing quantitative analysis in support of clinical trials and personalized patient care. This analysis provides the potential to impact clinical decision-making processes, including diagnosis and prognosis. In 2023, the well-established Brain Tumor Segmentation (BraTS) challenge presented a substantial expansion with eight tasks and 4,500 brain tumor cases. In this paper, we present a deep learning-based ensemble strategy that is evaluated for newly included tumor cases in three tasks: pediatric brain tumors (PED), intracranial meningioma (MEN), and brain metastases (MET). In particular, we ensemble outputs from state-of-the-art nnU-Net and Swin UNETR models on a region-wise basis. Furthermore, we implemented a targeted post-processing strategy based on a cross-validated threshold search to improve the segmentation results for tumor sub-regions. The evaluation of our proposed method on unseen test cases for the three tasks resulted in lesion-wise Dice scores for PED: 0.653, 0.809, 0.826; MEN: 0.876, 0.867, 0.849; and MET: 0.555, 0.6, 0.58; for the enhancing tumor, tumor core, and whole tumor, respectively. Our method was ranked first for PED, third for MEN, and fourth for MET, respectively.

Keywords: Brain tumor segmentation · MRI · Deep learning · Pediatric brain tumors · Meningioma · Metastases

---

D. Capellán-Martín, Z. Jiang and A. Parida—These authors contributed equally.

1 Introduction

The brain tumor segmentation (BraTS) challenge held in conjunction with the International Conference on Medical Image Computing and Computer Assisted Intervention (MICCAI) conference, established in 2012, has generated a benchmark dataset for the segmentation of adult brain gliomas [4–7,21]. The BraTS 2023 challenge has expanded to a cluster of challenges, encompassing a variety of tumor types alongside augmentation tasks [1,10,15,17,19,25]. Herein, we propose a segmentation technique for newly introduced tasks featuring smaller datasets or new types of tumors. Particularly, these tasks include pediatric brain tumors (PED) [16], intracranial meningioma (MEN) [18], and brain metastasis (MET) [22]. This paper presents the methodology primarily developed for PED tumor segmentation, which was also adapted for MEN and MET segmentation tasks.

Brain cancer has become the leading cause of cancer death among children in the United States [8]. Although rare, pediatric high-grade brain tumors can be aggressive. For example, the median overall survival was reported to be less than one year for pediatric diffuse mid-line gliomas (DMGs, which replaced the formerly known diffuse intrinsic pontine gliomas (DIPGs) to emphasize that the disease may affect areas other than the pons) [24]. Multi-parametric magnetic resonance imaging (mpMRI) is essential in pediatric brain tumor diagnosis and monitoring of tumor progression. While adult and pediatric brain tumors share certain similarities, their locations in the brain and imaging characteristics may be different. For DMGs, necrosis is rare or unclear and the tumor may or may not present enhancement on post-gadolinium T1-weighted MRI. Hence, imaging tools specially designed to analyze pediatric brain tumors are necessary to improve clinical management. Automatic tumor segmentation is usually the first and most important step for the success of such analysis. Over the years, several methods have been presented for adult brain tumor segmentation using the BraTS dataset, however, efforts are needed to develop methods more suitable for pediatric brain tumors. The recently introduced PED task in BraTS 2023 provided an opportunity to develop such methods.

Although, a few previous works addressed pediatric brain tumors [10,14,20], their automatic segmentation remains challenging. This is due to a lack of training data and variation in heterogeneous histologic sub-regions including peritumoral edematous/invaded tissue, necrotic core, and enhancing tumor. BraTS-PED 2023 provides these types of data for the first benchmarking initiative on pediatric brain tumor segmentation. The task provides the largest annotated publicly-available retrospective cohort of high-grade gliomas including astrocytomas and DMG/DIPG in children.

In this work, we developed an ensemble approach involving two state-of-the-art deep learning models. Our approach to segmenting pediatric tumors is tested on two additional tasks at BraTS 2023: the segmentation of meningiomas (MEN) and brain metastases (MET). Meningioma is the most common primary intracranial tumor in adults and can result in significant morbidity and mortality for affected patients. Brain metastases are the most common form of central nervous system (CNS) malignancy in adults. Accurate detection of small metastatic lesions is essential for patient prognosis, as missing even one lesion can lead to repeated interventions and treatment delays. For each task, training was performed only on the dataset provided by each sub-challenge.

2 Methods

The model ensemble technique is a widely recognized strategy used with machine learning methods and is aimed at increasing the stability and accuracy of model predictions. To harness the benefits inherent to both convolutional neural networks and vision transformers, we adopted an ensemble approach (see Fig. 1) involving two state-of-the-art models: nnU-Net ("no new U-Net", winner of BraTS 2020) [13] and Swin UNETR ("Swin U-Net transformers", top-performing model of BraTS 2021) [27]. Given that all tasks address the segmentation of multiple tumor sub-regions, our analysis and ensemble approach were conducted in a label-wise manner.

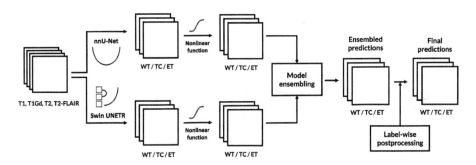

Fig. 1. Proposed method: model ensembling and post-processing pipeline. Outputs are obtained from two state-of-the-art deep learning models. These outputs are subjected to nonlinear activation functions and ensembling strategies. Finally, the ensembled predictions are subjected to a specifically tailored post-processing step.

2.1 Data Description

For all three sub-challenges, mpMRI data included pre- and post-gadolinium T1-weighted (T1 and T1CE), T2-weighted (T2), and T2-weighted fluid attenuated inversion recovery (T2-FLAIR) MRI. The mpMRI scans were pre-processed in a standardized fashion, including co-registration to the same anatomical template [25], re-sampling to an isotropic resolution, and skull-stripping. Each task provided three manual segmentation labels with slightly different definitions. For example, the labels for PED included enhancing tumor (ET), non-enhancing component (NCR - a combination of non-enhancing tumor, cystic component, and necrosis), and peritumoral edematous area (ED). The labels of MEN and

MET included enhancing tumor (ET), non-enhancing tumor core (NETC), and surrounding non-enhancing FLAIR hyperintensity (SNFH). Based on the three labels, three tumor sub-regions were defined to evaluate algorithm performance: enhancing tumor (ET), tumor coure (TC) and whole tumor (WT). The TC region included ET and NCR labels, and WT included all three labels. Figure 2 shows samples of training examples for the three tasks.

Imaging data for PED are split into training (n = 99), validation (n = 45), and additional testing subsets. Imaging data for MEN are split into training (n = 1,000), validation (n = 141), and testing datasets [18]. Imaging data for MET are split into training (n = 165), validation (n = 31), and testing datasets [22].

2.2 Deep Learning Models and Experimental Setup

nnU-Net. The nnU-Net, which is based on the U-Net architecture [26], is a self-configuring deep learning framework for semantic segmentation. According to the specific imaging modality and unique attributes of each dataset, the framework autonomously adjusts its internal configurations [13]. This results in an improved segmentation performance and generalization when compared to other state-of-the-art methods for biomedical image segmentation.

For each of the three tasks, we trained a full-resolution 3D nnU-Net (v2) model using a five-fold cross-validation approach. A preprocessing consisting

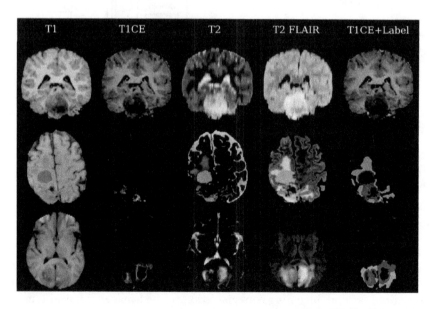

Fig. 2. Training examples in the PED, MEN, and MET tasks (from top to bottom) with the following tumor subregions: enhancing tumor ET (blue), a combination of nonenhancing tumor, cystic component, and necrosis NCR (red), and peritumoral edematous area ED in PED or surrounding nonenhancing FLAIR hyperintensity (SNFH) in MEN and MET (green). (Color figure online)

of a zero mean unit variance normalization was applied to input images. Each input image was divided into patches of 128 × 128 × 128 voxels for PED and 128 × 160 × 112 for MEN and MET. The model output consisted on three channels corresponding to the three tumor sub-regions. Region-based training was employed and the patch size was determined by the GPU memory allocation, favoring larger patches while remaining within the GPU's capacity [13]. We used a class-weight loss function that combined Dice loss and cross entropy loss. To optimize the loss function, we used the stochastic gradient descent (SGD) optimizer with Nesterov momentum with the following parameters: initial learning rate of 0.01, momentum of 0.99, and weight decay of 3e-05. Each of the five folds was trained for 100 epochs on an NVIDIA A100 (40 GB) GPU. At inference time, images were predicted using a sliding window approach. The window size matched the patch size used during training. The nnU-Net implementation is available in an open-source repository: https://github.com/MIC-DKFZ/nnUNet.

Swin UNETR. The Swin UNETR framework employs a vision transformer (ViT)-based [9] hierarchical structure for localized self-attention using non-overlapping windows [11,12,27]. Swin UNETR's innovative local window self-attention outperforms traditional ViT, which is well suited to multiscale tasks. The framework includes a 3D Swin transformer encoder with window-shifting for extended receptive fields, and it connects to a multiscale residual U-Net-like decoder to perform tasks like 3D medical image segmentation.

For each of the three tasks, we trained a full-resolution 3D Swin UNETR model using a five-fold cross-validation approach. A preprocessing consisting of a zero mean unit variance normalization was applied to input images. Each input image was sampled four times using patches of 96 × 96 × 96 voxels to fully utilize the GPU's memory. The model output was 4 channels corresponding to the three labels and background. We used a class-weight loss function that combined Dice loss and focal loss. To optimize the loss function, we used the AdamW optimizer with an initial learning rate of 0.0001, momentum of 0.99, and weight decay of 3e-05. Each of the folds were trained for 600 epochs on an NVIDIA A5000 (24 GB) GPU and NVIDIA A6000 (48GB) GPU. The Swin UNETR implementation is part of the PyTorch-based framework MONAI:[1]. Hyper-parameter optimization was carried out using Optuna [2]:[2].

2.3 Model Ensembling

To enhance the accuracy and robustness of the segmentation outcome, we propose a model ensembling strategy. This approach (see Fig. 1) involves harnessing the complementary strengths of the two models described, nnU-Net and Swin UNETR, to collectively address the task of pixel classification.

---

[1] https://monai.io.
[2] optuna.readthedocs.io/.

The ensembling strategy was optimized for each task based on each model's performance. For the PED task, we trained an nnU-Net solely on the ET region and ensembled its predictions with a Swin UNETR, which was trained on all labels, for ET region prediction. For TC and WT, we ensembled predictions from nnU-Net and Swin UNETR (as described previously), both trained on all labels. For MEN, predictions from both implementations, trained on all labels, were combined to generate ET, TC, and WT regions. Finally, for the MET task, only nnU-Net, trained on all labels, was used after experimental evaluation, as Swin UNETR showed inferior performance in this scenario.

When using a combination of nnU-Net and Swin UNETR, we ensembled the outputs (after applying the corresponding nonlinear activation functions) from each fold obtained during cross-validation ($k = 5$) training of both models. This allowed us to leverage the advantages of both approaches.

2.4 Post-processing

New performance metrics were introduced in this year's BraTS challenge to assess segmentation models at a lesion-wise level rather than over the entire/multiple tumor region(s). We developed a post-processing strategy to adapt to the lesion-wise scores. This post-processing (see Fig. 3) was applied on the ensembled predictions and, first, removed disconnected regions (which contributed to undesired noise) smaller than 130 voxels for PED, 110 voxels for MEN, and 15 voxels for MET (Fig. 4). These optimal threshold values were determined by experimenting with the cross-validation data.

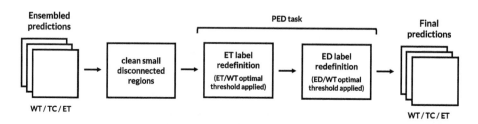

Fig. 3. Post-processing strategy. The ensemble predictions were first cleaned of small disconnected regions. Then, for the PED task, ET and ED labels were redefined based on ET/WT and ED/WT thresholds, respectively.

Subsequently, given the nature of pediatric brain tumors, in the PED task, numerous cases had empty ground truth annotations for the ET and the ED labels. Therefore, redefining these labels in cases where they fell below a certain threshold with respect to the WT volume was particularly useful. For example, if the ET/WT ratio fell below the threshold, the ET label would be redefined to either NCR or ED, which corresponds to the TC region. Figure 5a displays the lesion-wise Dice score *vs.* ET/WT threshold curve obtained from the optimal threshold search process performed on the cross-validation sets. For ET, we

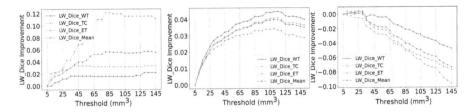

Fig. 4. Threshold search on the cross-validation set for identifying small disconnected regions in PED, MEN and MET, respectively. LW refers to lesion-wise metrics.

obtained an optimal threshold of 0.04. On the other hand, Fig. 5b displays the lesion-wise Dice score vs ED/WT threshold curve obtained from the same process but applied to the ED label, which yielded an optimal threshold of 1.00. These optimal threshold values were also determined by experimenting with the cross-validation data.

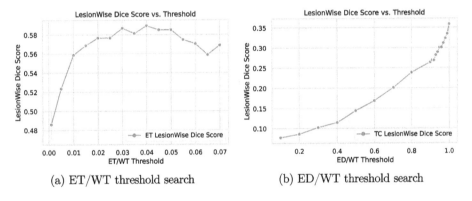

Fig. 5. Threshold search on the cross-validation set. Abbreviations: ED, Peritumoral edematous; ET, enhancing tumor; WT, whole tumor.

By carrying out these post-processing steps, we aimed for a balance between maintaining the integrity of the original predictions and enhancing the final scores by mitigating potential misclassifications.

3 Results

Table 1 provides a comprehensive overview of the performance evaluation of our models across the validation datasets for each task. This performance evaluation was performed automatically by the challenge's digital platform, with no access to the validation ground truth data. Additionally, Fig. 6 shows qualitative results on some cases of the validation datasets for PED, MEN, and MET tasks.

Table 2 provides quantitative evaluation of our proposed solution across the test datasets for each task.

Table 1. Quantitative results on the validation datasets of PED, MEN and MET. Lesion-wise (LW) Dice coefficients and 95% Hausdorff distances (HD95) were computed for enhancing tumor (ET), tumor core (TC), and whole tumor (WT), respectively. Numbers in bold indicate the best results for each task.

Task	Model	LW Dice			LW HD95 (mm)		
		ET	TC	WT	ET	TC	WT
PED	nnU-Net	0.462	0.731	0.798	224.71	30.41	26.08
	Swin UNETR	0.362	0.641	0.716	191.47	82.51	63.33
	Ensemble	0.466	0.73	0.797	158.89	39.34	35.11
	Post-processing	**0.733**	**0.782**	**0.817**	**75.93**	**25.54**	**24.18**
MEN	nnU-Net	0.818	0.799	0.794	51.06	55.74	55.59
	Swin UNETR	0.64	0.644	0.59	117.85	114.43	135.63
	Ensemble	0.833	0.832	0.804	45.94	43.68	53.26
	Post-processing	**0.852**	**0.846**	**0.832**	**37.98**	**38.68**	**42.9**
MET	nnU-Net	0.565	0.614	0.545	117.53	110.88	115.5
	Swin UNETR	0.341	0.378	0.343	204.33	191.12	200.05
	Ensemble	0.533	0.594	0.539	123.18	110.28	115.38
	Post-processing	0.559	0.604	0.565	110.07	105.12	102.77
	Without Swin	**0.608**	**0.649**	**0.587**	**91.62**	**91.29**	**95.7**

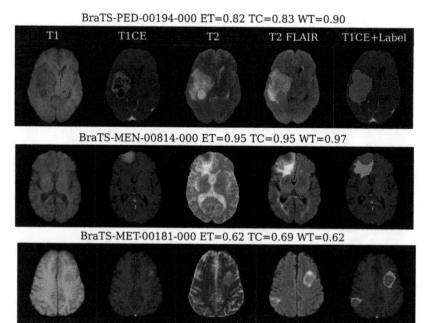

Fig. 6. Qualitative results on the validation datasets of PED, MEN, and MET. The selected cases show the median of the averaged lesion-wise Dice over three tumor regions for each task (NCR-red, ED-green, ET-blue). (Color figure online)

Table 2. Quantitative results on the testing datasets of PED, MEN and MET and ranks obtained in the competition. Lesion-wise (LW) Dice coefficients and 95% Hausdorff distances (HD95) were computed for enhancing tumor (ET), tumor core (TC), and whole tumor (WT), respectively.

Task	Statistic	LW Dice			LW HD95 (mm)		
		ET	TC	WT	ET	TC	WT
PED	Mean	0.653	0.809	0.826	43.89	21.82	20.86
	(Standard deviation)	(0.32)	(0.185)	(0.183)	(108.59)	(75.15)	(75.31)
1st rank	25th quantile	0.569	0.809	0.840	1.41	2.96	2.96
	Median	0.741	0.856	0.875	3.67	5.26	4.24
	75th quantile	0.916	0.888	0.895	8.98	9.17	6.76
MEN	Mean	0.876	0.867	0.849	30.04	31.69	35.17
	(Standard deviation)	(0.217)	(0.227)	(0.231)	(80.9)	(83.53)	(86.77)
3rd rank	25th quantile	0.907	0.885	0.863	1.00	1.00	1.00
	Median	0.968	0.968	0.953	1.00	1.00	1.62
	75th quantile	0.985	0.985	0.975	2.91	3.61	4.36
MET	Mean	0.555	0.6	0.58	113.96	112.84	108.17
	(Standard deviation)	(0.279)	(0.3)	(0.289)	(122.53)	(121.6)	(122.13)
4th rank	25th quantile	0.312	0.370	0.342	1.66	1.29	2.45
	Median	0.638	0.691	0.644	75.78	75.60	9.49
	75th quantile	0.813	0.863	0.826	202.39	189.43	189.03

4 Discussion

Overall, the combination of ensemble models and post-processing procedures yielded clear improvements in the performance for the PED, MEN, and MET tasks. With our approach, we are able to synergize the capabilities of nnU-Net and Swin UNETR models based on the validation scores to effectively generate more accurate and robust segmentation. Our strategy minimized undesired smaller contributions, which would negatively impact lesion-wise performance.

Despite the consistent labeling of the three tumor sub-regions (ET, TC, WT) across all tasks, the lesions' morphology and spatial location are variable across subjects and tasks. Among these three sub-regions, ET identification was the most challenging in the PED task, as evidenced by the lowest Dice coefficient for this region. For the MEN and MET tasks, a better balance between label segmentation was achieved. This confirms the importance of applying label-wise post-processing techniques tailored to each task. Consequently, binary metrics disproportionately penalize false positive predictions. Moreover, the novel metrics centered on lesions result in severe penalties for isolated volumes that do not correspond to actual lesions. All of this accentuates the necessity for post-processing strategies to address disconnected and small components.

Each task's training process was restricted to the usage of task-specific data, adhering to the predefined guidelines of the BraTS 2023 challenge. Outside of the scope of this challenge, it would be beneficial to enhance the model's capacity with additional pre-training to ensure it generalizes effectively.

Our intention was to tackle the diversity in the challenge data from both the perspective of the model and that of the data. Towards this, we argue that self supervised learning strategies and the concept of foundation model [3,23] holds the potential to augment model's generalizability, thus making it suitable for a more extensive range of clinical applications. The PED and MET tasks were conducted with limited available data, which is not surprising given the rarity of brain tumors. To overcome this limitation, the incorporation of generative artificial intelligence could also be a potential solution to augment the training set with synthetic data.

5 Conclusion

The segmentation of rare tumors from radiology images using deep learning techniques is challenging given the limited available data. We developed a model ensemble technique to address the segmentation of three types of brain tumors included in the BraTS 2023 challenge: i.e., pediatric, meningioma, and metastases. The ensemble prediction from nnU-Net and Swin UNETR provided better segmentation accuracy for all tumor types. Furthermore, our targeted post-processing strategy based on cross-validated thresholding search improved the performance in all tasks, being more noticeable in pediatric tumor segmentation due to the label-wise targeted post-processing steps. Through this work, we explored ensembling techniques that leverage the generalizability of deep learning models and strategies across diverse data distributions and tasks. The success of our method is demonstrated by the challenge ranking positions on unseen test cases, being the winner in PED task, ranked third for MEN, and fourth for MET task.

Acknowledgements. Partial support for this work was provided by the National Cancer Institute (UG3 CA236536) and by the Spanish Ministerio de Ciencia e Innovación, the Agencia Estatal de Investigación and NextGenerationEU funds, under grants PDC2022-133865-I00 and PID2022-141493OB-I00. The authors gratefully acknowledge the Universidad Politécnica de Madrid (www.upm.es) for providing computing resources on Magerit Supercomputer.

References

1. Adewole, M., Rudie, J.D., Gbadamosi, A., et al.: The Brain Tumor Segmentation (BraTS) Challenge 2023: Glioma Segmentation in Sub-Saharan Africa Patient Population (BraTS-Africa) (2023)
2. Akiba, T., Sano, S., Yanase, T., Ohta, T., Koyama, M.: Optuna: a next-generation hyperparameter optimization framework. In: Proceedings of the 25th ACM SIGKDD International Conference on Knowledge Discovery and Data Mining (2019)

3. Anwar, S.M., Parida, A., Atito, S., et al.: SS-CXR: multitask representation learning using self supervised pre-training from chest x-rays. arXiv:2211.12944 (2022)
4. Baid, U., Ghodasara, S., Mohan, S., et al.: The RSNA-ASNR-MICCAI BraTS 2021 benchmark on brain tumor segmentation and radiogenomic classification. arXiv preprint arXiv:2107.02314 (2021)
5. Bakas, S., Akbari, H., Sotiras, A., et al.: Advancing the cancer genome atlas glioma MRI collections with expert segmentation labels and radiomic features. Sci. Data **4**(1), 170117 (2017). https://doi.org/10.1038/sdata.2017.117
6. Bakas, S., Akbari, H., Sotiras, A., et al.: Segmentation labels and radiomic features for the pre-operative scans of the TCGA-GBM collection. The Cancer Imaging Archive (2017). https://doi.org/10.7937/K9/TCIA.2017.KLXWJJ1Q
7. Bakas, S., Akbari, H., Sotiras, A., et al.: Segmentation labels and radiomic features for the pre-operative scans of the TCGA-LGG collection. The Cancer Imaging Archive (2017). https://doi.org/10.7937/K9/TCIA.2017.GJQ7R0EF
8. Curtin, S., Minino, A., Anderson, R.: Declines in cancer death rates among children and adolescents in the united states, 1999-2014. National Center for Health Statistics Data Brief (2016)
9. Dosovitskiy, A., Beyer, L., Kolesnikov, A., et al.: An image is worth 16x16 words: transformers for image recognition at scale. arXiv preprint arXiv:2010.11929 (2020)
10. Fathi Kazerooni, A., Arif, S., Madhogarhia, R., et al.: Automated tumor segmentation and brain tissue extraction from multiparametric MRI of pediatric brain tumors: a multi-institutional study. Neuro-Oncol. Adv. **5**(1), vdad027 (2023)
11. Hatamizadeh, A., Nath, V., Tang, Y., et al.: Swin UNETR: Swin transformers for semantic segmentation of brain tumors in MRI images. In: Crimi, A., Bakas, S. (eds.) Brainlesion: Glioma, Multiple Sclerosis, Stroke and Traumatic Brain Injuries, pp. 272–284. Springer, Cham (2022). https://doi.org/10.1007/978-3-031-08999-2_22
12. Hatamizadeh, A., Tang, Y., Nath, V., et al.: UNETR: transformers for 3D medical image segmentation. In: IEEE/CVF Winter Conference on Applications of Computer Vision (WACV), pp. 574–584 (2022)
13. Isensee, F., Jaeger, P.F., Kohl, S.A., et al.: nnU-Net: a self-configuring method for deep learning-based biomedical image segmentation. Nat. Methods **18**(2), 203–211 (2021)
14. Jiang, Z., Parida, A., Anwar, S.M., et al.: Automatic visual acuity loss prediction in children with optic pathway gliomas using magnetic resonance imaging. In: 2023 45th Annual International Conference of the IEEE Engineering in Medicine & Biology Society (EMBC), pp. 1–5 (2023)
15. Karargyris, A., Umeton, R., Sheller, M., et al.: Federated benchmarking of medical artificial intelligence with MedPerf. Nat. Mach. Intell. **5**, 799–810 (2023)
16. Kazerooni, A.F., Khalili, N., Liu, X., et al.: The Brain Tumor Segmentation (BraTS) Challenge 2023: Focus on Pediatrics (CBTN-CONNECT-DIPGR-ASNR-MICCAI BraTS-PEDs) (2023)
17. Kofler, F., Meissen, F., Steinbauer, F., et al.: The Brain Tumor Segmentation (BraTS) Challenge 2023: Local Synthesis of Healthy Brain Tissue via Inpainting (2023)
18. LaBella, D., Adewole, M., Alonso-Basanta, M., et al.: The ASNR-MICCAI Brain Tumor Segmentation (BraTS) Challenge 2023: Intracranial Meningioma (2023)
19. Li, H.B., Conte, G.M., Anwar, S.M., et al.: The Brain Tumor Segmentation (BraTS) Challenge 2023: Brain MR Image Synthesis for Tumor Segmentation (BraSyn) (2023)

20. Liu, X., Bonner, E., Jiang, Z., et al.: Automatic segmentation of rare pediatric brain tumors using knowledge transfer from adult data. In: 20th IEEE International Symposium on Biomedical Imaging (2023)
21. Menze, B.H., Jakab, A., Bauer, S., et al.: The multimodal brain tumor image segmentation benchmark (BRATS). IEEE Trans. Med. Imaging **34**(10), 1993–2024 (2015). https://doi.org/10.1109/TMI.2014.2377694
22. Moawad, A.W., Janas, A., Baid, U., et al.: The Brain Tumor Segmentation (BraTS-METS) Challenge 2023: Brain Metastasis Segmentation on Pre-treatment MRI (2023)
23. Parida, A., Capellan-Martin, D., Atito, S., et al.: DiCoM–diverse concept modeling towards enhancing generalizability in chest X-ray studies. arXiv:2402.15534 (2024)
24. Rashed, W.M., Maher, E., Adel, M., et al.: Pediatric diffuse intrinsic pontine glioma: where do we stand? Cancer Metastasis Rev. **38**(4), 759–770 (2019)
25. Rohlfing, T., Zahr, N.M., Sullivan, E.V., Pfefferbaum, A.: The SRI24 multichannel atlas of normal adult human brain structure. Hum. Brain Mapp. **31**(5), 798–819 (2010)
26. Ronneberger, O., Fischer, P., Brox, T.: U-Net: convolutional networks for biomedical image segmentation. In: Navab, N., Hornegger, J., Wells, W.M., Frangi, A.F. (eds.) MICCAI 2015. LNCS, vol. 9351, pp. 234–241. Springer, Cham (2015). https://doi.org/10.1007/978-3-319-24574-4_28
27. Tang, Y., Yang, D., Li, W., Roth, H.R., et al.: Self-supervised pre-training of swin transformers for 3D medical image analysis. In: Proceedings of the IEEE/CVF Conference on Computer Vision and Pattern Recognition, pp. 20730–20740 (2022)

Synthesis of Healthy Tissue Within Tumor Area via U-Net

Juexin Zhang, Ke Chen, and Ying Weng(✉)

University of Nottingham Ningbo China, Ningbo 315100, China
`ying.weng@nottingham.edu.cn`

Abstract. This paper demonstrates our contributions to the task of 'Synthesis (Local) - Inpainting, BraTS 2023 Challenge'. We propose a U-Net like model for synthesizing the healthy 3D brain tissue from the masked input with the aim to synthesize the healthy brain magnetic resonance imaging (MRI) scans from the pathological ones. To enhance our model's generalizability and robustness, we work out a coherent strategy for data augmentation by generating randomly masked healthy images during the training phase. Our model is trained on the BraTS-Local-Inpainting training set and has achieved an overall performance with an SSIM score of 0.811946, a PSNR score of 21.445863 and an MSE score of 0.009317 on the BraTS-Local-Inpainting validation set computed by the online evaluation platform Synapse. Meanwhile, our model also has relatively low standard deviations for these three evaluation metrics, i.e. 0.113501 for SSIM score, 3.444001 for PSNR score and 0.006453 for MSE score. Our approach has ranked the first place in the testing phase on the outstanding performance with an SSIM score of 0.885162, a PSNR score of 23.849556, and an impressively low MSE score of 0.005523. The standard deviations for these three evaluation metrics in the test dataset are 0.102514 for SSIM score, 3.921114 for PSNR score, and 0.004766 for MSE score, respectively.

Keywords: Healthy Tissue Synthesis · BraTS 2023 · U-Net · Inpainting

1 Introduction

Brain is a vital organ containing 100 billion nerve cells, or neurons. According to data collected by Global Cancer Statistics 2022 [3], brain tumors are one of the deadliest cancers worldwide with a death rate at about 80% and also one of the most common type of cancers [4]. Brain tumors also result in significantly high cost at treatment. According to [6], the average cost of a craniotomy is $10,042 and the total cost of imaging for the duration of brain tumor care reaches a mean value at $2788 ± 3719 depending on the imaging technique used. Moreover, the surgery cost of the recurrent disease has an average value at $27,442 ± 18,992.

J. Zhang and K. Chen—Contribute equally to this work.

© The Author(s), under exclusive license to Springer Nature Switzerland AG 2024
U. Baid et al. (Eds.): crossMoDA 2023/BraTS 2023, LNCS 14669, pp. 233–240, 2024.
https://doi.org/10.1007/978-3-031-76163-8_21

For the diagnosis and monitoring of the treatment of brain tumors, medical imaging is one of the most promising and fastest way, where magnetic resonance imaging (MRI) is the most preferred one among medical imaging methods as it produces precise and detailed images [1]. With the rapid development of artificial intelligence (AI), there are many AI-based methods developed to assist clinicians in the brain tumor care. The Brain Tumor Segmentation (BraTS) Challenge is held annually by the Medical Image Computing and Computer Assisted Intervention Society (MICCAI) [2,10], which also leads the brain tumor segmentation to be one of the most popular research directions for AI-based methods applied to brain tumors.

Though there are lots of AI-based methods applied to brain tumors, these methods mostly rely on the standard input, equivalently the standard pre-processed images. A large number of automatic brain MRI analysis tools can be used to pre-process the raw images, for instance, FMRIB's Software Library (FSL) [7], Statistical parametric mapping (SPM) [11], FreeSurfer [5], etc. These tools are developed based on healthy brain scans while for patients with brain tumors, the time serial image acquisition process usually begins with scans that are already pathological, which might lead to bias in the image pre-processing and cannot guarantee images of lesions [9]. More specifically, the direct usage of brain pathological images can affect the pre-process results by introducing bias in procedures including but not limited to brain registration to standard space, skull removal, brain anatomy segmentation, tissue segmentation and brain extraction, which would further affect the latter prediction made by AI-based methods as well as clinicians' decision making.

A more reasonable way is to synthesize healthy brain images from the pathological images and further use the synthesized healthy images to obtain the parameters and masks to apply into the pathological images. In this paper, we propose a U-Net like model to synthesize 3D healthy brain tissue in the area affected by glioma. The problem is casted as inpainting within the tumor area according to the 'Synthesis (Local) - Inpainting, BraTS 2023 Challenge' [9]. In summary, our major contributions are:

- We proposed a U-Net like model to synthesizing 3D healthy brain tissue in the area affected by glioma.
- We applied a variety of data augmentation methods to enhance the model's generalizability.

The remainder of the paper is organized as follows: The BraTS dataset and the methodologies related to the U-Net like model are described in Sect. 2. Section 3 presents the experimental methods of the proposed model, whereas the paper is concluded in Sect. 4.

2 Methods

2.1 Dataset

The dataset used for training, validating, and testing our model is the BraTS-Local-Inpainting dataset [9] from the BraTS Challenge 2023. This dataset contains only T1 MRI scans from the multi-modal BraTS 2022 segmentation challenge. It includes 1251 scans along with truth annotations of tumorous regions approved by expert neuroradiologists. The sub-regions are united to a single area of interest and dilated to account for mass effect. Healthy regions are determined by a mask generation algorithm described in [9]. It is worth noting that the healthy masks are transformed using random mirroring and rotation. The resultant MRI volumes and associated masks are of shape $240 \times 240 \times 155$. There are four different types of data in the training set:

- t1n: The ground truth image, which includes all tissue.
- t1n-voided: Images that have had the healthy and unhealthy tissue removed.
- healthy mask: A mask that identifies the healthy tissue in the t1n image.
- unhealthy mask: A mask that identifies the tumor region in the t1n image.
- mask: A mask that combines the healthy and unhealthy masks.

2.2 Pre-processing

The BraTS 2022 dataset underwent basic preprocessing steps, including co-registration to the same anatomical template, isotropic resampling to $1\,\mathrm{mm}^3$ resolution, and skull-stripping. In our method, we further cropped the MRI scans and masks to a size of $128 \times 128 \times 96$. Notably, we integrate our model's inferences on cropped patches with the original t1-weighted MRI image through a stitching process to obtain the final output. We first normalized the images to $[0, 1]$ by dividing each image by its maximum value, and then normalized them to $[-1, 1]$.

2.3 Data Augmentation

Deep learning models with a large number of parameters are prone to overfitting and may generalize poorly to unseen data. To overcome these problems, we generated five healthy masks for each MRI scan according to the healthy inpainting mask generation algorithm in [9]. It is worth noting that the mask generation algorithm employs random mirroring and rotation to augment the data. Random mirroring is applied independently to each dimension with a 50% probability, and a random angle between 0° and 360° is used for both the X-Y and Y-Z planes. Despite some overlap between different healthy masks of each MRI scan, the augmented data helps train a more generalized model because of the variation in mask shape, location, and size.

2.4 Network Architecture

To synthesize healthy tissues, we used the U-Net architecture [12] as our model. The architecture of our U-Net is presented in Fig. 1. The model consists of three types of blocks: downsampling blocks, bridge blocks, and upsampling blocks. Each block contains two 3D convolutional layers with a kernel size of 3. The

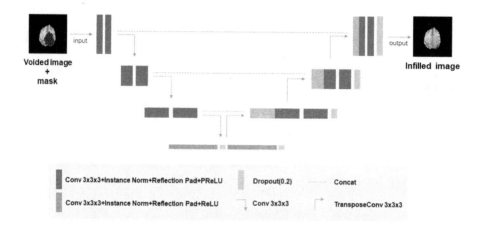

Fig. 1. U-Net

activation functions are ReLU in the bridge block and PReLU in the downsampling/upsampling blocks. Instance normalization is used to normalize the data for each MRI scan. Both bridge block and upsample block contains dropout to prevent overfitting issue. Our model has three downsampling/upsampling blocks and one bridge block. The first downsampling block has 32 channels, and the number of channels doubles in each subsequent downsampling block. In contrast, the number of channels in each upsampling block is half the number of channels in the corresponding downsampling block. We also applied skip connections to pass different levels of features from the downsampling blocks to the upsampling blocks. Our model takes t1n-voided images and masks as input and output infilled images. There are two loss functions applied to train our model: mean absolute error (MAE) and structural similarity index measure (SSIM) [13] loss. We only compute the MAE between the healthy regions of the ground truth image GT and the infilled image I, while the SSIM is computed for the entire images. The loss functions are defined as follow:

$$MAE(x,y) = \frac{1}{m}\sum_{i=1}^{m}|y_i - f(x_i)| \qquad (1)$$

$$SSIM(x,y) = \frac{(2\mu_x\mu_y + c_1)(2\sigma_{xy} + c_2)}{(\mu_x^2 + \mu_y^2 + c_1)(\sigma_x^2 + \sigma_y^2 + c_2)} \qquad (2)$$

$$Loss(I, GT) = \lambda_1 \times MAE(I, GT) + \lambda_2 \times SSIM(I, GT) \qquad (3)$$

3 Experiment Results

3.1 Evaluation Metrics

To measure the performance of our model, we evaluate the generated healthy regions using three metrics: structural similarity index measure (SSIM), peak-signal-to-noise-ratio (PSNR), and mean-square-error (MSE). It is worth noting that we only evaluate the healthy regions against the ground truth data.

3.2 Experiment Settings

In our experiments, we use 5-fold cross-validation to select hyperparameters during training. We set the maximum number of epochs to 500 and early stop training when the validation loss no longer decreases. We set the dropout rate equal to 0.2 in the bridge block and upsample block. In validation phase, we applied Adam optimizer with initial learning rate $1e^{-4}$ and betas $(0.9, 0.999)$ and we set λ_1 and λ_2 to 1 in our loss function. In testing phase, we also train models with λ_1 set to 1 and λ_2 set to 0. We normalize the healthy mask region to a range of $[0, 1]$ based on the maximum value of the healthy and unhealthy regions of the ground truth image in validation phase, as well as by clipping to the 0.5–99.5 percentile value of the region outside the healthy mask of the ground truth image when calculating an MAE loss in testing phase. The model is implemented with PyTorch and all experiments are conducted on a single Nvidia RTX 3090 with 24GB VRAM. The top five model checkpoints for each setting are saved. We only use the best model to generate infilled images in validation phase, while we average the infilled images generated by all saved models in testing phase.

3.3 Validation Phase

We present the overall results of our model on the BraTS-Local-Inpainting validation dataset in Table 1. The evaluation metric values were computed by the online evaluation platform of Sage Bionetworks Synapse (Synapse). We also visualize the best, median, and worst infilled results of our model on the validation set in Fig. 2. However, the ground truth data is not visible in the validation phase or test phase, so we cannot visualize the ground truth data to compare with our infilled images. Additionally, the orange areas are mask areas that include both healthy and unhealthy tissues, but our aim is to only infill the healthy tissues, so only the healthy areas are evaluated. From the visualization, we have found that our model is able to capture low-level textures and synthesize brain tissues well. The structure of the infilled areas also very similar to the surrounding areas. However, the infilled areas appear blurry, especially in the low-intensity areas in Fig. 2(c) and 2(c). The blurry problem may be caused by the MAE loss, which averages the error over the entire image. This can lead to the model smoothing out the image in order to minimize the error, even if this means sacrificing detail.

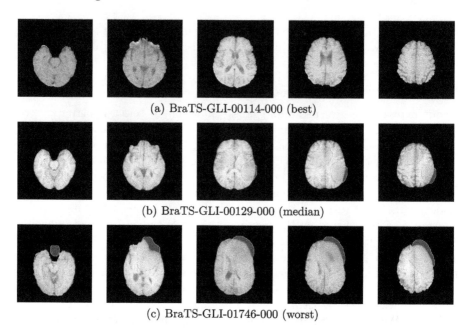

Fig. 2. Visualization of the infilled validation MRI scans. In the images, the orange portions represent the masked regions containing both healthy and unhealthy tissues, since they were not explicitly labeled in the validation dataset. During the validation phase, our model's performance has been exclusively assessed using healthy tissue segments. (a) has achieved an SSIM score of 0.998026252, a PSNR score of 33.18456268 and an MSE score of 0.000480335. (b) has achieved an SSIM score of 0.756804347, a PSNR score of 20.88445473 and an MSE score of 0.00815745. (c) has achieved an SSIM score of 0.671889424, a PSNR score of 14.22145939 and an MSE score of 0.037831534. In (b) and (c), we selected the scans with the median and lowest values of MSE and PSNR scores, which are not corresponding to the median and lowest values of SSIM scores.

Table 1. Overall validation data results

	MSE	PSNR	SSIM
Mean	0.00931688	21.4458628	0.811946301
Standard deviation	0.006452887	3.444001017	0.113501218
25 quantile	0.004899009	18.47534084	0.697519034
Median	0.00815745	20.88445473	0.820237577
75 quantile	0.012397069	23.689291	0.890722066

3.4 Test Phase

As shown in Table 2, we report our model's overall performance on the test set. The results of the top 3 teams are shown in Table 3 and our approach has achieved the first place in the BraTS 2023 inpainting challenge. It is worth mentioning that the specific scores for individual files are not disclosed. Additionally, due to the restricted access to the test dataset, we have executed our model's inferences through the MedPerf platform [8]. Hence, we do not have the infilled images of test data and cannot provide visualizations of the results. Despite the lack of visual evidence for the test dataset's results, it is evident that our model exhibits strong performance and generalizability on unseen inputs.

Table 2. Overall test data results

	MSE	PSNR	SSIM
Mean	0.00552301584925574	23.849555907115132	0.8851618572649821
Standard deviation	0.00476571414306412	3.9211143702311837	0.10251383295001223
25 quantile	0.00213325023651117	21.185830593109127	0.8240863978862762
Median	0.0043738612439483	23.323928833007812	0.9143267273902893
75 quantile	0.00731270492542527	26.154579162597656	0.969466969370842

Table 3. Top 3 of the BraTS 2023 inpainting Challenge. Our approach has ranked the first place in the testing phase.

	MSE	PSNR	SSIM
Ying-Weng-Team (Ours)	**0.00552302**	**23.84955591**	**0.88516186**
Domaso	0.01147546	20.17632638	0.82712242
MedSegCTRL	0.01737461	18.79448767	0.83428928

4 Conclusion

This paper presents our contributions to the task of 'Synthesis (Local) - Inpainting, BraTS 2023 Challenge'. A U-Net like model has been proposed to synthesize the healthy 3D brain tissue. Multiple data augmentations have been applied, including random healthy mask generation, random mirroring and rotation. Our derived model is trained on the BraTS-Local-Inpainting training set and its performance on the BraTS-Local-Inpainting validation set computed by the online evaluation platform Synapse has been shown in Table 1. Remarkably, our method has achieved an SSIM score of 0.811946, a PSNR score of 21.445863 and an MSE score of 0.009317. Meanwhile, our model also has a relatively low standard deviation for the three evaluation metrics, i.e., 0.113501 for SSIM score, 3.444001 for PSNR score and 0.006453 for MSE score. Our proposed solution has secured the top place in the test phase, and achieved the outstanding results with an SSIM score of 0.885162, a PSNR score of 23.849556, and a minuscule MSE score of 0.005523. It is noteworthy that the respective standard deviations for these three evaluation metrics in the test set are 0.102514 for SSIM score, 3.921114 for PSNR score, and 0.004766 for MSE score, respectively.

Acknowledgements. This work was supported by Ningbo Major Science & Technology Project under Grant 2022Z126.

References

1. Agravat, R.R., Raval, M.S.: A survey and analysis on automated glioma brain tumor segmentation and overall patient survival prediction. Arch. Comput. Methods Eng. **28**, 4117–4152 (2021)
2. Bakas, S., et al.: Advancing the cancer genome atlas glioma MRI collections with expert segmentation labels and radiomic features. Sci. Data **4**(1), 1–13 (2017)
3. Chhikara, B.S., Parang, K.: Global cancer statistics 2022: the trends projection analysis. Chem. Biol. Lett. **10**(1), 451–451 (2023)
4. Das, S., Nayak, G.K., Saba, L., Kalra, M., Suri, J.S., Saxena, S.: An artificial intelligence framework and its bias for brain tumor segmentation: a narrative review. Comput. Biol. Med. **143**, 105273 (2022)
5. Fischl, B.: Freesurfer. Neuroimage **62**(2), 774–781 (2012)
6. Goel, N.J., Bird, C.E., Hicks, W.H., Abdullah, K.G.: Economic implications of the modern treatment paradigm of glioblastoma: an analysis of global cost estimates and their utility for cost assessment. J. Med. Econ. **24**(1), 1018–1024 (2021)
7. Jenkinson, M., Beckmann, C.F., Behrens, T.E., Woolrich, M.W., Smith, S.M.: FSL. Neuroimage **62**(2), 782–790 (2012)
8. Karargyris, A., et al.: Federated benchmarking of medical artificial intelligence with medperf. Nat. Mach. Intell. **5**(7), 799–810 (2023)
9. Kofler, F., et al.: The brain tumor segmentation (brats) challenge 2023: local synthesis of healthy brain tissue via inpainting. arXiv preprint arXiv:2305.08992 (2023)
10. Menze, B.H., et al.: The multimodal brain tumor image segmentation benchmark (brats). IEEE Trans. Med. Imaging **34**(10), 1993–2024 (2014)
11. Penny, W.D., Friston, K.J., Ashburner, J.T., Kiebel, S.J., Nichols, T.E.: Statistical parametric mapping: the analysis of functional brain images. Elsevier (2011)
12. Ronneberger, O., Fischer, P., Brox, T.: U-Net: convolutional networks for biomedical image segmentation. In: Navab, N., Hornegger, J., Wells, W.M., Frangi, A.F. (eds.) MICCAI 2015. LNCS, vol. 9351, pp. 234–241. Springer, Cham (2015). https://doi.org/10.1007/978-3-319-24574-4_28
13. Wang, Z., Bovik, A.C., Sheikh, H.R., Simoncelli, E.P.: Image quality assessment: from error visibility to structural similarity. IEEE Trans. Image Process. **13**(4), 600–612 (2004)

Bridging the Gap: Generalising State-of-the-Art U-Net Models to Sub-Saharan African Populations

Alyssa R. Amod[1,2]( ), Alexandra Smith[3], Pearly Joubert[4],
Confidence Raymond[5,6], Dong Zhang[7], Udunna C. Anazodo[5,6,8,9],
Dodzi Motchon[4], Tinashe E. M. Mutsvangwa[4], and Sébastien Quetin[10,11]

[1] Brain Behaviour Unit, Neuroscience Institute, University of Cape Town, Cape Town, South Africa
amdaly001@myuct.ac.za
[2] ShockLab, Department of Mathematics and Applied Mathematics, University of Cape Town, Cape Town, South Africa
[3] Applied Mathematics Division, Stellenbosch University, Stellenbosch, South Africa
[4] Division of Biomedical Engineering, Neuroscience Institute, University of Cape Town, Cape Town, South Africa
[5] Medical Artificial Intelligence Lab, Lagos, Nigeria
[6] Lawson Health Research Institute, London, ON, Canada
[7] Department of Electrical and Computer Engineering, University of British Columbia, Vancouver, Canada
[8] Montreal Neurological Institute, McGill University, Montréal, Canada
[9] Department of Medicine and Department of Clinical and Radiation Oncology, University of Cape Town, Cape Town, South Africa
[10] Medical Physics Unit, Department of Oncology, McGill University, Montréal, Canada
[11] Montreal Institute for Learning Algorithms, Montréal, Canada

Abstract. A critical challenge for tumour segmentation models is the ability to adapt to diverse clinical settings, particularly when applied to poor quality neuroimaging data. The uncertainty surrounding this adaptation stems from the lack of representative datasets, leaving top-performing models without exposure to common artefacts found in MRI data throughout Sub-Saharan Africa (SSA). We replicated a framework that secured the 2nd position in the 2022 BraTS competition to investigate the impact of dataset composition on model performance and pursued four distinct approaches through training a model with various combinations of the BraTS-Africa and BraTS-Adult Glioma datasets. Notably, training on the smaller low-quality BraTS-Africa dataset alone yielded subpar results, and training on the larger high-quality BraTS-Adult Glioma dataset alone struggled to delineate oedematous tissue in the low-quality validation set. The most promising approach involved pre-training a model on high-quality neuroimages and then fine-tuning it on the smaller low-quality dataset. This approach took second place in the MICCAI BraTS Africa global challenge external testing phase. These findings underscore the significance of larger sample sizes and broad exposure to data in improving segmentation performance. Furthermore, we demonstrated there is potential for improving such models by fine-tuning them with a wider range of data locally.

Keywords: Sub-Saharan Africa · Brain Tumour Segmentation · MRI · Deep Learning · U-Net

1 Introduction

The burden of cancer continues to rise each year, disproportionately affecting low and middle-income countries (LMICs) due to limited access to imaging technologies as well as specialists, which are crucial for early diagnosis and successful treatment [1, 2]. Accurate tumour segmentation provides essential information for treatment decisions, thereby impacting patient survival rate [3, 4]. Among intracranial tumours, gliomas are highly heterogeneous, and their prognosis remains poor despite considerable progress in the field of neuro-oncology [5–7]. Gliomas have varied shapes, sizes, boundaries, intensity distributions, and volume fluctuations, which all pose a challenge for accurate segmentation using magnetic resonance imaging (MRI) [8]. MRI is the standard of care and preferred modality for brain tumor imaging [9].

Despite its advantages, various challenges still need to be addressed in low-resource settings, specifically, within sub-Saharan Africa (SSA), such as limited access to highfield MRI scanners and a shortage of qualified experts to acquire, analyze, and interpret MRI data, which leads to delayed tumour diagnosis [5, 10]. This, coupled with the relatively poor healthcare systems, socio-economic status, and the usual late presentation of disease in SSA, worsens prognosis and sustain the high mortality rates in SSA [1]. These factors continue to drive the growing demand for access to early diagnosis and timely interventions for intracranial tumours. The development of accurate automatic brain tumour segmentation models that can perform well across varying clinical settings therefore holds significant importance on a global scale.

The field of brain tumour segmentation has evolved considerably in recent decades, aiming to overcome limitations such as reliance on domain expertise, subjectivity, or sensitivity to noise and intensity non-homogeneity [12, 13]. Machine learning techniques, specifically deep learning, are at the forefront of this domain, demonstrating significant improvement in terms of segmentation precision between the tumorous tissue, surrounding oedema and normal tissue [14–16]. A combination of convolutional neural networks (CNNs) and autoencoders is currently the best approach and has gradually reduced the dependence on domain expertise and complex feature extraction methods [17]. Specifically, the U-Net model has established itself as a gold-standard in automated brain tumour segmentation tasks [18, 19]. Several adaptations of the U-Net have been proposed to further improve efficiency, accuracy, and generalisability [20–23]. However, large neuroimaging datasets required for the generalisation of deep learning models are limited in the medical field, due to both ethical concerns, and data privacy regulations [24].

Since its establishment, the Brain Tumour Segmentation (BraTS) Challenge[1] has witnessed a remarkable surge in globally contributed brain patient data derived from multi-parametric (mp-)MRI scans; comprising the largest annotated publicly available

---

[1] Initiated 2012, in collaboration with the Medical Image Computing and Computer Assisted Interventions (MICCAI) Society.

brain tumour dataset in 2023, with ~4,500 cases [25]. The community-developed benchmark for automated brain tumour segmentation fostered through this collaboration has significantly contributed to the development of novel architectures and refined training procedures within the domain [3, 14, 23, 26]. However, despite promising performance, it is still uncertain whether these top performing methods can be effectively applied to data obtained from SSA populations, where the quality of MR images remain poor [11, 29]. This is largely due to a lack of representative datasets compounded by vast differences in image acquisition parameters across settings, which create challenges for generalisation [17]. Current benchmarks are primarily based on high-resolution brain MRI obtained in standard resource-rich clinical settings in high-income countries, incorporating image pre-processing steps that may not expose models to artefacts commonly seen in routine clinical scans from SSA [30].

A key framework currently at the forefront is the nnU-Net developed by Isensee and colleagues [27], which provides a robust tumour segmentation pipeline capable of adapting to various imaging modalities and anatomical structures [28]. This framework demonstrates improved efficacy through ensembling predictions from different U-Net based architectures, with emphasis on the importance of modelling decisions such as pre-processing, data augmentation pipelines, and hyper-parameter tuning approaches. Recently, Zeineldin and colleagues [31] demonstrated that an expectation-maximisation ensemble of the DeepSeg, the nnU-Net, and the Deep-SCAN U-Net based pipelines performs well on a small external test dataset from SSA; achieving Dice score coefficients (DSC) of 0.9737, 0.9593, and 0.9022, for the whole tumour (WT), tumour core (TC) and enhancing tumour (ET), respectively, and Hausdorff distance (95%) (HD95) scores below 3.32 for all sub-regions. However, testing on an external dataset with similar characteristics to the training data did not perform as well, and the difference between validation results for their ensemble approach and the independent run of a nnU-Net based model was minuscule (~0.005, $U = 6.0$, $p = 0.7$). This may further emphasise that a simpler framework with more aggressive data augmentations and carefully selected post-processing methods are likely to play a significant role in developing models that achieve similar performance across a variety of datasets and that can be applied readily in low-resource settings. The former is particularly important for increasing relevant data representations during model training [32].

This year for the first time, the BraTS challenge was expanded to include multimodal MRI training data from low-resource settings. In this work, we examined the extent to which established U-Net tumour segmentation frameworks can train with and generalize to MRI data from low-resource settings to their lower resolution and data quality, and the feasibility of implementing such frameworks with limited resources. Given the challenge's goal of creating a versatile benchmark model, we prioritised establishing comparable metrics with top performing methods as a reference point rather than introducing complex augmentations. Our strategy was to replicate a BraTS Challenge benchmark model [37] to investigate the influence of training data composition on the segmentation predictions of an external dataset comprised solely of low-resolution data.

2 Methods

2.1 Data Description

The datasets used in this study were derived from the BraTS 2023 Challenge data. The training, validation and testing datasets comprised of mp-MRI scans from a total 1565 pre-operative adult glioma patients with 1470 from pre-exiting BraTS data (BraTS-Adult Glioma) as described in previous works [3, 25, 26, 30], and an additional 95 cases from SSA (BraTS-Africa) [11]. These are typical clinical scans obtained from various institutions as part of standard care, leading to significantly diverse imaging quality. Each case included a T1-weighted (T1), post-gadolinium contrast T1-weighted (T1Gd), T2-weighted (T2) and T2 Fluid Attenuated Inversion Recovery (T2-FLAIR). Figure 1 illustrates sample slices obtained from volumes of a patient from each dataset, emphasising the substantial variations in data quality between BraTS-Adult Glioma and BraTS-Africa. The BraTS-Africa dataset was collected through a collaborative network of imaging centres in Africa, with support from the Consortium for Advancement of MRI Education and Research in Africa (CAMERA)[2] and funding from the Lacuna Fund in Health Equity[3]. In each case, image-based ground truth annotations of the tumour sub-regions were generated and approved through an iterative process [11]. Refinement occurred through manual review by volunteers, two expert radiologists, and final approval for release was provided by an expert neuro-radiologist. These tumour sub-regions are radiological features and do not reflect strict biological entities [11, 25]. They include enhancing tumour (ET; label = 3), peritumoral oedematous tissue (ED; label = 2), and the necrotic core (NCR; label = 1), while the voxels not annotated are considered as background (label = 0).

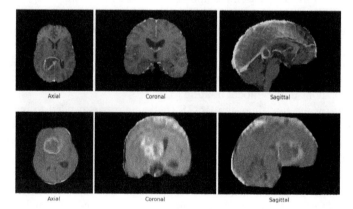

Fig. 1. Axial, coronal, and sagittal slices of T1Gd MRIs from the high-resolution BraTS-Adult Glioma dataset (*top*) and the low-resolution BraTS-Africa dataset (*bottom*).

---

[2] https://www.cameramriafrica.org/.
[3] https://lacunafund.org.

2.2 Selecting a Framework

Since the development of the nnU-Net pipeline [27], it has undergone several revisions which primarily focused on the training parameters rather than the architecture itself. Table 1 (rows 1–3) shows challenge results for the original nnU-Net model from 2017, and revised models submitted by Isensee et al. in subsequent BraTS challenges, where it placed 2nd in 2018 [33] and 1st in 2020 [34]. The nnU-Net effectively addresses the challenges of manually accounting for co-dependencies when making design changes and selecting the best performing ensemble (see further [28]). However, some teams participating in the BraTS challenge in 2021 [35, 36] and 2022 [31, 37] demonstrated that the basic 3D U-Net component of nnU-Net could be optimised to achieve good performance on brain tumour segmentation tasks, without the need to run the full ensemble of networks encompassed in the nnU-Net pipeline. A comparison of results (see Table 1, rows 4–7 showing external validation results) produced by these teams primarily shows that there is minor difference in overall model performance when sample size remains the same. In comparison to the varied performance seen in the three nnU-Net submissions trained with different smaller sample sizes, this may further highlight the importance of the sample size used for training segmentation models and its effect on model performance.

Table 1. BraTS Challenge results: final test scores for nnU-Net trained with different samples, and validation set scores for nnU-Net based models trained with the same sample[a].

Year [ref.][b]	N	Model	Ave DSC (*HD95*)	WT DSC (*HD95*)	TC DSC (*HD95*)	ET DSC (*HD95*)
2017 [27]	285	nnU-Net	82.1 *(-)*	85.8 *(-)*	77.5 *(-)*	64.7 *(-)*
2018 [33]	285[c]	nnU-Net	84.33 *(5.64)*	87.81 *(6.03)*	80.62 *(5.08)*	77.88 *(2.90)*
2020 [34]	369	nnU-Net	85.35 *(14.55)*	88.95 *(8.50)*	85.06 *(17.34)*	82.03 *(17.81)*
2021 [35]	1251	3D U-Net	91.56 *(1.72)*	94.86 *(1.41)*	94.25 *(1.73)*	90.81 *(2.00)*
2021 [36]	1251	3D U-Net + attention	88.36 *(10.61)*	92.75 *(3.47)*	87.81 *(7.62)*	84.51 *(20.73)*
2022 [31]	1251	Ensemble	88.21 *(9.54)*	92.71 *(3.60)*	87.53 *(7.53)*	84.38 *(17.50)*
2022 [37]	1251	3D U-Net	88.25 *(7.96)*	92.92 *(3.59)*	88.02 *(5.84)*	83.81 *(14.46)*

[a]Results obtained from published papers, except [35], which is obtained from the Synapse online evaluation platform for 2021; [b] Year of BraTS challenge and citation. [c] Final model submitted was co-trained with external dataset ($N = 484$).

Our selection took into account both simplicity and efficacy, as easy replication in resource-limited environments would be more beneficial for translation to local settings in the long term. In addition to sample size, Futrega et al. [35] demonstrated that alterations to network architecture make little difference in terms of overall tumour segmentation performance. Specifically, they show that varying network layers (e.g., residual connections, multi-head self-attention) or integrating different architectures (e.g., a residual U-Net with an autoencoder or a vision transformer with basic U-Net) remain comparable with a basic 3D U-Net architecture (mean Dice score across sub-regions ranging ~0.002) [35]. This is further supported by a comparison of the ensemble models in [31] and [36], which show no significant difference between the nnU-Net pipeline and their ensemble results ($p > 0.7$). We therefore chose to implement the framework outlined by Futrega and colleagues from their 2022 BraTS challenge participation and we refer the reader to both their original paper [35], and their recently released paper [37], which details the full pipeline of the framework.

2.3 Data Pre-processing

All data were provided after initial pre-processing by the challenge organisers to ensure the removal of all protected health information prior to the public sharing of data. The BraTS standardised pipeline detailed in [3, 25] was used, and pre-processing steps included conversion of the DICOM files to NifTI format, to strip all personal patient metadata from headers; skull stripping, to deface neuroimaging scans; co-registration to the SRI24 anatomical template; and finally, resampling to a uniform 1mm3 isotropic resolution (see also [11]). We then implemented several additional pre-processing steps as outlined by the OptiNet pipeline [35]. These steps included: stacking the volumes from all modalities; cropping the redundant background voxels, to reduce computational cost; normalisation of the non-zero regions; and, adding a foreground one hot encoding channel, to differentiate between tumorous and non-tumorous regions. This resulted in a final input tensor of shape (5,240,240,155) with channels representing the four modalities and the one-hot encoding layer.

2.4 OptiNet Pipeline and Experiments

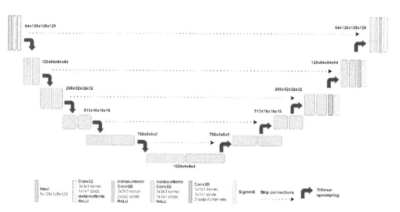

Fig. 2. Tuned OptiNet model architecture replicated from [37].

OptiNet primarily adjusts the nnU-Net framework in terms of modelling choices related to pre-processing of data, data augmentations implemented, loss function applied (region-based, summing binary cross-entropy and Dice loss), and several post-processing steps. Data augmentations applied included both spatial transforms (random crop of size 128 × 128 × 128, random flip) and intensity related transforms (Gaussian noise, Gaussian blur, changes in brightness) and were implemented during training. Yousef et al.

[38] provides a detailed review of the basic U-Net architecture: briefly, it consists of a contracting (encoder) and an expansive (decoder) path that are used for down sampling and up sampling, respectively. In the OptiNet version, the encoder, made up of a standard CNN, partners with a decoder that combines feature maps from convolutional layers and trilinear up-sampling. Cropped volumes of size 128 × 128 × 128 with preserved context undergo skip connections to reduce information loss between the encoder and decoder, aiding the decoder in restoring image resolution and spatial structure. Figure 2 depicts the model architecture used in our experiments, reproduced from the open access notebooks provided[4]. Futrega et al. [37] include minor architectural changes (e.g., channel sizes, up sampling technique) to the default U-Net architecture from nnU-Net. A full review of all architectural and non-architectural tweaks explored by Futrega and colleagues are detailed in their 2021 [35] and 2022 [37] papers. Notably, their results showed only a slight increase in mean Dice score when combining some of these changes with the additional one-hot encoding channel (~0.0026, $p = 0.5$; see Table 3 in [35]).

We ran four experiments using the OptiNet pipeline by varying the composition of the training dataset. We trained these models with 1) BraTS-Africa data only (*train_SSA*, N = 60), 2) BraTS-Adult Glioma data only (*train_GLI*, N = 1251), 3) both datasets together (*train_ALL*, N = 1311), and 4) through further training the *train_GLI* model with BraTS-Africa data (*train_ftSSA*). The *train_ftSSA* model was included to obtain an estimate of the feasibility of exporting pre-trained benchmark models for fine-tuning locally in Africa. All trainings and validations were conducted with Pytorch 1.9 on a high-performance computing cluster provided by Compute Canada, using one GPU of either NVIDIA T4 Turing (16 GB GDDR6 memory) or NVIDIA V100 Volta (16 GB/32 GB HBM2 memory), depending on the availability on the cluster. All trainings were performed with an internal validation procedure, using a split of the training dataset. Due to time and computational constraints, we trained models containing the larger BraTS-Adult Glioma dataset for 100 epochs on one-fold each. For models containing only the smaller BraTS-Africa dataset (*train_SSA* and *train_ftSSA*), training was set for a maximum of 150 epochs per fold with a 5-fold cross validation and an early stopping strategy when there was no improvement in DSC on internal validation in 100 epochs. Checkpoints giving best overall mean DSC on the internal validation set of each fold were used for external validation predictions for each experiment (Table 2).

3 Results

Below we describe the performance metrics obtained for each of the 4 training variations, with validation scores computed through the challenge online evaluation system. Metrics provided by the system (see Table 3) are lesion-wise dice score coefficients (DSC) and Hausdorff distance (95%) (HD95) averaged across the 15 patient samples provided for the BraTS-Africa 2023 validation phase. No ground truth segmentations are provided; however, the small size of the dataset allowed for a more detailed review of the generated segmentation masks for all validation subjects. The figures presented in this section show the segmentations we generated from our models on selected validation cases. All

---

[4] https://github.com/NVIDIA/DeepLearningExamples/tree/master/PyTorch/Segmentation/nnUNet.

Table 2. Mean Dice scores across sub-regions from 5-fold cross validation comparing training results of OptiNet models [35, 37] and our models.

5-fold CV	OptiNet 2021	OptiNet 2022	train_SSA	train_ALL	train_GLI	train_ftSSA
Fold 0	91.18	91.48	93.48	90.64	90.18	89.83
Fold 1	91.41	91.5	88.64	-	-	92.62
Fold 2	91.76	92.17	89.35	-	-	95.04
Fold 3	92.68	92.74	89.62	-	-	93.64
Fold 4	90.76	91.05	82.15	-	-	87.30
Mean Dice	**91.56**	**91.79**	**88.65**	**90.64**	**90.18**	**91.69**

segmentations are represented by the non-biological labels provided for annotation as described earlier, where ED is green, ET is blue, NCR is red.

Table 3. Segmentation performance on BraTS-Africa validation set ($N = 15$)[a].

Model	DSC				HD95			
	Average	WT	TC	ET	Average	WT	TC	ET
train_SSA	59.11 (31.65)	61.34 (31.52)	58.94 (31.70)	57.05 (31.74)	130.15 (126.56)	126.31 (128.30)	126.34 (127.46)	137.80 (123.92)
train_ALL	78.93 (24.14)	77.43 (28.53)	79.71 (22.45)	79.65 (21.45)	45.21 (88.18)	66.76 (111.23)	35.25 (76.39)	33.62 (76.92)
train_GLI	80.04 (20.89)	74.68 (25.04)	82.18 (21.10)	83.27 (16.54)	39.75 (74.17)	77.13 (94.61)	23.07 (63.99)	19.05 (63.92)
train_ftSSA	82.18 (21.68)	90.81 (12.59)	79.58 (24.78)	76.14 (27.67)	38.65 (76.77)	14.66 (47.99)	42.26 (82.57)	59.04 (99.73)

[a] Metrics reported as mean (*standard deviation*) among different cases of the validation set.

As expected, training a model with only 60 samples (*train_SSA*) is not sufficient, and most validation segmentations were obtained at a chance level (50%). To provide performance estimates on similar data as well as a comparison for other training set compositions, the low-resolution naive *train_GLI* model was submitted for validation in both Task 1 (BraTS-Adult Glioma) and Task 2 (BraTS-Africa). Despite being trained only for 100 epochs on one-fold, this model performed relatively well on the Task 1 validation dataset comprised of 219 glioma patients in terms of performance metrics (mean DSC of 79.81, 82.12, 78.48 and HD95 of 54.04, 28.80, 42.90 for WT, TC and ET, respectively). Average performance metrics across tumour sub-regions achieved on Task 2 validation data were good. As the intention was to use this as a pre-trained base to further train with SSA data, and inspection of internal validation loss indicated it was stabilising, we deemed the model sufficient for subsequent fine-tuning with BraTS-Africa data. Fine-tuning of the trained BraTS-Adult Glioma data with the BraTS-Africa data across a 5-fold training procedure resulted in a similar mean Dice score across sub-regions.

Further investigation of sub-region performance showed that despite the same mean DSC, the *train_GLI* and *train_ftSSA* models had varied performance for different sub-regions. The *train_GLI* model struggled with delineating the WT from non-tumour tissue, with 40% of cases achieving below chance DSCs. Conversely, the *train_ftSSA* model appeared to do well in this region, but struggled with the ET regions, with 26% of subjects scoring below chance. The ET sub-region is traditionally the most difficult to precisely segment given its size and overlap with surrounding sub-regions. The HD95 also provides a clearer indication of a model's ability to delineate sub-regions, as it better estimates performance on small or low-quality segmentations and when contours are important. Looking at differences in these scores, we see that the *train_ftSSA* model on average was able to predict the whole tumour boundary much better (HD95~63 units lower) than the *train_GLI* model. Conversely, the *train_GLI* model is, on average, better able to delineate ET sub-region than *train_ftSSA* does (HD95~40 units lower). Figure 3 shows two cases where these differences are clearly seen.

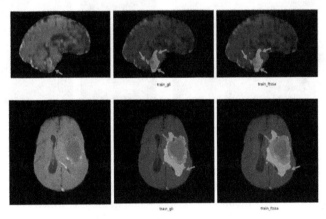

Fig. 3. T1Gd of two cases highlighting segmentation differences in ED (green) and ET (blue). (Color figure online)

Two outlier cases were identified. In the first case, all models struggled to accurately segment the TC sub-region (mean DSC ranging 22.33–49.04) likely due to the confounding presence of ET and TC like voxel intensities within the oedematous tissue in the posterior region of the cortex. This case heavily influenced the *train_ftSSA* scores more than the other models: removing this outlier resulted in DSC increases by 4.13 and 3.43 (with a corresponding drop in HD95 by 13.04 and 8.04) for ET and TC sub-regions, respectively (see Table 4). Furthermore, this outlier also demonstrated improvements in sub-region performance of both ET and TC for the *train_SSA* and *train_ALL* models, albeit weaker than with *train_ftSSA*. Only performance in the TC sub-region was impacted in the *train_GLI* model. The second case consistently demonstrated extremely poor segmentation results for all models with mean DSC across sub-regions ranging 35.40–37.02 and HD95 229.37–229.89, as shown in Fig. 4.

Table 4. Differences in Dice (DSC) and Hausdorff95 (HD95) after excluding outlier case.

Model	DSC				HD95			
	Ave	WT	TC	ET	Ave	WT	TC	ET
train_SSA	1.01	−2.43	2.62	2.84	−1.51	8.82	−5.94	−7.41
train_ALL	1.05	−1.26	2.19	2.23	1.10	4.57	−0.66	−0.61
train_GLI	**0.25**	−1.43	**2.38**	−0.20	**1.67**	5.31	**−1.50**	1.21
train_ftSSA	**2.40**	−0.35	**3.43**	**4.13**	**−11.61**	0.87	**−8.04**	**−13.04**

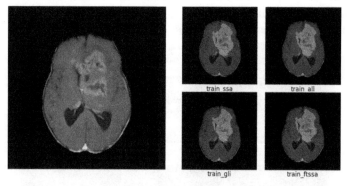

Fig. 4. T1Gd of outlier case where poor performance was seen across models for all labels.

Figure 5 depicts a subject for which extremely good scores were obtained on the ET and TC segmentations (mean DSC > 89 and HD95 < 2.00) but not for the WT region. Traditionally, it is more difficult to precisely segment the ET, which is usually a small region. The whole tumour itself should be more easily identifiable. Mean DSC (HD95) achieved was 72.22 (9.273), 0.125 (285.335), 41.33 (190.082) and 89.49 (1.414) for each model depicted in panel 1 from left to right, respectively. Visually we see that most models primarily struggled with delineating oedematous tissue (ED), of which there is very little.

In reviewing the performance of all models, we also considered that the whole tumour comprises oedematous tissue, which is harder to differentiate in low-resolution scans. It is likely that without being exposed to the low-quality data from SSA, the *train_GLI* model struggled to precisely identify the boundaries of tumours with extensive oedema. We therefore submitted the model pre-trained with the larger BraTS-Adult Glioma dataset and further trained on the smaller SSA dataset (*train_ftSSA*)[5].

---

[5] The code and docker file used for final submission can be found at: https://github.com/CAMERA-MRI/SPARK2023/tree/main/SPARK_UNN.

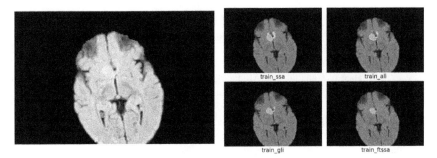

Fig. 5. T2-FLAIR showing varied ED (green) segmentation across all models.

This model performed well on an unseen external test dataset comprised of 20 patients with scans from SSA, ranking 2nd globally. Final mean DSC (and HD95) scores achieved in the testing phase were 84.37 (48.33), 80.65 (55.79), and 78.12 (60.66) for the WT, TC and ET sub-regions, respectively. The model demonstrated exceptional performance with nearly 100% specificity across all sub-regions, showcasing its robust ability to accurately identify tumour regions. However, sensitivity indices indicated challenges were observed in accurately delineating the TC (88.16%) and ET (88.37%) sub-regions, in comparison to the WT (94.25%). These results highlight the model's effectiveness in overall segmentation, with notable performance variations across different tumor sub-regions.

4 Discussion

Taken together, the results from our experiments emphasise that current state-of-the-art models cannot be implemented directly to SSA data, as the limited training data available will result in overfitting the model. Our final model performed extremely well with a single pre-training fold of 100 epochs and fine-tuning with a 5-fold cross-validation. Futrega et al. [37] demonstrated that a 10-fold cross validation allows for more accurate segmentation performance. We only validated 5 folds for *train_SSA* and *train_ftSSA* and did not run cross-validation on the *train_ALL* and *train_GLI* models. It is therefore likely that more extensive cross-validation could yield a more accurate comparison between each model. Yet, the high-ranking performance of our final model reiterates what has been previously demonstrated in simulated cases [39]: state-of-the-art models can be improved with a wider range of data through federated learning, providing opportunity for institutes in low-resource setting to re-train on a smaller set of local data without the need for obtaining data from external sources. However, these results need to be interpreted with caution, as they may be confounded by the limited sample size of the BraTS-Africa training and validation datasets. Furthermore, going forward, future works should involve both integrating more extensive datasets sourced from various regions within Africa and implementing stronger data augmentations related to scanner artefacts when training on high quality MRI scans. These steps are vital to the development of a model capable of generalising across image qualities seen in varied clinical settings.

Acknowledgements. This work was supported by the Lacuna Fund for Health and Equity (PI: Udunna Anazodo, 0508-S-001) and the National Science and Engineering Research Council of Canada (NSERC) Discovery Launch Supplement (PI: Udunna Anazodo, DGECR-2022-00136). The authors gratefully acknowledge the computational infrastructure support provided by the Digital Research Alliance of Canada (The Alliance) and the knowledge translation support through the McGill University Doctoral Internship program. The authors would like to express their appreciation to the global instructors who contributed to the Sprint AI Training for African Medical Imaging Knowledge Translation (SPARK) Academy and Africa-BraTS BrainHack2023 training initiatives. Special thanks go to Linshan Liu for administrative support to the SPARK Academy training and capacity building activities, from which the authors benefited. Finally, the authors extend their gratitude to the McMedHacks team for their continuous support throughout the program, including the provision of foundational programming material and their efforts in enabling in-person training.

Author Contributions. ARA & AS: Conceptualisation, Methodology, Software, Validation, Formal Analysis, Investigation, Writing, Visualisation; PJ: Writing - Review & Editing, Visualisation, Statistics; CR, DZ, & UA: Funding Acquisition, Project Administration, Resources, Data Curation, Conceptualisation, Writing - Review & Editing; DM & TEMM: Resources, Writing - Review & editing; SQ: Supervision, Conceptualisation, Software, Writing - Review & Editing.

References

1. Shah, S.C., Kayamba, V., Peek, R.M., Heimburger, D.: Cancer control in low- and middle-income countries: is it time to consider screening? JGO 1–8 (2019). https://doi.org/10.1200/JGO.18.00200
2. Pramesh, C.S., et al.: Priorities for cancer research in low- and middle-income countries: a global perspective. Nat. Med. **28**, 649–657 (2022). https://doi.org/10.1038/s41591-022-01738-x
3. Bakas, S., et al.: Advancing the cancer genome atlas glioma MRI collections with expert segmentation labels and radiomic features. Sci. Data **4**, 170117 (2017). https://doi.org/10.1038/sdata.2017.117
4. Williams, S., et al.: Artificial intelligence in brain tumour surgery—an emerging paradigm. Cancers **13**, 5010 (2021). https://doi.org/10.3390/cancers13195010
5. Aderinto, N., AbdulBasit Opeyemi, M., Opanike, J., Afolayan, O., Sakaiwa, N.: Navigating the challenges of neuro-oncology in Africa: addressing diagnostic and treatment barriers in the region: a correspondence. Int. J. Surg. Glob. Health **6**, e136–e136 (2023). https://doi.org/10.1097/GH9.0000000000000136
6. Bray, F., et al.: Cancer in sub-Saharan Africa in 2020: a review of current estimates of the national burden, data gaps, and future needs. Lancet Oncol. **23**, 719–728 (2022). https://doi.org/10.1016/S1470-2045(22)00270-4
7. Soomro, T.A., et al.: Image segmentation for MR brain tumor detection using machine learning: a review. IEEE Rev. Biomed. Eng. **16**, 70–90 (2023). https://doi.org/10.1109/RBME.2022.3185292
8. Naser, M.A., Deen, M.J.: Brain tumor segmentation and grading of lower-grade glioma using deep learning in MRI images. Comput. Biol. Med. **121**, 103758 (2020). https://doi.org/10.1016/j.compbiomed.2020.103758
9. Ranjbarzadeh, R., Caputo, A., Tirkolaee, E.B., Jafarzadeh Ghoushchi, S., Bendechache, M.: Brain tumor segmentation of MRI images: a comprehensive review on the application of

artificial intelligence tools. Comput. Biol. Med. **152**, 106405 (2023). https://doi.org/10.1016/j.compbiomed.2022.106405
10. Anazodo, U.C., et al.: The consortium for advancement of MRI education and research in Africa (CAMERA): a framework for advancing sustainable magnetic resonance imaging access in Africa. NMR Biomed. **36**, e4846 (2023). https://doi.org/10.1002/nbm.4846
11. Adewole, M., et al.: The Brain Tumor Segmentation (BraTS) Challenge 2023 (2023)
12. Wadhwa, A., Bhardwaj, A., Singh Verma, V.: A review on brain tumor segmentation of MRI images. Magn. Reson. Imaging **61**, 247–259 (2019). https://doi.org/10.1016/j.mri.2019.05.043
13. Fawzi, A., Achuthan, A., Belaton, B.: Brain image segmentation in recent years: a narrative review. Brain Sci. **11**, 1055 (2021). https://doi.org/10.3390/brainsci11081055
14. Aggarwal, M., Tiwari, A.K., Sarathi, M.P.: Comparative analysis of deep learning models on brain tumor segmentation datasets: BraTS 2015–2020 datasets. RIA **36**, 863–871 (2022). https://doi.org/10.18280/ria.360606
15. Shal, K., Choudhry, M.S.: Evolution of deep learning algorithms for MRI-based brain tumor image segmentation. Crit. Rev. Biomed. Eng. **49**, 77–94 (2021). https://doi.org/10.1615/CritRevBiomedEng.2021035557
16. Wagner, M.W., Namdar, K., Biswas, A., Monah, S., Khalvati, F., Ertl-Wagner, B.B.: Radiomics, machine learning, and artificial intelligence—what the neuroradiologist needs to know. Neuroradiology **63**, 1957–1967 (2021). https://doi.org/10.1007/s00234-021-02813-9
17. Jyothi, P., Singh, A.R.: Deep learning models and traditional automated techniques for brain tumor segmentation in MRI: a review. Artif. Intell. Rev. **56**, 2923–2969 (2023). https://doi.org/10.1007/s10462-022-10245-x
18. Magadza, T., Viriri, S.: Deep learning for brain tumor segmentation: a survey of state-of-the-art. J. Imaging **7**, 19 (2021). https://doi.org/10.3390/jimaging7020019
19. Krishnapriya, S., Karuna, Y.: A survey of deep learning for MRI brain tumor segmentation methods: trends, challenges, and future directions. Health Technol. **13**, 181–201 (2023). https://doi.org/10.1007/s12553-023-00737-3
20. Armstrong, T.R.E., Manimegalai, P., Abinath, A., Pamela, D.: Brain tumor image segmentation using deep learning. In: 2022 6th International Conference on Devices, Circuits and Systems (ICDCS), pp. 48–52. IEEE, Coimbatore, India (2022). https://doi.org/10.1109/ICDCS54290.2022.9780707
21. Cheng, J., Liu, J., Kuang, H., Wang, J.: A fully automated multimodal MRI-based multi-task learning for glioma segmentation and IDH genotyping. IEEE Trans. Med. Imaging **41**, 1520–1532 (2022). https://doi.org/10.1109/TMI.2022.3142321
22. Battalapalli, D., Rao, B.V.V.S.N.P., Yogeeswari, P., Kesavadas, C., Rajagopalan, V.: An optimal brain tumor segmentation algorithm for clinical MRI dataset with low resolution and non-contiguous slices. BMC Med Imaging **22**, 89 (2022). https://doi.org/10.1186/s12880-022-00812-7
23. Mehta, R., et al.: QU-BraTS: MICCAI BraTS 2020 challenge on quantifying uncertainty in brain tumor segmentation – analysis of ranking scores and benchmarking results. Melba **1**, 1–54 (2022). https://doi.org/10.59275/j.melba.2022-354b
24. Cirillo, M.D., Abramian, D., Eklund, A.: What is the best data augmentation for 3D brain tumor segmentation? In: 2021 IEEE International Conference on Image Processing (ICIP), pp. 36–40. IEEE, Anchorage, AK, USA (2021). https://doi.org/10.1109/ICIP42928.2021.9506328
25. Baid, U., et al.: The RSNA-ASNR-MICCAI BraTS 2021 benchmark on brain tumor segmentation and radiogenomic classification (2021). http://arxiv.org/abs/2107.02314
26. Menze, B.H., et al.: The multimodal brain tumor image segmentation benchmark (BRATS). IEEE Trans. Med. Imaging. **34**, 1993–2024 (2015). https://doi.org/10.1109/TMI.2014.2377694

27. Isensee, F., Kickingereder, P., Wick, W., Bendszus, M., Maier-Hein, K.H.: Brain Tumor Segmentation and Radiomics Survival Prediction: Contribution to the BRATS 2017 Challenge (2018). http://arxiv.org/abs/1802.10508
28. Isensee, F., Jaeger, P.F., Kohl, S.A.A., Petersen, J., Maier-Hein, K.H.: nnU-Net: a self-configuring method for deep learning-based biomedical image segmentation. Nat. Methods **18**, 203–211 (2021). https://doi.org/10.1038/s41592-020-01008-z
29. Mollura, D.J., et al.: Artificial intelligence in low- and middle-income countries: innovating global health radiology. Radiology **297**, 513–520 (2020). https://doi.org/10.1148/radiol.2020201434
30. Bakas, S., et al.: Identifying the best machine learning algorithms for brain tumor segmentation, progression assessment, and overall survival prediction in the BRATS Challenge (2019). http://arxiv.org/abs/1811.02629
31. Zeineldin, R.A., Karar, M.E., Burgert, O., Mathis, F.: Multimodal CNN networks for brain tumor segmentation in MRI: A braTS 2022 challenge solution (2022)
32. Atya, H.B., Rajchert, O., Goshen, L., Freiman, M.: Non parametric data augmentations improve deep-learning based brain tumor segmentation. In: 2021 IEEE International Conference on Microwaves, Antennas, Communications and Electronic Systems (COMCAS), pp. 357–360. IEEE, Tel Aviv, Israel (2021). https://doi.org/10.1109/COMCAS52219.2021.9629083
33. Isensee, F., Kickingereder, P., Wick, W., Bendszus, M., Maier-Hein, K.H.: No New-Net (2019). http://arxiv.org/abs/1809.10483. https://doi.org/10.48550/arXiv.1809.10483
34. Isensee, F., Jaeger, P.F., Full, P.M., Vollmuth, P., Maier-Hein, K.H.: nnU-Net for brain tumor segmentation http://arxiv.org/abs/2011.00848 (2020)
35. Futrega, M., Milesi, A., Marcinkiewicz, M., Ribalta, P.: Optimized U-Net for brain tumor segmentation, http://arxiv.org/abs/2110.03352 (2021)
36. Luu, H.M., Park, S.-H.: Extending nnU-Net for brain tumor segmentation, http://arxiv.org/abs/2112.04653 (2021)
37. Futrega, M., Marcinkiewicz, M., Ribalta, P.: Tuning U-Net for brain tumor segmentation. In: Bakas, S., et al. (eds.) Brainlesion: Glioma, Multiple Sclerosis, Stroke and Traumatic Brain Injuries, pp. 162–173. Springer, Cham (2023)
38. Yousef, R., et al.: U-Net-based models towards optimal MR brain image segmentation. Diagnostics **13**, 1624 (2023). https://doi.org/10.3390/diagnostics13091624
39. Zhang, D., Confidence, R., Anazodo, U.: Stroke lesion segmentation from low-quality and few-shot MRIs via similarity-weighted self-ensembling framework. In: Wang, L., Dou, Q., Fletcher, P.T., Speidel, S., Li, S. (eds.) Medical Image Computing and Computer Assisted Intervention – MICCAI 2022. MICCAI 2022. Lecture Notes in Computer Science, vol. 13435. Springer, Cham (2022). https://doi.org/10.1007/978-3-031-16443-9_9

nnUNet for Brain Tumor Segmentation in Sub-Saharan Africa Patient Population

Valeriia Abramova[✉], Uma M. Lal-Trehan Estrada, Cansu Yalçın, Rachika E. Hamadache, Albert Clèrigues, Francisco Aarón Tovar Sáez, Marc Guirao, Joaquim Salvi, Arnau Oliver, and Xavier Lladó

Computer Vision and Robotics Group, University of Girona, Girona, Spain
`valeriia.abramova@udg.edu`

Abstract. Glioma is one of the most dangerous and aggressive brain tumor types. These tumors are difficult to diagnose, and they require careful and precise identification and delineation of different tumor subtypes. Currently, magnetic resonance imaging (MRI) is the gold standard for glioma detection. However, not all the territories are equipped with up-to-date medical devices and highly skilled professionals, and it is important to develop glioma segmentation methods for the images acquired in such low-resource settings. Therefore, BraTS-Africa challenge was announced in 2023 to provide researchers the opportunity to develop segmentation algorithms using brain MRI glioma cases from Sub-Saharan Africa population. In this paper, we present our submission to this challenge. We based our approach on the well-known nnUNet model, which won original BraTS 2020 and 2021 challenges. Within our work, we studied the impact of using pretrained and fine-tuned models, different image input modalities, ensemble of different models, and the application of specific region based strategies. Obtained results on the unseen testing data showed promising results, having good Dice values for all 3 classes and a small HD95 distance.

Keywords: Brain tumor segmentation · nnUNet · Sub-Saharan Africa

1 Introduction

Brain tumors rank among the most aggressive types of cancer. Specifically, glioma is the most common brain tumor type, comprising nearly 80% of malignant brain tumors [8]. Such tumors are hard to diagnose and treat, and patients with glioma have an average prognosis of 15 months following standard treatment [3]. Currently, magnetic resonance imaging (MRI), including T2-weighted, T2-weighted fluid-attenuated inversion recovery (FLAIR) and 3D T1-weighted sequences before and after application of a gadolinium-based contrast agent, is considered the gold standard for detecting brain tumors [14]. Useful pathological features, which are helpful in detecting and analyzing glioma, can be extracted from these images. Therefore, it is crucial to accurately identify and segment the different sub-regions of the brain tumor for precise patient diagnosis.

Computer-aided diagnosis (CAD) tools for automatic brain tumor segmentation are rapidly developing and evolving, showing promising results [8]. Since 2012, the Brain Tumor Segmentation (BraTS) Challenge focus on improving automatic glioma segmentation state-of-the-art algorithms, linking researchers from all over the world to the solution of this problem [3,4,10]. Each year, a big open-source dataset of multiparametric MRI images together with the ground-truth annotations is provided to the participants for developing their research and comparing their algorithms.

Globally, such automated solutions can be a great help for low-resource settings, e.g. in territories with limited technical resources or with lack of highly skilled experts. Specifically, the development of these techniques can be very beneficial for low- and middle-income countries, like the region of Sub-Saharan Africa (SSA), where the above limitations are mostly observed. However, the current BraTS dataset mainly consists of high quality images acquired from major clinical and research institutions in high-income countries. Therefore, it is interesting to find out if the methods developed using this dataset can be transferred to the SSA, considering that images acquired there have typically lower resolution and contrast, and also that the disease might be present in late advanced stages, presenting unique characteristics inherent in the SSA population [1].

For this reason, in 2023 one of the tracks of BraTS challenge is the so called BraTS-Africa Challenge, which provides an opportunity to use brain MRI glioma cases from Sub-Saharan Africa to develop and evaluate lesion segmentation methods in resource-limited settings, where the potential for CAD tools to transform healthcare is higher [2].

In this work we present an approach based on the well-known nnUNet framework [5]. We started studying the impact of using pretrained and fine-tuned models from the work of [9], the use of different image input modalities, the creation of ensemble of different models, and the development of specific region based strategies. Our evaluation done with a 5-fold cross-validation on the training set and the results obtained on the online validation set produced promising results, providing competitive Dice values for all the classes and some of the smallest HD95 distances.

2 Methods

2.1 Data

The dataset provided for the challenge consists of pre-operative multiparametric MRI scans of glioma acquired using conventional brain tumor imaging protocols; the images were acquired from different institutions and scanners, hence the dataset is of heterogeneous image quality and characteristics [1].

The provided MRI scans for BraTS-Africa 2023 challenge include 4 modalities 1: T1-weighted (T1), post gadolinium contrast T1-weighted (T1Gd), T2-weighted (T2), and T2 Fluid Attenuated Inversion Recovery (T2-FLAIR). The preprocessing protocol follows the same steps as original BraTS challenge, comprising conversion of the images to NIfTI format, registration of all images to

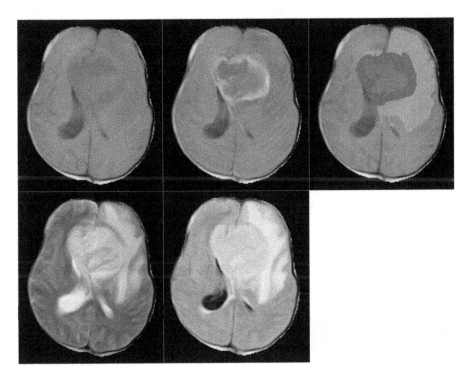

Fig. 1. An example of a patient from the BraTS-Africa dataset. The following MRI modalities are included in the challenge (from left to right): top row: T1-weighted (T1), post-contrast T1-weighted (T1Gd), T1 with groundtruth labels overlayed. Bottom row: T2-weighted (T2), T2 Fluid Attenuated Inversion Recovery (T2-FLAIR). The groundtruth labels are: enhancing tumor (ET, blue), non-enhancing tumor core (NETC, red), and surrounding non-enhancing FLAIR hyperintensity (SNFH, green). (Color figure online)

a template, resampling to a uniform isotropic resolution ($1mm^3$), and finally skull-stripped [1]. The ground truth annotations were done in a semi-automatic way, where initial segmentations were generated from an nnUNet pretrained on BraTS 2021 dataset [12], and then were manually refined by expert radiologists. The labelling of the challenge is consistent with the one of BraTS 2023, and includes 3 labels (Fig. 1): the enhancing tumor, which includes tumor areas that have noticeable increase in T1 signal on postcontrast images compared to precontrast images; the non-enhancing tumor core, which includes the part of tumor core that does not enhance; and the surrounding non-enhancing FLAIR hyperintensity, which is the entire extent of FLAIR signal abnormality around the tumor that is not part of the tumor core.

BraTS-Africa 2023 also allows its participants to use the dataset from the original BraTS glioma segmentation challenge for the development of the algorithms. This dataset contains 1251 multiparametric MRI scans of the same

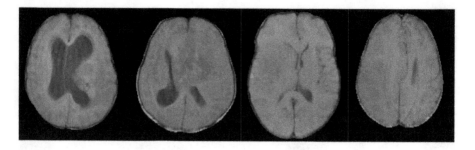

Fig. 2. Examples of MRI imaging artifacts on T1 images from BraTS-Africa 2023.

modalities and preprocessing steps as the BraTS-Africa dataset. As this dataset is much bigger, it can be beneficial to use it for pretraining a segmentation model, which can be then fine-tuned to the BraTS-Africa problem. In our approach, we check if this helps the model to better convergence to an optimal solution for BraTS-SSA dataset, or in contrast, it moves the gradients away from an optimal solution, due to the intrinsic differences of the datasets. As mentioned by the challenge organizers [1], the images of the BraTS-Africa challenge are of lower quality and resolution; moreover, a lot of cases of this dataset include imaging artifacts, as shown in Fig. 2, which makes the problem even more challenging. However, in this work we do not put our main effort into preprocessing the images and improving their quality, even though this could be a point for consideration in future work.

2.2 Model

U-Net architecture [11,13] proved itself effective in biomedical segmentation problems. It also showed great potential in different segmentation challenges, including BraTS, where the majority of top-ranked or winning submissions were based on the U-Net model [7]. nnUNet [5] is an extension of the traditional U-Net architecture and it was also extensively used for the glioma segmentation problem within the BraTS challenge, providing winning solutions for BraTS 2020 and 2021 [6,9].

Following these results, we also decided to utilize nnUNet as our main approach. We used the same baseline nnUNet configuration as in [9]. Online data augmentation was applied, and consisted of random rotation and scaling, gamma scaling, elastic deformation, and additive brightness augmentation. The loss function used was the sum of the binary cross-entropy loss and the batch Dice loss, which was calculated over all samples in the batch for better regularization, as proposed in [6]. The nnUNet was optimized with stochastic gradient descent with Nesterov momentum of 0.99 and with initial learning rate set to 0.01, which was decayed following a polynomial schedule as in [9]. The number of epochs in each training was set to 1000.

In our work, we analyzed different settings for the nnUNet. Firstly, we started applying a pretrained nnUNet model for the original task of glioma segmentation from the winners of 2021 challenge [9] and ran inference directly on our provided dataset. Moreover, we also used the nnUNet pretrained on original BraTS glioma dataset and fine-tuned the last convolution layer using the BraTS-Africa dataset. We also trained from scratch a nnUNet model using only the provided BraTS-SSA dataset. Apart from these approaches, we also explored the use of different image modalities for training in order to improve the representation of the three classes. In addition, we tried to improve results for the individual NETC class by training a specific model only on this label. All this set of experiments were performed using a 5-fold cross-validation scheme and for inference in the online validation platform we submitted the ensemble of the resulting 5 models for generating our final predictions.

All the implementation of the approaches and the experiments were conducted using PyTorch 1.13.1 on NVIDIA A30 GPU with 24 GB RAM.

3 Results

3.1 Metrics

The BraTS-Africa 2023 challenge utilizes new performance metrics called lesion-wise Dice score and lesion-wise Hausdorff distance-95 (HD95) compared with previous BraTS. The goal of evaluating segmentation performance on a lesion level rather than the patient level is to understand how well can models distinguish between individual lesions within one patient and segment them. Therefore, the Dice score and HD95 are calculated individually per lesion and then averaged per particular patient. Moreover, prior to averaging, False Positives and False Negatives are penalized with 0 for Dice score and 374 for HD95. The lesion tissue sub-regions are isolated into the following labels: ET, corresponding to the initial ET, TC, which is enhancing tumor + non-enhancing tumor core, and WT, which incorporates all the provided labels.

3.2 Quantitative Results

As described before, different experimental tests were performed to choose the best configuration of the models and the final approach used for the testing phase of the BraTS-SSA challenge. The results obtained when using a 5-fold cross-validation over the training set are shown on the top rows of Table 1, while middle rows show the results obtained when testing the validation set, that were computed by averaging the outputs from the 5 models.

From these initial results, we observed that fine-tuned models provided better predictions for validation cases, whereas the opposite applied to the training cases. Moreover, we noticed that the Dice score was significantly lower for the TC class compared to the other labels, while its HD95 was also much higher.

With the idea to improve the performance on the TC class, we considered two different approaches: 1) providing better inputs for the models, so that TC class could be better distinguishable in the images, and 2) training a separated

Table 1. Results of training nnUNet with different configurations for training cases (5-fold cross-validation), for validation dataset (results obtained after submission), and for test set.

	Lesion-wise Dice score ↑			Lesion-wise HD95 ↓		
	5-fold cross-validation on 60 training cases					
	ET	TC	WT	ET	TC	WT
Trained from scratch	0.67 ± 0.32	0.19 ± 0.31	0.83 ± 0.23	86.93 ± 122.32	294.18 ± 122.49	43.72 ± 86.21
Fine-tuned model	0.62 ± 0.32	0.05 ± 0.09	0.77 ± 0.30	93.14 ± 128.09	351.20 ± 37.48	68.73 ± 114.836
	Inference on validation cases					
Trained from scratch	0.74 ± 0.32	0.31 ± 0.33	0.79 ± 0.29	72.27 ± 125.90	249.08 ± 134.45	64.56 ± 114.62
Fine-tuned model	0.79 ± 0.24	0.28 ± 0.36	0.80 ± 0.23	11.24 ± 32.60	230.90 ± 166.81	28.17 ± 64.86
Separate models for TC and ET&SNFH	0.79 ± 0.24	0.79 ± 0.25	0.80 ± 0.23	11.09 ± 32.61	13.83 ± 32.60	28.16 ± 64.86
	Inference on test cases					
Separate models for TC and ET&SNFH	0.77 ± 0.26	0.82 ± 0.27	0.84 ± 0.23	34.86 ± 97.00	33.81 ± 90.78	42.01 ± 90.45

and specific model only able to detect and segment the non-enhancing tumor core class and then combine the predictions with the ET and SNFH predictions from another model.

The challenge description paper [1] gives information about the input modalities and the different target classes (see also Fig. 1): enhancing tumor (ET) have noticeable signal increase in T1ce compared to T1, whereas for NETC it is the opposite - it does not enhance after admission of the contrast agent. Therefore, we could use the difference image of T1ce and T1 for learning these two classes, and it is also worth to mention that such subtraction image was provided to the expert radiologists for creating annotations for the challenge [1]. Moreover, SNFH is the extent of FLAIR signal abnormality, so this modality could be helpful in our experiments as well. Therefore, we trained an nnUNet model just using these two input modalities: T1ce-T1 and FLAIR. The results of these experiment showed that the Dice score increased for both TC and ET class, which suggested that the difference image was helpful for correctly identifying enhancing and non-enhancing tumor core. However, we observed a big drop in results for the HD95 metric. Therefore, this configuration of using only these two input modalities was not used for our final approach.

We also decided to train a separate nnUNet model for TC class only, specifically for the NETC class, using the initial notation of the challenge. As this class can contain many components (e.g. necrosis, cystic change, calcification, etc.), some of which can be very small and distant, we wanted to train a more sensitive model to obtain more TP voxels for this class. Hence, we trained the same nnUNet with all 4 provided image modalities, but only for the NETC class. An example of the obtained results can be seen in Fig. 3. The red arrow shows a sublesion of NETC class which exists in the ground truth and which was segmented by the model trained on this label separately. However, when the model

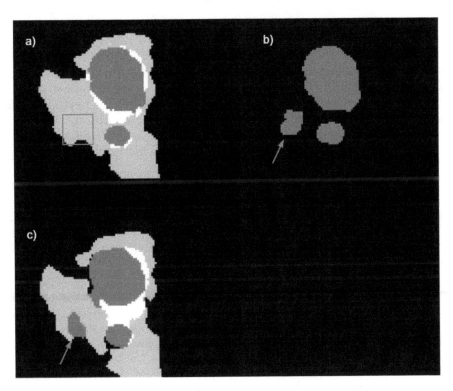

Fig. 3. Example of segmentation obtained by training on NETC label only. a) shows segmentation obtained when nnUNet is trained on all the provided labels; b) is the prediction of a model trained only on NETC class; and c) is the groundtruth image. The arrow shows the improvement of using the specific class-learning.

was trained on all the labels together, it missed this lesion part and assigned to another label. This suggested us that the separate prediction of NETC part could be helpful for improving overall results.

Considering all the experiments performed, we decided to combine the predictions from two different ensemble models to improve the performance for each of the classes. We used the specific nnUNet model to get the NECT region and the outputs of an nnUNet trained on BraTS-glioma dataset [9] fine-tuned on the BraTS-SSA data to provide the predictions of the ET together with SNFH. This was actually the approach that provided better performance overall, achieving more robust results in all measures, especially HD95, and for all classes in the online validation dataset (see Table 1), with the mean Dice scores in validation set of 0.79, 0.79 and 0.80 for ET, TC and WT, respectively. Finally, we chose this configuration for the final evaluation on the unseen test set, obtaining the results presented in the last row of Table 1.

4 Discussion

In this work, we described our approach used for the BraTS-Africa 2023 challenge. We observed that the images provided for the challenge differ a lot from the cases of the original BraTS challenge, noticing also a strong intra-class variability in the images. The problem becomes even more difficult due to the fact that most of the images had poor quality and contained imaging artifacts. Therefore, working on the image quality improvement could also be an interesting point to improve results, however we did not focus on this line for the solution presented in this work.

As nnUNet has proven itself as a very effective medical image segmentation approach, being a winner in a lot of challenges, we chose it as a main model for our solution without trying to improve the architecture by adding new blocks. We mostly focused our solution on the way to feed the data to the network so to produce better segmentation results. We studied training with different modalities, training for a specific class and pretraining the network with a large dataset of glioma cases from the original BraTS challenge, being the best approach a combination of a specific nnUNet model for the NETC class with the results of a fine-tuned model from the BraTS-glioma dataset to provide the predictions of the ET together with SNFH. Our final approach produced robust results not only in the online validation phase but also in the unseen test evaluation both in terms of Dice and HD95 values.

Acknowledgements. Valeriia Abramova holds FPI grant from the Ministerio de Ciencia, Innovación y Universidades with reference number PRE2021-099121. Uma Maria Lal-Trehan Estrada holds an IFUdG2022 grant from Universitat de Girona. Cansu Yalçın holds an FI grant from the Catalan Government with reference number 2023 FI-1 00096. This work has been supported by DPI2020-114769RB-I00 from the Ministerio de Ciencia, Innovación y Universidades and also by the ICREA Academia program.

References

1. Adewole, M., et al.: The brain tumor segmentation (brats) challenge 2023: Glioma segmentation in sub-saharan Africa patient population (brats-africa) (2023). https://doi.org/10.48550/ARXIV.2305.19369. https://arxiv.org/abs/2305.19369
2. Anazodo, U.C., Adewole, M., Dako, F.: AI for population and global health in radiology. Radiology: Artif. Intell. **4**(4) (2022). https://doi.org/10.1148/ryai.220107
3. Baid, U., et al.: The rsna-asnr-miccai brats 2021 benchmark on brain tumor segmentation and radiogenomic classification (2021). https://doi.org/10.48550/ARXIV.2107.02314. https://arxiv.org/abs/2107.02314
4. Bakas, S., et al.: Advancing the cancer genome atlas glioma MRI collections with expert segmentation labels and radiomic features. Sci. Data **4**(1) (2017). https://doi.org/10.1038/sdata.2017.117
5. Isensee, F., Jaeger, P.F., Kohl, S.A.A., Petersen, J., Maier-Hein, K.H.: nnU-net: a self-configuring method for deep learning-based biomedical image segmentation. Nat. Methods **18**(2), 203–211 (2020). https://doi.org/10.1038/s41592-020-01008-z

6. Isensee, F., Jäger, P.F., Full, P.M., Vollmuth, P., Maier-Hein, K.H.: nnU-Net for brain tumor segmentation. In: Crimi, A., Bakas, S. (eds.) BrainLes 2020. LNCS, vol. 12659, pp. 118–132. Springer, Cham (2021). https://doi.org/10.1007/978-3-030-72087-2_11
7. Jiang, Z., Ding, C., Liu, M., Tao, D.: Two-stage cascaded U-Net: 1st place solution to BraTS challenge 2019 segmentation task. In: Crimi, A., Bakas, S. (eds.) BrainLes 2019. LNCS, vol. 11992, pp. 231–241. Springer, Cham (2020). https://doi.org/10.1007/978-3-030-46640-4_22
8. Luo, J., Pan, M., Mo, K., Mao, Y., Zou, D.: Emerging role of artificial intelligence in diagnosis, classification and clinical management of glioma. Semin. Cancer Biol. **91**, 110–123 (2023). https://doi.org/10.1016/j.semcancer.2023.03.006
9. Luu, H.M., Park, S.H.: Extending nn-UNet for brain tumor segmentation. In: Brainlesion: Glioma, Multiple Sclerosis, Stroke and Traumatic Brain Injuries, pp. 173–186. Springer, Heidelberg (2022). https://doi.org/10.1007/978-3-031-09002-8_16
10. Menze, B.H., et al.: The multimodal brain tumor image segmentation benchmark (BRATS). IEEE Trans. Med. Imaging **34**(10), 1993–2024 (2015). https://doi.org/10.1109/tmi.2014.2377694
11. Ronneberger, O., Fischer, P., Brox, T.: U-net: convolutional networks for biomedical image segmentation (2015). https://doi.org/10.48550/ARXIV.1505.04597. https://arxiv.org/abs/1505.04597
12. Sheller, M.J., et al.: Federated learning in medicine: facilitating multi-institutional collaborations without sharing patient data. Sci. Rep. **10**(1) (2020). https://doi.org/10.1038/s41598-020-69250-1
13. Çiçek, Ö., Abdulkadir, A., Lienkamp, S.S., Brox, T., Ronneberger, O.: 3d u-net: learning dense volumetric segmentation from sparse annotation (2016). https://doi.org/10.48550/ARXIV.1606.06650. https://arxiv.org/abs/1606.06650
14. Weller, M., et al.: EANO guidelines on the diagnosis and treatment of diffuse gliomas of adulthood. Nat. Rev. Clin. Oncol. **18**(3), 170–186 (2020). https://doi.org/10.1038/s41571-020-00447-z

Advanced Tumor Segmentation in Medical Imaging: An Ensemble Approach for BraTS 2023 Adult Glioma and Pediatric Tumor Tasks

Fadillah Maani[1]([✉]), Anees Ur Rehman Hashmi[1], Mariam Aljuboory[1,2], Numan Saeed[1], Ikboljon Sobirov[1], and Mohammad Yaqub[1]

[1] Mohamed bin Zayed University of Artificial Intelligence, Abu Dhabi, UAE
{fadillah.maani,anees.hashmi}@mbzuai.ac.ae
[2] Northwestern University, Evanston, IL, USA

Abstract. Automated segmentation proves to be a valuable tool in precisely detecting tumors within medical images. The accurate identification and segmentation of tumor types hold paramount importance in diagnosing, monitoring, and treating highly fatal brain tumors. The BraTS challenge serves as a platform for researchers to tackle this issue by participating in open challenges focused on tumor segmentation. This study outlines our methodology for segmenting tumors in the context of two distinct tasks from the BraTS 2023 challenge: Adult Glioma and Pediatric Tumors. Our approach leverages two encoder-decoder-based CNN models, namely SegResNet and MedNeXt, for segmenting three distinct subregions of tumors. We further introduce a set of robust post-processing to improve the segmentation, especially for the newly introduced BraTS 2023 metrics. The specifics of our approach and comprehensive performance analyses are expounded upon in this work. *Our proposed approach achieves third place in the* `BraTS 2023 Adult Glioma Segmentation Challenge` with an average of 0.8313 and 36.38 Dice and HD95 scores on the test set, respectively.

Keywords: BraTS · MRI · Glioma · Tumor Segmentation · BraTS-PEDs · Challenge · BraTS-adult

1 Introduction

Cancerous brain tumors are one of the deadliest types of central nervous system tumors [1], and they account for the highest number of cancer-related deaths in pediatrics. Glioma is a brain tumor that originates from glial cells, which provide structure and support to the nerve cells. Astrocytoma is the type of glioma that occurs in the astrocytes (a type of glial cells), which are responsible for a healthy brain environment. The treatment options for brain tumors include surgery,

---

F. Maani and A. U. R. Hashmi—Equal contribution.

© The Author(s), under exclusive license to Springer Nature Switzerland AG 2024
U. Baid et al. (Eds.): crossMoDA 2023/BraTS 2023, LNCS 14669, pp. 264–277, 2024.
https://doi.org/10.1007/978-3-031-76163-8_24

chemotherapy, and radiation therapy. Neurologists, oncologists, and radiologists work together to develop the treatment plan for patients. Magnetic Resonance Imaging (MRI) scans provide information on the patient's internal structure, tissue, and organs. The scans are used for treatment plans and to assess the performance of the treatment [15].

Radiologists predict tumor classification and whereabouts from MRI scans. As a result of the shortage of healthcare workers in some countries, radiologists are often overworked and under constant pressure, which at times naturally leads to human error. Manual segmentation of the tumor can be very time-consuming for radiologists. Automatic segmentation can increase the accuracy of tumor classifications and improve the workload for radiologists by providing them with additional resources that can help them feel supported.

The annual Medical Image Computing and Computer Assisted Interventions (MICCAI) conference hosts medical imaging challenges for research teams to participate internationally. One of MICCAI's challenges is BraTS [13], the brain tumor segmentation that consists of nine tasks this year. Initially, BraTS started as a challenge that only aimed at adult glioma [3–5]; however, recently, it has expanded its dataset to increase the diversity of the segmentation tasks. The additional population in the expanded dataset includes sub-Saharan African patients, pediatrics, and meningioma tumors. The aim of expanding the dataset is to account for different brain tumors, a diverse range of image quality, and tumor sizes. This paper focuses on the adult and pediatric datasets.

Artificial intelligence uses neural networks to train on pre-existing data to learn the boundaries of brain tumors. Automatic segmentation is made possible by deep learning models that analyze the MRI dataset. As a result, physicians can use the algorithms to effectively and accurately identify tumors. This paper highlights the use of MedNeXt and SegResNet models for fully automated brain tumor segmentation. The training and validation occurred simultaneously when testing the different models on the dataset. BraTS provided researchers with the ground truth to accurately assess the performance of the models based on the predictions. The tumor segmentations were outlined by radiologists and reviewed by neurologists to ensure the accuracy of the data.

Manual segmentations are often time-consuming; semi-automated segmentation is a computer-based model with human contributions. Generally, the expert radiologist needs to manually guide the algorithm by providing the outlines for the segmentations. Then, the model uses the information imputed and automatically segments the region of interest in scans. This technique was one of the initial transitions to artificial intelligence segmentations [21]. Two-stage segmentation frameworks are fully automatic but consist of two steps: balancing the classes and refining to the proper proportions. For brain tumors, there are several different imbalance classes; balancing the classes allows for equal representation and prevents biased training. Refining the predictions can improve the segmentation results by matching the accurate class distribution [16]. While both the semi-automated and two-stage segmentations improve the workload in radiology, fully automated segmentations are the most efficient and consistent.

Our main contributions are the following:

- A proposed ensemble of deep learning models for adult and pediatric brain tumor segmentation from the BraTS 2023 challenge.
- An integration of the deep supervision component with the models and investigation of its effects on the performance.
- A thorough investigation and analysis of post-processing techniques for the brain tumor segmentation tasks.

2 Methods

2.1 Dataset

BraTS-Adult Glioma. The dataset contains multi-institutional structural MRI scans of four different contrasts: pre and post-gadolinium T1-weighted (T1 and T1CE), T2-weighted (T2), and T2-weighted fluid-attenuated inversion recovery (T2-FLAIR). The dataset was acquired from multiple institutions with high variance in many aspects, including brain shape, appearance, and tumor morphology. The dataset [2,9] comprises 1251 training and 219 validation brain MRI scans. Furthermore, the final model performance will be evaluated on the testing set that will not be released.

BraTS-PEDs. A total of 228 high-quality are acquired from 3 different institutions, including Children's Brain Tumor Network (CBTN), Boston's Children Hospital, and Yale University. The acquired MRI modalities are T1, T1Gd, T2, and T2-FLAIR. All the included pediatric subjects contain histologically-approved high-grade glioma, i.e., high-grade astrocytoma and diffuse midline glioma (DMG), including radiologically or histologically-proven diffuse intrinsic pontine glioma (DIPG) [9,10]. The released training and validation datasets comprise 99 and 45 subjects, respectively.

Segmentation Labels. The provided annotations consist of the GD-enhancing tumor (ET), the peritumoral edematous or invaded tissue (ED), and the necrotic tumor core (NCR). Instead of being evaluated on these labels, segmentation performance is assessed based on the different glioma sub-regions: enhancing tumor, tumor core (NCR + ET), and whole tumor (NCR + ET + ED).

Preprocessing. The provided MRI scans were preprocessed by co-registration of the four modalities to a standard SR124 template [17], isotropic interpolating to meet $1\,\text{mm}^3$ resolution and skull-stripping. All of the MRI image sizes are uniform $240 \times 240 \times 155$. We further preprocess each scan by cropping the foreground, normalizing voxels with non-zero intensities, and finally stacking the four modalities into a single image. Yet, we experienced a bottleneck when we applied the preprocessing steps on the fly. Thus, we preprocess all MRI scans and store them in the .npy format, and then load the *Numpy* arrays during training.

2.2 Models

We conducted a comprehensive performance analysis by comparing 2 different segmentation models with varying sets of hyper-parameters. Initially, we employed MedNeXt [19], a novel 3D segmentation network inspired by ConvNeXt architecture, recently introduced into the field. Alongside this, we utilized SegResNet [14], a CNN-based segmentation model developed by the winning team of the BraTs 2018 challenge. These models were trained to predict 3 classes in 3 different output channels (TC, WT, ET); however, we also conducted experiments where we trained the models separately for one underperforming class (ET). In addition, our model input size is $128 \times 128 \times 128$. The models are illustrated in Fig. 1 and Fig. 2. The details are mentioned in the sections below.

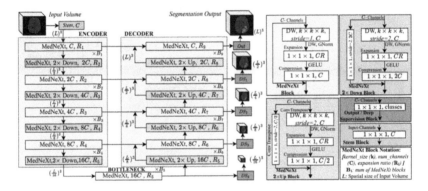

Fig. 1. The MedNeXt network [19].

MedNeXt. Architecture draws inspiration from vision transformer [6] and incorporates them into the kernel segmentation network design. This combines the benefits of ConvNeXT [11]-like structures in a UNet [18]-like design. Consequently, MedNeXt harnesses the inherent strengths of CNN models while integrating transformer-inspired ConvNeXt blocks tailored for 3D segmentation tasks. Notably, this design also implements deep supervision (DS) that can alleviate the problem of vanishing gradients, thus enhancing model training. Our experimentation encompassed two variants of the MedNeXt model: 'base' (B) and 'medium' (M) from the standard MedNeXt implementation[1].

SegResNet. Adopts a CNN-based encoder-decoder architecture that exhibits a relatively straightforward yet highly effective design for the 3D segmentation task. This architecture was originally introduced by the BraTs 2018 winning team, who achieved the highest dice score in segmenting tumor sub-regions by employing an ensemble of ten models. SegResNet has a ResNet-based [7] asymmetric architecture, containing UNet-like encoder-decoder blocks but with skip

---
[1] https://github.com/MIC-DKFZ/MedNeXt.

connections on both the encoder and decoder, allowing better gradient propagation. It also uses Group Normalization [20] that is suggested to work better by the authors, especially in small batch size scenarios.

Moreover, SegResNet incorporates an additional VAE (Variational Autoencoder) branch in the decoder during the training only. This VAE branch allows reconstructing the original image using features derived from the encoder bottleneck and does not contain skip connections from the encoder. This ensures a better regularization for the model training and allows the model to learn rich features for segmentation. During our experimentation, we conducted training iterations of both *with* and *without* the VAE regularization in order to assess its impact on the performance across the targeted tasks.

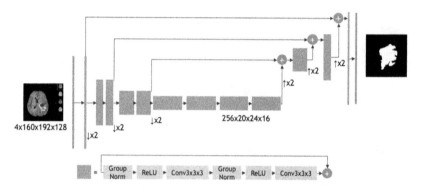

Fig. 2. The SegResNet network [14].

2.3 Inference

Prediction from a Single Network. Our model input size is $128 \times 128 \times 128$, smaller than the MR image size. We implement the sliding window inference technique with 0.5 overlaps to predict tumor probabilities for each voxel. We apply test-time-augmentation (TTA) by flipping an input image through all possible flip combinations (8 combinations) and aggregating the mean probabilities.

Ensemble. We train each model on the 5-fold CV setting, resulting in 5 trained networks for every training. To predict an input image during inference, we pass the image to each network to estimate tumor probabilities. Then, we aggregate the outputs from the 5-fold CV networks by taking the mean probabilities.

Ensembling multiple models can help improve overall performance [22] by leveraging the inherent strength of every model. In this work, we ensemble models output on probability level by weighted averaging to give importance to every model on each channel ($weight\_tc, weight\_wt, weight\_et$). The pseudocode of our model ensembling is given in Algorithm 1.

Postprocessing. The postprocessing step plays a crucial role in the overall performance, especially for this year's competition, as the organizer decided to change the evaluation focus from study-wise to lesion-wise performance, where False positive (FP) and negative (FN) are penalized severely with 0.0 Dice and 374 HD95 scores. Our experiments show that raw segmentation prediction contains many FPs due to small-size predicted lesions. To alleviate this, we do the following for each output channel (TC, WT, and ET);

1. Perform thresholding with a specific threshold for each channel.
2. Perform connected component analysis to group predicted connected tumor voxels into lesions.
3. Filter every group based on tumorous voxel count and the mean of tumorous voxel probabilities.

In short, we implement two postprocessing functions as described in Algorithm 2 and Algorithm 3.

Algorithm 1. Model Ensembling

Require: N models with each corresponding weighting for every channel (TC, WT, ET) and an input brain MRI scan $x \in \mathbb{R}^{3 \times H \times W \times D}$
$y \leftarrow \mathbf{0}^{3 \times H \times W \times D}$
$sum_w \leftarrow \mathbf{0}^3$
for $n = 1, 2, \ldots N$ **do**
    $y \leftarrow y + \texttt{models}[n](x) * \texttt{weightings}[n]$
    $sum_w \leftarrow sum_w + \texttt{weightings}[n]$
end for
$y \leftarrow y / sum_w$
return y

Algorithm 2. AsDiscrete(T_{TC}, T_{WT}, T_{ET})

Require: Threshold values for each channel (T_{TC}, T_{WT}, T_{ET}), and a predicted tumor heatmap $x \in \mathbb{R}^{3 \times H \times W \times D}$ where the channels correspond to TC, WT, and ET respectively
Ensure: $0 < T_{TC}, T_{WT}, T_{ET} < 1$
$y \leftarrow \mathbf{0}^{3 \times H \times W \times D}$
for $w, h, d = \texttt{range}(W), \texttt{range}(H), \texttt{range}(D)$ **do**
    if $x[1, w, h, d] \geq T_{TC}$ **then**
        $y[1, w, h, d] \leftarrow 1$
    end if
    if $x[2, w, h, d] \geq T_{WT}$ **then**
        $y[2, w, h, d] \leftarrow 1$
    end if
    if $x[3, w, h, d] \geq T_{ET}$ **then**
        $y[3, w, h, d] \leftarrow 1$
    end if
end for
return y

2.4 Experimental Setup

We follow the 5-fold CV training setting by partitioning the training data into five subsets, performing training on four of them, and validating one subset on each iteration. We train our networks based on the region-based training mechanism [8] for 150 epochs, batch size of 2, and apply on-the-fly data augmentation consisting of the random spatial crop to 128 × 128 × 128 size, random flips, and random intensity scaling as well as shifting. For the objective function, we apply batch dice loss and focal loss with 2.0 γ and then sum them to get the total loss. We optimize our networks using AdamW optimizer [12], and we use the cosine-annealing with linear-warmup scheduler. The optimizer and scheduler hyperparameters are 1e–4 base learning rate (LR), 1e–6 weight decay, 8 warmup epochs, 1e–7 initial LR, 1e–6 final LR, and 150 maximum epochs. In addition, we conducted some experiments involving deep supervision by additionally applying the loss at each decoder stage and giving lower importance weights on lower resolutions by a factor of 1/2.

Algorithm 3. FilterObjects($T_{s,u}$, $T_{s,l}$, $T_{p,u}$, $T_{p,m}$)

Require: A predicted tumor heatmap and binary map $x_p, x_b \in \mathbb{R}^{H \times W \times D}$, upper size threshold ($T_{s,u}$), lower size threshold ($T_{s,l}$), upper probability threshold ($T_{p,u}$), and mid probability threshold ($T_{p,m}$)
Ensure: $T_{s,u} \geq T_{s,l}$, $T_{s,l} \geq 0$, and $0 \leq T_{p,u}, T_{p,m} < 0$
    $y \leftarrow \mathbf{0}^{H \times W \times D}$
    $y_{cc} \leftarrow$ get_connected_components(x_b)
    $N_{cc} \leftarrow$ get_the_number_of_ccs(y_{cc})
    for $n \in$ range(N_{cc}) **do**
        size $\leftarrow$ count_tumor_pixels_of_nth_cc(y_{cc}, n)
        mean $\leftarrow$ get_mean_prob_of_nth_cc(x_p, y_{cc}, n)
        if size $\geq T_{s,u}$ **then**
            if mean $\geq T_{p,u}$ **then** $y \leftarrow$ insert_cc_to_y(y, y_{cc}, n)
        end if
        else if $T_{s,l} \leq$ size $< T_{s,u}$ **then**
            if mean $\geq T_{p,m}$ **then** $y \leftarrow$ insert_cc_to_y(y, y_{cc}, n)
        end if
        end if
    end for
    return y

We apply *AsDiscrete* (Algorithm 2) and *FilterObjects* (Algorithm 3) on each channel at the output prediction. The postprocessing hyperparameters are selected experimentally as we found that different model configurations have different output characteristics, leading to different suboptimum hyperparameters.

3 Results

We trained our pipeline using the 5-fold cross-validation (CV) on the training data and performed an evaluation using the internal validation set to select the

Table 1. Ablation study on post-processing using 5-fold CV. We utilize MedNeXt B-3 with deep supervision. Our post-processing steps significantly affect the BraTS 2023 Score, while the Legacy Score is not much affected. **Notes**: (a) Test-time augmentations (TTA), (b) Replace ET to TC if total predicted ET area is small, (c) Filter connected components (tumor objects) based on size, (d) Filter connected components based on mean confidence of each tumor object.

| | | | | BraTS 2023 Score | | | | | | | | Legacy Score | | | | | | |
| | | | | Dice | | | | HD95 | | | | Dice | | | | HD95 | | | |
a	b	c	d	ET	TC	WT	Avg	ET	TC	WT	Avg	ET	TC	WT	Avg	ET	TC	WT	Avg
				78.82	84.55	70.88	78.08	47.66	33.84	93.57	58.36	87.14	91.38	93.29	90.60	11.69	7.50	6.59	8.59
✓				79.99	86.30	77.45	81.25	43.25	26.62	67.94	45.94	87.24	91.40	93.46	90.70	11.82	**7.19**	6.54	8.52
✓	✓			80.91	86.30	77.45	81.55	41.26	26.62	67.94	45.27	88.08	91.40	93.40	90.98	11.06	**7.19**	6.54	8.26
✓		✓		85.51	88.63	89.06	87.74	21.83	19.28	22.96	21.36	88.29	91.10	93.34	90.91	10.49	9.89	7.02	9.13
✓			✓	84.94	88.42	**89.61**	87.66	24.47	**18.36**	**20.83**	21.22	88.19	**91.46**	**93.48**	**91.04**	**10.34**	7.47	**6.35**	**8.06**
✓		✓	✓	**86.01**	**88.70**	89.44	**88.05**	**20.59**	19.11	21.59	**20.43**	**88.38**	91.07	93.36	90.94	10.35	10.10	6.81	9.09

Table 2. Adult-glioma performance on the validation leaderboard. DS indicates using Deep Supervision during training. The postprocessing hyperparameters for each submission were selected experimentally. The final postprocessing steps (*) are AsDiscrete(0.5, 0.5, 0.4), FilterObjects(2000, 100, 0.85, 0.925) for WT, FilterObjects(95, 70, 0.71, 0.5) for ET, FilterObjects(350, 350, 0, 0) for TC. The final ensemble weightings are MedNeXt-DS=(0, 1, 1), SegResNet-DS=(0, 1, 0), SegResNet=(1, 0, 0).

Model	Dice				HD95			
	ET	TC	WT	Avg	ET	TC	WT	Avg
SegResNet	0.8280	0.8606	0.9044	0.8643	23.90	17.89	12.52	18.10
SegResNet-DS	0.8239	0.8595	0.9016	0.8617	27.46	16.24	13.48	19.06
MedNeXt	0.8400	0.8486	0.9059	0.8648	22.25	26.71	12.49	20.48
MedNeXt-DS	0.8363	0.8486	0.9051	0.8633	23.92	28.27	12.65	21.61
MedNeXt-DS + SegResNet-DS	0.8346	0.8622	**0.9063**	0.8677	23.70	18.71	**11.70**	18.04
*MedNeXt-DS + SegResNet-DS + SegResNet	**0.8432**	**0.8627**	**0.9063**	**0.8707**	**17.37**	**13.10**	**11.70**	**14.06**

Table 3. Performance on the test set in both tasks. Our final submission for the adult glioma segmentation task was ranked 3rd in the final test set leaderboard. DS indicates using Deep Supervision during training, and ET indicates the models specifically trained for class ET in the pediatric tumor segmentation task.

Task	Model	Dice				HD95			
		ET	TC	WT	Avg	ET	TC	WT	Avg
Adult Glioma	MedNeXt-DS + SegResNet-DS	0.8198	0.8233	0.8508	0.8313	35.15	39.86	34.12	36.38
Pediatric Tumors	SegResNet-ET + SegResNet	0.5522	0.77	0.7755	0.6992	45.32	30.35	30.45	35.37

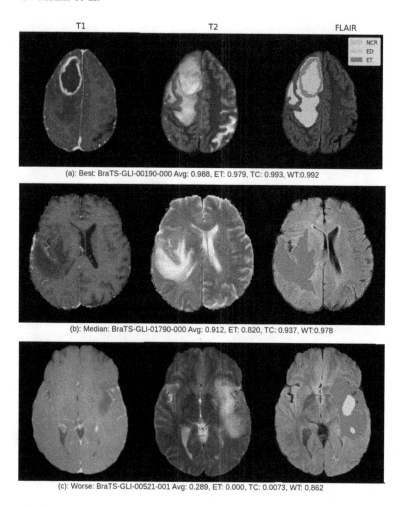

Fig. 3. The figure shows the qualitative results for the adult-glioma task on the validation sample for three cases.

best set of hyperparameters. We further utilized highly effective post-processing steps (see Sect. 2.3) on the model predictions to get the final output, which was submitted to the online leaderboard. After rigorous experimentation on different models on the internal validation set, we narrowed it down to two models for the external validation based on the online leaderboard. SegResNet and MedNeXt models are selected for the final submissions. The dice similarity coefficient (DSC) and 95% Hausdorff distance (HD95) from the online validation for the Adults-Glioma and Pediatrics task are mentioned in Table 2 and Table 4, respectively. Furthermore, the performance for both tasks on the final test set is given in Table 3.

Table 1 shows the effect of different post-processing steps on the performance evaluated using the local validation set. This ablations study used the MedNeXt-B-3 model with deep supervision (DS). The best-performing setting is achieved by using test-time augmentations (TTA) along with filtering connected components based on each tumor object's size and mean confidence. We achieved approximately a 10% increase in average Dice score using and a large drop in the HD95 distance, suggesting the effectiveness of the used post-processing.

Table 4. The table presents the validation results for BraTs-Pediatrics segmentation obtained from the leaderboard. In the WT (weighted-loss) training scheme, the focal loss weight is set to 2. Our final prediction is the result of various model combinations. Models specifically trained for class ET are marked as **-ET. The optimal performance was attained with a 5-Fold-CV of SegResNet (predicting WT and TC) and an additional 5-Fold-CV of SegResNet (predicting ET).

Model	Dice				HD95			
	ET	TC	WT	Avg	ET	TC	WT	Avg
MedNeXt	0.3338	0.7829	0.8291	0.6586	202.33	**16.76**	20.96	60.17
SegResNet	0.2674	**0.7930**	**0.8334**	0.6313	183.82	19.98	**19.32**	55.94
SegResNet-WL	0.3238	0.7588	0.8060	0.6295	204.02	24.75	26.18	63.90
SegFormer ET + MedNeXt	0.5015	0.7829	0.8291	0.7045	149.81	16.76	20.97	47.06
MedNeXt ET model + MedNeXt	0.4004	0.7765	0.8325	0.6698	189.98	17.14	19.61	56.85
SegResNet ET model + SegResNet-VAE	0.5595	0.7777	0.8018	0.7130	124.91	21.56	29.76	**44.23**
SegResNet ET model + SegResNet	**0.5595**	0.78106	0.8206	**0.7204**	124.91	25.30	24.77	58.32

We further report the performance metrics on the adult Glioma task in table 2. In the vanilla 5-fold CV, both baseline models (SegResNet and MedNeXt) achieve a similar performance of approx. 0.86 mean DSC. Moreover, using DS shows a slight positive trend in HD95 distance. Following this, we create an ensemble of MedNeXt-DS, SegResNet-DS, and SegResNet without DS to achieve the highest performance in terms of mean DSC and HD95, 0.871 and 14.06, respectively. Our best-performing setting is a weighted combination of all three used models, where we used MedNeXt-DS for class TC and WT, SegResNet-DS for class TC, and SegResNet for ET class only. We used this combination for the final submission. Table 3 shows the performance on the hidden test set, where our approach achieved 0.8313 and 36.38 mean DSC and HD95, respectively. The qualitative results for the best, median, and worst performing validation samples are shown in Fig. 3.

Following a similar experimental setting, we applied our proposed pipeline to the pediatric tumor segmentation task as well. Table 4 shows that the baseline MedNeXt and SegResNet models achieve a mean DSC of 0.65 and 0.63 and a

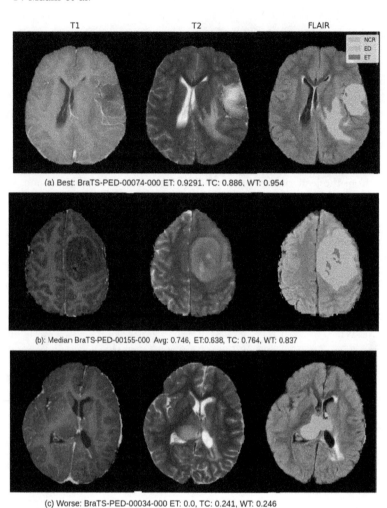

Fig. 4. The figure shows the qualitative results for the pediatric task on the validation sample for the best-performing model.

mean HD95 of 60.17 and 55.94, respectively, with sub-optimal performance for the ET class. We developed two techniques to tackle this issue: (i) a weighted loss (WL) based model that penalizes the ET class more than other classes and (ii) a standalone model for the ET class only. While SegResNet-WL showed some improvement in the ET class performance, it did not perform on par with approach (ii), where a separate network is trained for the ET class only. Our best-performing model for this task is a combination of a SegResNet-ET and a multi-class SegResNet model, achieving a mean DSC of 0.72 and HD95 of 58.32. We used our best-performing combination for the test set submission. Table 3 shows that our approach achieved 0.6992 and 35.37 mean DSC and HD95 on the hidden test set, respectively. The qualitative results for the best, median, and worst performing validation samples are shown in Fig. 4.

4 Discussion

In this paper, we summarize our proposed methodology for the BraTS 2023 adult and pediatrics glioma segmentation competition. Our pipeline is based on the two highly efficient segmentation models, namely; MedNeXt and SegResNet. Our work benefited from the power of DS and an ensemble strategy involving heterogeneous models to tackle a challenging real-life problem. The primary focus was based on integrating suitable post-processing steps with deep supervision and the ensemble of diverse models, resulting in substantial performance gains. We conducted comprehensive experiments to show the significance of understanding the clinical problem and implementing domain-specific processing steps to augment the efficiency of deep-learning models, ultimately providing a significant boost in performance. The post-processing steps stood very helpful in following this year's new scoring system that is designed carefully based on the clinical diagnosis and heavily penalizes missing even a small tumor region.

Furthermore, we used a similar approach for both tasks, motivated by the similarity between both tasks; however, the performance in both tasks remained significantly different. In the adult-glioma challenge, all three classes showed similar results, while the ET class in the pediatric dataset suffered much lower performance when compared to the other two classes. This discrepancy can potentially be due to the size of the ET regions as compared to the entire brain volume and other classes. The models find it hard to distinguish the regions, especially when one class is imbalanced, as in the case of the pediatric dataset. Another reason is that the ET class is a small area within the TC region, which itself is within the WT region. This suppresses the ET class significantly, affecting smooth model learning. Furthermore, the size of the available dataset for the pediatric task is significantly smaller than the adult-glioma dataset, which could also contribute to this performance difference in both tasks.

5 Conclusion

The paper studies different approaches to segmenting the tumor region in the brain. We used the BraTS 2023 challenge datasets for the adult glioma and pediatric tumor. Both datasets are multi-modal, multi-class segmentation tasks, with four modalities to input and three classes to predict. The automatic approach for segmenting tumor regions is highly beneficial for clinical practice, helping clinicians speed up their work. Our approach combines the advantages of deep supervision and an ensemble of models for the successful segmentation of the brain tumor from the MR images. To conclude, we achieve third place in the `BraTS 2023 Adult Glioma Challenge`.

References

1. Alexander, B.M., Cloughesy, T.F.: Adult glioblastoma. J. Clin. Oncol. **35**(21), 2402–2409 (2017)
2. Baid, U., et al.: The rsna-asnr-miccai brats 2021 benchmark on brain tumor segmentation and radiogenomic classification. arXiv preprint arXiv:2107.02314 (2021)
3. Bakas, S., et al.: Segmentation labels and radiomic features for the pre-operative scans of the tcga-gbm collection (2017). https://doi.org/10.7937K, 9
4. Bakas, S., et al.: Segmentation labels and radiomic features for the pre-operative scans of the tcga-lgg collection. Cancer Imaging Arch. **286** (2017)
5. Bakas, S., et al.: Advancing the cancer genome atlas glioma mri collections with expert segmentation labels and radiomic features. Sci. Data **4**(1), 1–13 (2017)
6. Dosovitskiy, A., et al.: An image is worth 16x16 words: transformers for image recognition at scale. arXiv preprint arXiv:2010.11929 (2020)
7. He, K., Zhang, X., Ren, S., Sun, J.: Identity mappings in deep residual networks. In: Leibe, B., Matas, J., Sebe, N., Welling, M. (eds.) ECCV 2016. LNCS, vol. 9908, pp. 630–645. Springer, Cham (2016). https://doi.org/10.1007/978-3-319-46493-0_38
8. Isensee, F., Jäger, P.F., Full, P.M., Vollmuth, P., Maier-Hein, K.H.: nnU-Net for brain tumor segmentation. In: Crimi, A., Bakas, S. (eds.) BrainLes 2020. LNCS, vol. 12659, pp. 118–132. Springer, Cham (2021). https://doi.org/10.1007/978-3-030-72087-2_11
9. Karargyris, A., Umeton, R., Sheller, M.J., et al.: Federated benchmarking of medical artificial intelligence with medperf. Nat. Mach. Intell. **5**, 799–810 (2023)
10. Kazerooni, A.F., et al.: The brain tumor segmentation (BraTS) challenge 2023: Focus on pediatrics (CBTN-CONNECT-DIPGR-ASNR-MICCAI BraTS-PEDs). arXiv preprint arXiv:2305.17033 (2023)
11. Liu, Z., Mao, H., Wu, C.-Y., Feichtenhofer, C., Darrell, T., Xie, S.: A convnet for the 2020s. In: Proceedings of the IEEE/CVF Conference on Computer Vision and Pattern Recognition, pp. 11976–11986 (2022)
12. Loshchilov, I., Hutter, F.: Decoupled weight decay regularization. In: 7th International Conference on Learning Representations, ICLR 2019, New Orleans, LA, USA, 6–9 May 2019. OpenReview.net (2019)
13. Menze, B.H., et al.: The multimodal brain tumor image segmentation benchmark (brats). IEEE Trans. Med. Imaging **34**(10), 1993–2024 (2014)
14. Myronenko, A.: 3D MRI brain tumor segmentation using autoencoder regularization. In: Crimi, A., Bakas, S., Kuijf, H., Keyvan, F., Reyes, M., van Walsum, T. (eds.) BrainLes 2018. LNCS, vol. 11384, pp. 311–320. Springer, Cham (2019). https://doi.org/10.1007/978-3-030-11726-9_28
15. Owrangi, A.M., Greer, P.B., Glide-Hurst, C.K.: Mri-only treatment planning: benefits and challenges. Phys. Med. Biol. **63**(5), 05TR01 (2018)
16. Pereira, S., Pinto, A., Alves, V., Silva, C.A.: Brain tumor segmentation using convolutional neural networks in mri images. IEEE Trans. Med. Imaging **35**(5), 1240–1251 (2016)
17. Rohlfing, T., et al.: The SRI24 multichannel atlas of normal adult human brain structure. Hum. Brain Mapp. **31**(5), 798–819 (2010)
18. Ronneberger, O., Fischer, P., Brox, T.: U-net: convolutional networks for biomedical image segmentation. In: Navab, N., Hornegger, J., Wells, W.M., Frangi, A.F. (eds.) MICCAI 2015. LNCS, vol. 9351, pp. 234–241. Springer, Cham (2015). https://doi.org/10.1007/978-3-319-24574-4_28

19. Roy, S., et al.: Mednext: transformer-driven scaling of convnets for medical image segmentation. arXiv preprint arXiv:2303.09975 (2023)
20. Wu, Y., He, K.: Group normalization. In: Proceedings of the European Conference on Computer Vision (ECCV), pp. 3–19 (2018)
21. Xie, K., Yang, J., Zhang, Z., Zhu, Y.: Semi-automated brain tumor and edema segmentation using mri. Eur. J. Radiol. **56**(1), 12–19 (2005)
22. Zeineldin, R.A., Karar, M.E., Burgert, O., Mathis-Ullrich, F.: Multimodal cnn networks for brain tumor segmentation in mri: A brats 2022 challenge solution. In: Bakas, S., et al. (eds.) Brainlesion: Glioma. Multiple Sclerosis, Stroke and Traumatic Brain Injuries, pp. 127–137. Springer, Cham (2023). DOI: https://doi.org/10.1007/978-3-031-33842-7_11

Multiscale Encoder and Omni-Dimensional Dynamic Convolution Enrichment in nnU-Net for Brain Tumor Segmentation

Sahaj K. Mistry[1(✉)], Aayush Gupta[1], Sourav Saini[1], Aashray Gupta[1], Sunny Rai[2], Vinit Jakhetiya[1], Ujjwal Baid[3], and Sharath Chandra Guntuku[2]

[1] Indian Institute of Technology Jammu, Jammu, India
sahajmistry005@gmail.com
[2] University of Pennsylvania, Philadelphia, PA, USA
[3] Indiana University, Bloomington, IN, USA

Abstract. Brain tumor segmentation plays a crucial role in computer-aided diagnosis. This study introduces a novel segmentation algorithm utilizing a modified nnU-Net architecture. Within the nnU-Net architecture's encoder section, we enhance conventional convolution layers by incorporating omni-dimensional dynamic convolution layers, resulting in improved feature representation. Simultaneously, we propose a multi-scale attention strategy that harnesses contemporary insights from various scales. Our model's efficacy is demonstrated on diverse datasets from the BraTS-2023 challenge. Integrating omni-dimensional dynamic convolution (ODConv) layers and multi-scale features yields substantial improvement in the nnU-Net architecture's performance across multiple tumor segmentation datasets. Remarkably, our proposed model attains good accuracy during validation for the BraTS Africa dataset. The ODconv source code (https://github.com/i-sahajmistry/nnUNet_BraTS2023/blob/master/nnunet/ODConv.py) along with full training code (https://github.com/i-sahajmistry/nnUNet_BraTS2023) is available on GitHub.

Keywords: BraTS-2023 · deep learning · brain · segmentation · Adult Glioma · BraTS-Africa · Meningioma · Brain Metastases and Pediatric Tumors · nnU-Net · ODConv3D · multiscale · lesion · medical imaging

1 Introduction

Glioblastomas (GBM) are the most prevalent and aggressive primary brain tumors in adults. The significant morphological and histological diversity of gliomas, encompassing distinct zones like active tumors, cystic and necrotic

---

S. K. Mistry, A. Gupta, S. Saini—Equal Contributors.
U. Baid and S. C. Guntuku—Senior authors.

structures, as well as edema and invasion areas, adds complexity to the precise identification of the tumor and its sub-regions. The manual segmentation of brain tumors demands substantial time and resources, while also being susceptible to errors originating from both inter and intra-observer variability [1]. Consequently, developing automated and accurate methods to locate gliomas and their sub-regions within MRI scans precisely is paramount for diagnosis and treatment purposes [2].

The BraTS datasets and challenges offer an extensive repository of labeled brain MR images in an open-source format, facilitating the development of cutting-edge solutions in the field of neuroradiology. The BraTS-2023 challenge includes 4 mpMRI scans from each patient, including native (T1N), post-contrast T1-weighted (T1C), T2-weighted (T2W), and T2 Fluid Attenuated Inversion Recovery (T2F) volumes. The label mask comprised three categories: Edema (ED), Enhancing Tumor (ET), and Necrosis (NE). The Tumor Core (TC) is defined as the combined value of ET and NE, while the sum of ED, ET, and NE forms the Whole Tumor (WT).

Prior BraTS challenges focused on adult brain diffuse astrocytoma [3–6]. The current edition of BraTS presents a series of challenges encompassing a range of tumor types, incomplete data, and technological factors. The focus of this paper will be mainly on two challenges, namely (a) Brain Metastases Dataset and, (b) the BraTS-Africa Dataset, where we achieved good performance in the validation phase of the BraTS 2023 Challenge.

Our proposed approach uses the modified nnU-Net [7] architecture and comprises (a) two encoders, both inspired by the nnU-Net [7] framework (See Fig. 2) and (b) Omni-dimensional Dynamic Convolution (ODConv-2D) [8] layers adapted to work with 3D images, which we refer as ODConv3D.

By integrating two encoders into the network architecture, we exploit the capability of simultaneously processing the same image at two distinct scales. This approach enables us to extract features spanning a wide range of complexities. ODConv utilizes an innovative multi-dimensional attention mechanism to acquire four distinct forms of attention for convolutional kernels, simultaneously encompassing all four dimensions of the kernel space. This enriched, dynamic convolution design enables the model to effectively capture intricate spatial, channel-wise, and temporal information. The results demonstrate the superiority of ODConv3D over the conventional convolutional layers in nnU-Net [7]. For submitting the code for evaluation purposes, we use MedPerf's MLCube [9].

2 Materials

2.1 Datasets

BraTS 2023 introduces five diverse challenges, each encompassing a distinct aspect of Brain Tumor Segmentation. Each challenge corresponds to datasets targeting specific types of brain tumors, namely: Adult Glioma, BraTS-Africa (Glioma from Sub-Saharan Africa), Meningioma, Brain Metastases, and Pediatric Tumors.

The BraTS dataset comprises retrospective multi-parametric magnetic resonance imaging (mpMRI) scans of brain tumors gathered from diverse medical institutions. These scans were acquired using varied equipment and imaging protocols, leading to a broad spectrum of image quality that reflects the diverse clinical approaches across different institutions. Annotations outlining each tumor sub-region were meticulously reviewed and validated by expert neuroradiologists.

Following the customary methodology for evaluating machine learning algorithms, the BraTS 2023 challenge follows a division of the dataset into training, validation, and testing sets. The training data includes the provided ground truth labels. Participants are given access to the validation data, which lacks associated ground truth labels. The testing data, kept confidential during the challenge, serves as an evaluation benchmark.

2.1.1 Adult Glioma

The dataset comprises a comprehensive collection of 5,880 MRI scans from a cohort of 1,470 patients diagnosed with brain diffuse glioma [6]. Among these scans, 1,251 have been designated for training purposes, while an additional 219 scans are allocated for validation. This dataset is consistent with the data meticulously compiled for the BraTS 2021 Challenge. This dataset focuses on glioblastoma (GBM), which stands out as the most prevalent and aggressive form of brain-originating cancer. With a grade classification of IV, GBMs display an extraordinary degree of heterogeneity in terms of their appearance, morphology, and histology. Typically originating in the cerebral white matter, these tumors exhibit rapid growth and can attain considerable sizes before manifesting noticeable symptoms. Given the challenging nature of GBM and its dire prognosis, with a median survival rate of approximately 15 months, the comprehensive dataset is a vital resource for advancing research, diagnosis, and treatment strategies in the field.

2.1.2 BraTS-Africa

With a total training cohort size of 60 cases, the Sub-Saharan Africa dataset [10] represents a specialized collection of glioma cases among patients from the Sub-Saharan Africa region. This dataset stands out due to its distinct characteristics, arising from the utilization of lower-grade MRI technology and the limited availability of MRI scanners in the region. Consequently, the MRI scans included exhibit diminished image contrast and resolution. This reduction in clarity poses a challenge by obscuring the distinct features present in the aforementioned dataset and introducing intricacies in the segmentation process. Notably, patients within this dataset from the Sub-Saharan Africa region often present with comorbidities like HIV/AIDS, malaria, and malnutrition. These underlying health conditions influence the appearance of brain tumors in MRI scans, further complicating the diagnostic process.

2.1.3 Meningioma

The dataset contains an extensive collection of cases, comprising 1,000 instances designated for training and an extra 141 cases set aside for validation. These cases are centered around meningiomas [11], a specific type of tumor that originates from the meninges. These meninges are protective layers that cover the brain and spinal cord. Meningiomas are noteworthy since they represent the most frequently occurring primary tumors within the brain of adults. Their significant risks emphasize the clinical importance of these tumors in terms of health complications and mortality. This dataset was introduced as part of the BraTS challenge in 2023.

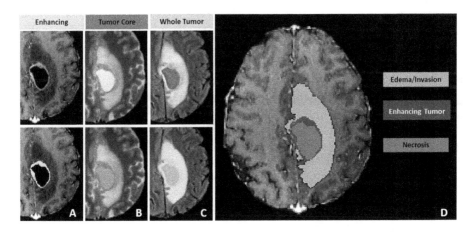

Fig. 1. Tumor Sub-regions Annotations Depicted various annotated tumor sub-regions across different multi-parametric MRI scans. Image panels A-C illustrate the areas designated for assessing algorithm performance, highlighting the enhancing tumor (ET - indicated in yellow) as seen in a T1C scan. This region encompasses the cystic/necrotic components of the core in panel A. In panels B and C, the tumor core (TC - magenta) and the entire tumor (WT - cyan) are delineated, respectively, in corresponding T2W and T2F scans. Panel D provides an overview of the merged segmentations forming the comprehensive tumor sub-region labels given to participants in the BraTS 2021 challenge. These labels comprise the enhancing core (yellow), necrotic/cystic core (red), and edema/invasion (green). The image is obtained from [6]. (Color figure online)

2.1.4 Brain Metastases

The Brain Metastases dataset's [12] training segment comprises 165 samples. In comparison, an additional 31 samples are included in the validation set, providing a comprehensive collection of multiparametric MRI (mpMRI) scans focusing on brain tumors. Diverging from the characteristics of gliomas, which tend to be more readily detectable in their initial scans due to their larger size, brain metastases exhibit a distinctive heterogeneity in their dimensions. These metastatic tumors manifest across a spectrum of sizes, often presenting as smaller lesions within the brain. Notably, these metastatic growths possess the capacity to emerge at various locations throughout the brain, contributing to the diversity of their appearances.

A noteworthy aspect of this dataset is the prevalence of brain metastases measuring less than 10 mm in diameter. These smaller lesions stand out in terms of their frequency, underscoring their clinical significance. Unlike their larger counterparts, these diminutive metastases have been observed to surpass others in terms of occurrence.

2.1.5 Pediatric Tumor

Despite certain similarities between pediatric tumors [13] and adult tumors, notable differences exist in their appearance in both imaging and clinical contexts. Both high-grade gliomas, such as GBMs, and pediatric diffuse midline gliomas (DMGs) have limited survival rates. Interestingly, DMGs are roughly three times rarer than GBMs. While GBMs typically emerge in the frontal or temporal lobes in the age of 60 s, DMGs are predominantly found within pons and are frequently identified in the age range of 5 and 10.

GBMs are typically characterized by the presence of an enhancing tumor region in post-gadolinium T1-weighted MRI scans, accompanied by necrotic regions. In contrast, these imaging characteristics are less pronounced or distinct in DMGs. Pediatric brain tumors are more inclined to be low-grade gliomas, generally displaying slower growth rates compared to those in adults. The dataset at hand comprises 99 training samples and 45 validation samples.

2.2 Annotation Methtod

The dataset is established via a meticulous process for annotating tumor subregions, combining automated segmentation and manual refinement by expert neuroradiologists. The methodology involves initial automated segmentations using established methodsDeepMedic [14–16], which are then fused through the STAPLE label fusion [17] technique to address errors. Expert annotators meticulously enhance these segmentations using multimodal MRI scans and ITK-SNAP [18] software. Senior neuroradiologists review the refined segmentations, ensuring accuracy. This iterative process results in annotations conforming to BraTS-defined sub-regions: enhancing tumor (ET), tumor core (TC), and whole tumor (WT) as described in Fig. 1. The process acknowledges challenges in radiological tumor boundary definition, providing a standardized, dependable ground truth for assessing segmentation algorithms.

3 Proposed Algorithm

In this section, we introduce our innovative methodology designed to precisely segment brain tumors using a multi-modal attention-based model. The proposed algorithm leverages a combination of data preprocessing, model architecture, and attention mechanisms to enhance the segmentation accuracy on 3D brain scans.

3.1 Preprocessing

3.1.1 Data Augmentation

Before inputting the data into our model, we apply multiple data augmentation techniques to enhance the robustness of the model. These random augmentations within a specific range include crop, zoom, flip, noise, blur, brightness, and contrast. This ensures that the model can generalize better to various spatial transformations and variations in the input data.

3.1.2 Patch Extraction

We extract patches of size $5 \times 128 \times 128 \times 128$ from the original brain scan images. These patches capture localized features and enable the model to focus on specific regions of interest. This patch-based approach also aids in reducing memory requirements and computational complexity during training and inference.

3.2 Model Architecture

3.2.1 Encoder

Our proposed model architecture consists of two encoder layers, each inspired by the nnU-Net [7] framework. Instead of using conventional Conv3D layers, we employ Omni-dimensional Dynamic Convolution 2D (ODConv2D) layers, which we extend for use with 3D images and refer to as ODConv3D. ODConv3D integrates a multi-dimensional attention mechanism utilizing a parallel strategy. This empowers us to acquire complementary attention patterns for convolutional kernels across all four dimensions of the kernel space. This enriched dynamic convolution design enables the model to effectively capture intricate spatial, channel-wise, and temporal information.

3.2.2 Multi-modal Attention

Our multi-modal attention strategy enhances the model's ability to leverage complementary information from different scales. We provide the original input image and a downsampled version of the same image as inputs to the model. This enables the model to capture fine-grained details and broader contextual information simultaneously. Separate encoders process each of these inputs, and the attention mechanism is then applied to fuse the encoded features. This approach encourages the model to focus on informative regions across scales, contributing to enhanced feature representation.

3.2.3 Decoder

The decoder of our model is similar to the nnU-Net's decoder architecture. It reconstructs the fused encoded features to generate a comprehensive feature map that preserves spatial information. This map is then processed to yield the final predicted segmentation.

3.3 Segmentation Process

3.3.1 Post-processing

Post-processing is applied to the output feature map to refine the predicted segmentation. This includes steps such as thresholding, morphological operations, and connected component analysis to remove noise and ensure coherent tumor regions.

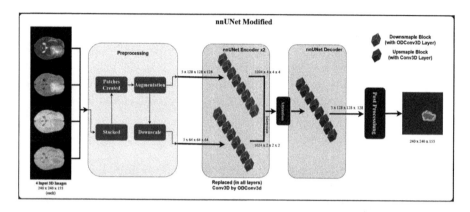

Fig. 2. nnU-Net with the addition of Multi-Scale and ODConv3D Layers: The architecture comprises a pair of identical encoders, responsible for extracting features from the input at distinct scales. These feature vectors undergo cross-attention processing, and the output is subsequently channeled into a decoder. The decoder's role involves upscaling the features to their original dimensions, effectively generating segmentations

3.3.2 Performance Metrics

To evaluate the accuracy and efficacy of our proposed model, we employ two performance metrics i.e., Dice coefficient and Hausdorff distance. These metrics provide quantitative measures of the segmentation quality and the model's ability to delineate tumor boundaries accurately.

3.4 Experimental Setup

We validate the performance of our proposed algorithm on the Brain Metastases dataset of brain scans containing instances of brain tumors. Each dataset instance consists of four 3D images of size $240 \times 240 \times 155$, along with corresponding ground truth segmentations. We divide the dataset into training and validation sets, and test on the synapse page, ensuring an unbiased evaluation of the model's performance.

4 Results

In this section, we present the results of our proposed attention-based tumor segmentation model on two distinct datasets: the Brain Metastases Dataset and the BraTS-Africa Dataset. We compare our model's performance against several baselines, including the original nnU-Net architecture, variations incorporating ODConv3D and multiscale strategies, and a data processing combination approach.

4.1 Evaluation Metrics

We evaluate the segmentation accuracy using a set of standard performance metrics, including the Dice coefficient for overall segmentation, as well as specific metrics for lesion subregions, namely Lesion ET (Enhancing Tumor), Lesion TC (Tumor Core), and Lesion WT (Whole Tumor).

4.2 BraTS-Africa Dataset

4.2.1 Baseline Models
We evaluate the baseline performance of the nnU-Net architecture on the BraTS-Africa Dataset. As shown in Table 1, the nnU-Net achieves a Dice coefficient of 0.8980 for overall segmentation. Lesion ET, TC, and WT achieve Dice coefficients of 0.8354, 0.8485, and 0.6578, respectively.

4.2.2 Multiscale and ODConv3D Integration
We investigate the effects of integrating the Multiscale and ODConv3D into the nnU-Net architecture on the BraTS-Africa Dataset. The nnU-Net + Multiscale + ODConv3D model achieves an enhanced Dice coefficient of 0.9092 for overall segmentation. However, individual lesion subregions show varying outcomes, with Lesion ET experiencing a slightly decreased Dice coefficient.

Table 1. Results of the different algorithms on BraTS-Africa validation dataset. Here a + b is taking best of a and b

Algorithm	Training Dice*	Lesion ET	Lesion TC	Lesion WT
nnU-Net (a)	0.8980	0.8354	0.8485	0.6578
nnU-Net + Multiscale + ODConv3D (b)	0.9092	0.8082	0.7634	**0.7872**
a + b		**0.8354**	**0.8485**	0.7564

* The models are trained on Glioma Dataset

Table 2. Results comparison of the different teams on BraTS-Africa validation dataset

Algorithm	Lesion ET	Lesion TC	Lesion WT
SPARC	0.7478	0.7649	0.7515
@harshi	0.7537	0.7051	0.5991
@ntnu40940111s	0.7603	0.7695	0.8403
blackbean	0.8264	0.8464	0.5690
@nic-vicorob	0.8029	0.7985	0.7487
BraTS2023_SPARK_UNN	0.7577	0.7907	**0.8647**
Ours	**0.8354**	**0.8485**	0.7564

4.2.3 Additional Post Processing

When we replace the labels of the nnU-Net model by the nnU-Net + Multiscale + ODConv3D model's Label 2 for the BraTS-Africa Dataset, this leads to an increase in Lesion WT from 0.65 to 0.75 as shown in Table 1, improving the overall accuracy. Our model's performance is highlighted in Table 2, demonstrating competitive results. Across all lesion subtypes, our model achieves Lesion ET scores of 0.8354, Lesion TC scores of 0.8485, and Lesion WT scores of 0.7564.

4.3 Brain Metastases Dataset

4.3.1 Baseline Models

We begin by evaluating the baseline performance of the nnU-Net architecture on the Brain Metastases Dataset. As depicted in Table 3, the nnU-Net achieves a Dice coefficient of 0.7675 for overall segmentation. The performance varies across lesion subregions, with Lesion ET, Lesion TC, and Lesion WT achieving Dice coefficients of 0.5157, 0.5105, and 0.4656, respectively.

4.3.2 Impact of ODConv3D

We assess the effectiveness of Omni-dimensional Dynamic Convolution (ODConv3D) by introducing the nnU-Net + ODConv3D model. This model replaces traditional Conv layers with ODConv3D layers for enhanced feature extraction. The results in Table 3 demonstrate that ODConv3D leads to an improved Dice coefficient of 0.7953 for overall segmentation. This improvement extends to lesion subregions, with Lesion ET, Lesion TC, and Lesion WT achieving Dice coefficients of 0.5364, 0.5451, and 0.5141, respectively.

4.3.3 Multiscale Strategy

We explore the benefit of a multiscale strategy by introducing the nnU-Net + Multiscale model. This approach leverages multiple scales of the input data to improve feature representation. As indicated in Table 3, the multiscale strategy yields a Dice coefficient of 0.7771 for overall segmentation. Lesion TC substantially improves with a Dice coefficient of 0.5737, compared to other subregions.

4.3.4 Combined Approach

The culmination of our model's innovation comes with the nnU-Net + Multiscale + ODConv3D configuration. Combining the multiscale strategy and ODConv3D layers yields exceptional results, evident in the overall Dice coefficient of 0.8188. This combined approach significantly enhances the segmentation performance across lesion subregions, with Dice coefficients of 0.5896, 0.6406, and 0.5555 for Lesion ET, Lesion TC, and Lesion WT, respectively. Table 4 showcases our model's performance, underscoring its competitive results. Our model consistently achieves good scores across all lesion subtypes, including Lesion ET with a score of 0.5896, Lesion TC with a score of 0.6406, and Lesion WT with a score of 0.5648.

Table 3. Results of the different algorithms on Brain Metastases validation dataset

Algorithm	Training Dice	Lesion ET	Lesion TC	Lesion WT
nnU-Net	0.7675	0.5157	0.5105	0.4656
nnU-Net + ODConv3D	0.7953	0.5364	0.5451	0.5141
nnU-Net + Multiscale	0.7771	0.5354	0.5737	0.5008
nnU-Net + Multiscale + ODConv3D	**0.8188**	**0.5896**	**0.6406**	**0.5555**

Table 4. Results comparison of the different teams on Brain Metastases validation dataset

Algorithm	Lesion ET	Lesion TC	Lesion WT
SPARC	0.4133	0.4378	0.4698
MIA_SINTEF	0.4433	0.4774	0.4832
DeepRadOnc	0.4575	0.4913	0.4665
@jeffrudie	0.4119	0.5171	0.5168
@parida12	0.5592	0.6039	0.5650
CNMC_PMI2023	**0.608**	**0.649**	**0.587**
Ours	0.5896	0.6406	0.5555

Table 5. Scores of modified nnU-Net on validation datasets in Brats 2023 Challenge

Challenge	Training Dice	Lesion ET	Lesion TC	Lesion WT
Adult Glioma Segmentation	0.909	0.798	0.826	0.789
BraTS-Africa Segmentation	0.909	0.835	0.849	0.756
Meningioma Segmentation	0.889	0.783	0.780	0.756
Brain Metastases Segmentation	0.819	0.590	0.641	0.556
Pediatric Tumors Segmentation	0.805	0.565	0.764	0.813

Table 6. Scores of modified nnU-Net on testing datasets in Brats 2023 Challenge

Challenge	Lesion ET	Lesion TC	Lesion WT
Adult Glioma Segmentation	0.798	0.826	0.789
BraTS-Africa Segmentation	0.818	0.775	0.845
Meningioma Segmentation	0.799	0.773	0.763
Brain Metastases Segmentation	0.491	0.534	0.483
Pediatric Tumors Segmentation	0.480	0.320	0.347

4.4 Comparison Across Diverse Datasets

To comprehensively assess our proposed multi-modal attention-based tumor segmentation model, we conducted evaluations on a diverse range of challenges: Adult Glioma Segmentation, BraTS-Africa Segmentation, Meningioma Segmentation, Brain Metastases Segmentation, and Pediatric Tumors Segmentation. As summarized in Tables 5 and 6, the results offer a comparison of the achieved Dice coefficients across different datasets in the validation and testing phase of the BraTS 2023 challenge.

Moreover, to provide visual clarity on the model's performance, we present figures in Table 7. These figures visually represent the segmentation outcomes on representative examples from each challenge. These visual insights enrich our understanding of how the model's capabilities translate into actual segmentations in various clinical scenarios.

5 Discussion

Across both the Brain Metastases Dataset and the BraTS-Africa Dataset datasets, the results highlight the effectiveness of the proposed multi-modal attention-based tumor segmentation model, particularly when leveraging multi-scale inputs and Omni-dimensional Dynamic Convolution. The combination of these approaches improves the segmentation accuracy and performance of lesion subregions. The data processing combination further refines results. These findings contribute to more accurate and reliable tumor segmentation.

Table 7. This table displays input data, which comprises T2W, T2F, T1N, and T1C images. We compare these input images with corresponding ground truth data and our predictions. Specifically, (a, b) represent data for Adult Glioma, (c, d) for BraTS-Africa, (e, f) for Meningioma, (g, h) for Brain Metastases, and (i, j) for Pediatric Tumor

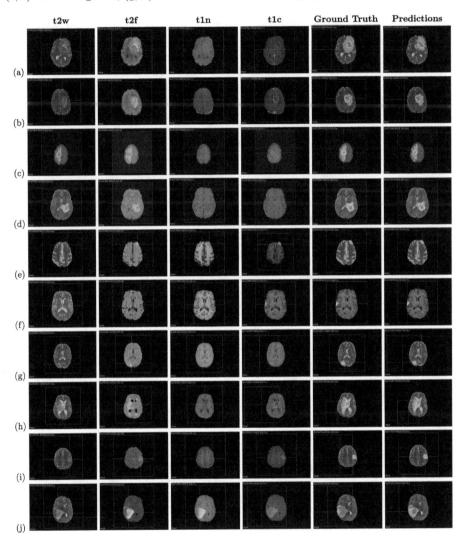

6 Conclusion

This paper has provided an in-depth exploration of our proposed model's performance across distinct datasets. The combined utilization of multiscale inputs, ODConv techniques, and strategic data processing leads to enhanced segmentation accuracy, showcasing the potential for more accurate and reliable tumor segmentation across various medical imaging scenarios.

References

1. Pereira, S., Pinto, A., Alves, V., Silva, C.A.: Brain tumor segmentation using convolutional neural networks in mri images. IEEE Trans. Med. Imaging **35**(5), 1240–1251 (2016)
2. Weller, M., et al.: Eano guidelines on the diagnosis and treatment of diffuse gliomas of adulthood. Nat. Rev. Clin. Oncol. **18**(3), 170–186 (2021)
3. Menze, B.H., et al.: The multimodal brain tumor image segmentation benchmark (brats). IEEE Trans. Med. Imaging **34**(10), 1993–2024 (2014)
4. Bakas, S., et al.: Advancing the cancer genome atlas glioma mri collections with expert segmentation labels and radiomic features. Sci. Data **4**(1), 1–13 (2017)
5. Bakas, S., et al.: Identifying the best machine learning algorithms for brain tumor segmentation, progression assessment, and overall survival prediction in the brats challenge. arXiv preprint arXiv:1811.02629 (2018)
6. Baid, U., et al.: The rsna-asnr-miccai brats 2021 benchmark on brain tumor segmentation and radiogenomic classification. arXiv preprint arXiv:2107.02314 (2021)
7. Isensee, F., et al.: Abstract: nnU-Net: self-adapting framework for U-net-based medical image segmentation. In: Bildverarbeitung für die Medizin 2019. I, pp. 22–22. Springer, Wiesbaden (2019). https://doi.org/10.1007/978-3-658-25326-4_7
8. Li, C., Zhou, A., Yao, A.: Omni-dimensional dynamic convolution (2022). arXiv preprint arXiv:2209.07947
9. Karargyris, A., et al.: Medperf: open benchmarking platform for medical artificial intelligence using federated evaluation. arXiv preprint arXiv:2110.01406 (2021)
10. Adewole, M., et al.: The brain tumor segmentation (brats) challenge 2023: Glioma segmentation in sub-saharan africa patient population (brats-africa). arXiv preprint arXiv:2305.19369 (2023)
11. LaBella, D., et al.: The asnr-miccai brain tumor segmentation (brats) challenge 2023: Intracranial meningioma. arXiv preprint arXiv:2305.07642 (2023)
12. Moawad, A.W., et al.: The brain tumor segmentation (brats-mets) challenge 2023: Brain metastasis segmentation on pre-treatment mri. arXiv preprint arXiv:2306.00838 (2023)
13. Kazerooni, A.F., et al.: The brain tumor segmentation (brats) challenge 2023: Focus on pediatrics (cbtn-connect-dipgr-asnr-miccai brats-peds). arXiv preprint arXiv:2305.17033 (2023)
14. Kamnitsas, K.: Efficient multi-scale 3d cnn with fully connected crf for accurate brain lesion segmentation. Med. Image Anal. **36**, 61–78 (2017)
15. McKinley, R., Meier, R., Wiest, R.: Ensembles of densely-connected CNNs with label-uncertainty for brain tumor segmentation. In: Crimi, A., Bakas, S., Kuijf, H., Keyvan, F., Reyes, M., van Walsum, T. (eds.) BrainLes 2018. LNCS, vol. 11384, pp. 456–465. Springer, Cham (2019). https://doi.org/10.1007/978-3-030-11726-9_40
16. Isensee, F., Jaeger, P.F., Kohl, S.A., Petersen, J., Maier-Hein, K.H.: nnu-net: a self-configuring method for deep learning-based biomedical image segmentation. Nat. Methods, 1–9 (2020)
17. Warfield, S.K., Zou, K.H., Wells, W.M.: Simultaneous truth and performance level estimation (staple): an algorithm for the validation of image segmentation. IEEE Trans. Med. Imaging **23**(7), 903–921 (2004)
18. Yushkevich, P.A., et al.: User-guided 3D active contour segmentation of anatomical structures: significantly improved efficiency and reliability. Neuroimage **31**(3), 1116–1128 (2006)

MenUnet: An End-to-End 3D Neural Network for Meningioma Segmentation from Multiparametric MRI

Hui Lin[1](✉), Xi Cheng[2], and Ziru Chen[3]

[1] Department of Electrical and Computer Engineering, Northwestern University, Evanston, IL 60208, USA
huilin2023@u.northwestern.edu
[2] Department of Civil, Materials, and Environmental Engineering, University of Illinois Chicago, Chicago, IL 60607, USA
[3] College of Computing, Georgia Institute of Technology, Atlanta, GA 30332, USA

Abstract. Meningioma is one of the most common and serious intracranial tumors. Multiparametric MRI (mpMRI) has been shown to provide significant information for precise tumor diagnosis. Manual segmentation of the meningioma is both lengthy and challenging. Automatic segmentation with high accuracy is of high interest. However, the state-of-art studies investigating automatic meningioma segmentation are unsatisfying in accuracy. An end-to-end network, MenUnet, is proposed to directly segment the whole 3D volume of MRIs. It captures the correlation among the surrounding slices in the 3D volume for accurate meningioma segmentation. It is validated in the public Brain Tumor Segmentation (BraTS) 2023 Meningioma Challenge, achieving the 5th in the validation phase. The dice scores of Enhancing Tumor (ET), Tumor core (TC), and whole tumor (WT), respectively, are 82.62%, 82.21%, and 83.00%. In the testing phase, the dice scores of Enhancing Tumor (ET), Tumor core (TC), and whole tumor (WT), respectively, are 83.01%, 82.01%, and 76.05%. The results show that MenUnet has the potential to assist the clinical practice of meningioma diagnosis.

Keywords: Tumor segmentation · Meningioma segmentation · Multiparametric MRI · Unet · Deep learning

1 Introduction

Meningiomas stand as one of the most frequently encountered intracranial tumors in clinical practice [16, 18]. Approximately 20% of all primary intracranial tumors are meningiomas [14]. Arising from the meninges, the protective layers surrounding the brain and spinal cord, these tumors can manifest with varying degrees of aggressiveness and symptoms. Their prevalence underscores the importance of accurate and efficient segmentation to enhance our understanding of their behavior, optimize early detection, and refine treatment strategies.

The multiparametric MRI data encapsulates crucial information about the tumor's location, size, and texture characteristics, which are essential for precise delineation. Since multiparametric MRI offers a diverse range of imaging sequences, each highlighting distinct tissue properties such as T1-weighted, T2-weighted, diffusion-weighted, and perfusion imaging. This enables a comprehensive assessment of anatomical structures and pathophysiological changes.

Automatic meningioma segmentation from multiparametric MRI holds prominent significance in clinical practice. Manual meningioma segmentation requires intensive labor, which can result in significant variance [3,12,19]. By automating this segmentation process, clinicians and radiologists can expedite the assessment of tumor growth, infiltration, and response to therapy. This advancement not only enhances diagnostic accuracy but also streamlines the workflow, enabling healthcare professionals to make well-informed decisions promptly. Moreover, the automation of meningioma segmentation reduces the potential for inter-observer variability, ensuring consistent and reliable results across different medical experts.

Convolutional neural networks (CNNs) have presented a promising performance in multiple applications [9,13,15]. A multiparametric deep-learning model (DLM) is proposed based on the DeepMedic architecture by Laukamp et al. [6]. It archives an average Dice score of 0.81 in the whole tumor segmentation. Their multiparametric MRI includes T1/T2-weighted, T1-weighted post-contrast T1-weighted, and T2 FLAIR from diverse institutions. The accuracy is still too preliminary to be applied in clinical diagnosis.

Unet [17] demonstrated promising performance in medical image segmentation [10,11] due to the skip connections in the Unet architecture. These connections not only recover spatial information for fine-grained segmentation but also alleviate the potential vanishing gradient problem during training.

In this work, an end-to-end network based on Unet architecture, MenUnet, is proposed to prevent error propagation caused by sub-optimal two-stage training. It captures the correlation among the surrounding slices in the 3D volume for accurate meningioma segmentation. MenUnet is validated in the public Brain Tumor Segmentation (BraTS) 2023 Meningioma Challenge, achieving the 5th in the validation phase. MenUnet has the potential to aid in the clinical practice of automatic meningioma segmentation from multiparametric MRI.

The remainder of the paper is organized as follows: The details of the proposed network are given in Sect. 2, including information on architecture, data augmentation, and loss function. Datasets, metrics, and implement details are shown in Sect. 3. Experimental results are shown in Sect. 4. Section 5 presents the conclusions and future directions.

2 Methods

2.1 NetworkspsArchitecture

The proposed Unet-based segmentation model, MenUnet, is depicted in Fig. 1. Like the classical Unet architecture, MenUnet comprises encoder and decoder networks on the left and right sides, respectively. The encoder network extracts high-level features from the input volume and gradually decreases the size of feature maps, while the decoder network gradually reconstructs these features to produce the segmentation maps at the original size. To improve spatial accuracy, skip connections are used to connect high-level and low-level features. MenUnet consists of six convolutional stages in both the encoder and decoder, each of which includes two convolutional layers and a max pooling or upsampling layer. Each layer is doing a 3D calculation in a 3D kernel.

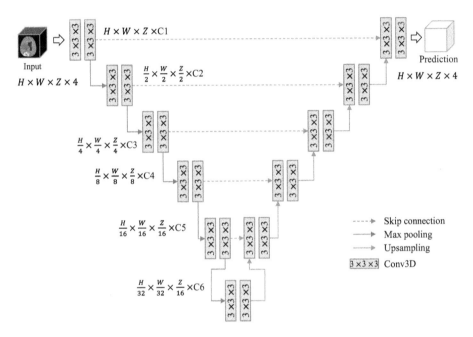

Fig. 1. The proposed MenUnet for end-to-end meningioma segmentation. MenUnet is based on a Unet architecture. $H \times W \times Z$ represents the size of a 3D MRI scan, and 4 indicates four types of modalities. The size of the output is $H \times W \times Z \times 4$, and 4 indicates four categories. The reader is referred to Sect. 2 for more details of MenUnet

2.2 Data Augmentation

Data augmentation was employed to prevent overfitting and improve generalizability. Three transformation methods- scaling, rotation, and translation- were applied to each axial plane with a probability of 50% for data augmentation. The scaling factor, rotation angle, and translation were randomly selected within $(0.5, 1.5)$, $(-25°, 25°)$, and $(-10, 10)$ pixels for the two axes in the axial plane, respectively. Our experiments presented that data augmentation increased the 3D dice score by around 2%.

2.3 Loss Function

The total segmentation loss $\mathcal{L}_{seg}$ is calculated as the weighted sum of binary cross entropy loss (BCE) and dice loss [1,2], using Eq. 1. The BCE loss $\mathcal{L}_{seg}^{BCE}$ treats all pixels' loss equally, but the foreground pixels' contributions to the training process are hampered due to the significant class imbalance between the foreground and background. On the other hand, the dice loss $\mathcal{L}_{seg}^{dice}$ is area-based and remains constant regardless of the background's size, addressing the class imbalance issue in the Meningioma segmentation dataset [5]. However, if only the dice loss is used, the training process becomes unstable when the foreground is small since minor changes can cause significant changes in the dice loss. Therefore, $\mathcal{L}_{seg}$ combines both losses to achieve a stable and effective training process. $\mathcal{L}_{seg}$ is given by:

$$\mathcal{L}_{seg} = \lambda \mathcal{L}_{seg}^{BCE} + \mathcal{L}_{seg}^{dice}$$
$$= -\lambda(Y \log \hat{Y} + (1-Y)\log(1-\hat{Y})) + (1 - \frac{2Y \cap \hat{Y}}{Y \cup \hat{Y}}) \quad (1)$$

where Y is the ground truth, $Y \in \{0,1,2,3\}$ and $\hat{Y}$ is the model output, $\hat{Y} \in [0,1,2,3]$, where 0, 1,2,3 represents the background, Enhancing Tumor (ET), Non-enhancing tumor core (NCR), and vasogenic EDema (ED), respectively.

To determine the weight of BCE loss, λ, MenUnet was trained with varying λ from the value list [0, 0.01 0.1, 1, 10], and the evaluation results are listed in Tables 1. We observed that MenUnet achieved the best 3D dice score when λ is 0.01. Thus, λ is set as 0.01 in the following experiments.

Table 1. Evaluation of the proposed MenUnet using different λ in the validation phase.

λ	Dice_ET (%)	Dice_TC (%)	Dice_WT (%)
0	75.33	74.29	75.67
0.01	**82.62**	**82.21**	**83.00**
0.1	81.67	80.84	80.23
1	80.00	81.47	80.24
10	78.21	79.16	78.21

3 Experiments

3.1 Dataset

The MRI data in the BraTS 2023 Meningioma Challenge [7,8] is utilized to validate the effectiveness of our method, MenUnet, in this study. This dataset was provided by major academic medical centers across the United States (e.g.,

Duke University). All cases include multiparametric MRI (mpMRI) comprised of 1) pre-contrast T1-weighted (T1), 2) post-contrast T1-weighted (T1Gd), 3) T2-weighted (T2), and 4) T2-weighted Fluid Attenuated Inversion Recovery (T2-FLAIR) series. One example with annotations is provided in Fig. 2. The annotations use a 3-label system, i.e., Enhancing Tumor (ET), Non-enhancing tumor core (NCR), and vasogenic EDema (ED), respectively, in blue, red, and green in Fig. 2. Different modalities might contribute to segmenting different categories. T1Gd might be suitable for segmenting the NCR and ETregion. T2-FLAIR might be suitable for segmenting the ED region.

Precise meningioma segmentation from mpMRI is challenging. Meningiomas can exhibit heterogeneous textures, shapes, and intensities, making it difficult to consistently delineate their boundaries. Moreover, factors like image artifacts, noise, and variations in imaging protocols further complicate accurate segmentation. Additionally, the presence of adjacent anatomical structures and potential overlaps with other brain tissues demand a robust and adaptable segmentation approach to ensure reliable and clinically meaningful results. The 3D visualization of the ground truth in Fig. 2 shows that the region of interest is complex in shapes with a lot of narrows. Especially the NCR region is too tiny to be segmented correctly.

The dataset has 1000 cases with available annotation for training in the validation phase. The training set is randomly divided into training and validation sets at a ratio of 4:1. 800 cases from the training set for training and 200 for validation.

3.2 Metrics

The dice score and Hausdorff Distance (HD) are two of the most commonly used metrics for meningioma segmentation. Enhancing Tumor (ET) and Non-enhancing tumor core (NCR) form tumor core (TC). Tumor core (TC) and vasogenic EDema (ED) form the whole tumor (WT). The dice score and Hausdorff Distance of ET, TC, and WT are independently calculated and ranked in the validation phase for evaluation and comparison. The dice score for each individual case in 3D and HD are calculated using Eqs. 2 and 3, respectively. The average 3D dice score and HD across all cases in the validation set are then used to evaluate the model's accuracy.

$$Dice = \frac{2TP}{2TP + FN + FP} \quad (2)$$

where TP, FN, TN, and FP represent respectively the number of true positives, false negatives, true negatives, and false positives over each patient's entire volume.

$$HD = \max \left\{ \begin{array}{l} \max_{p \in P} \min_{g \in G} d(p,g), \\ \max_{g \in G} \min_{p \in P} d(p,g) \end{array} \right\} \quad (3)$$

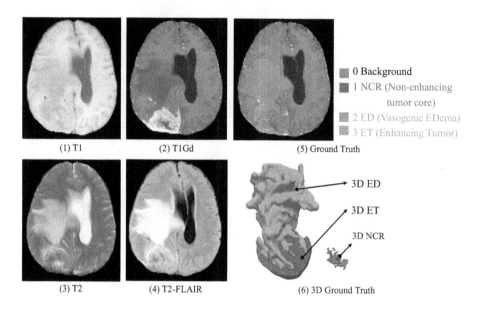

Fig. 2. Axial view of an example multiparametric MRI (mpMRI) and its corresponding ground truth from the challenge dataset. (1) Pre-contrast T1-weighted (T1); (2) post-contrast T1-weighted (T1Gd) (3) T2-weighted (T2) (4) T2-weighted Fluid Attenuated Inversion Recovery (T2-FLAIR). (5) 2D visualization of the corresponding ground truth. (6) 3D visualization of the ground truth. Annotations include Enhancing Tumor (ET), Non-enhancing tumor core (NCR), vasogenic EDema (ED), and background, respectively, in blue, red, green, and grey. (Color figure online)

where P and G denote surfaces of prediction and ground truth volumes, respectively. p and g are surface voxels in P and G. $d(\cdot)$ represents the distance between two voxels.

3.3 Implementation Details

The convolutions performed in the MenUnet use 3D kernels with size $3 \times 3 \times 3$ followed by a max pooling layer using kernels with size $2 \times 2 \times 2$. The Channel numbers C1, C2, C3, C4, C5, and C6 are, respectively, 32, 64, 128, 256, 320, and 320 to gradually improve the model's representation ability. MenUnet is implemented in a self-configuring framework, nnU-Net [4]. The batch size used for training is 32.

In our work, all experiments were conducted on a workstation equipped with a single NVIDIA A100-PCI GPU card with 40 GB memory. The MenUnet model was trained using the Stochastic Gradient Descent (SGD) optimizer. For the learning rate schedule, the cosine annealing learning rate schedule was adopted, with an initial learning rate set to 0.001 since the cosine annealing learning rate schedule has a smoother learning rate curve, which can contribute to more stable and reliable convergence during training.

4 Results and Discussion

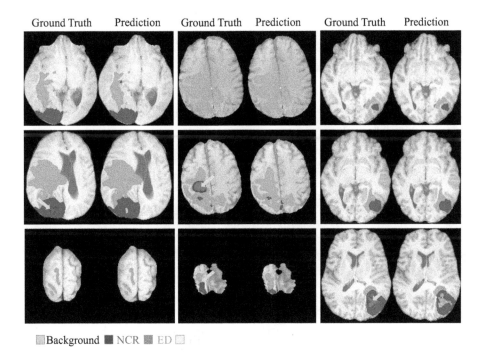

Fig. 3. Vislualization of example meningioma segmentation results on the challenge dataset by the proposed method. Arrows indicate the errors in the NCR region

The quantitative results of the validation set are listed in Tables 2 and 3. The results of the test set are shown in Table 4. It shows that data augmentation boots the performance of MenUnet on the validation set of the 2023 challenge. The performance of MenUnet-DA is ranked 5th in the validation phase. Figure 3 shows the 2D visualization of our meningioma segmentation results in the axial view. Each column displays two example slices of a scan. Figure 3 presents that our proposed method has promising performance in meningioma segmentation even though a large variation exists in shapes and sizes among patients. The predictions are generally smooth and accurate. The main errors are in the NCR.

Table 2. Evaluation of the proposed MenUnet with data augmentation (MenUnet-DA) and without data augmentation (MenUnet) in terms of 3D dice. The performance of MenUnet-DA is ranked 5th in the validation phase

Methods	Dice_ET (%)	Dice_TC (%)	Dice_WT (%)
MenUnet	80.11	80.95	81.40
MenUnet-DA	**82.62**	**82.21**	**83.00**

Table 3. Evaluation of the proposed MenUnet with data augmentation (MenUnet-DA) and without data augmentation (MenUnet) in terms of Hausdorff Distance. The performance of MenUnet-DA is ranked 5th in the validation phase

Methods	Hausdorff_ET (mm)	Hausdorff_TC (mm)	Hausdorff_WT (mm)
MenUnet	56.19	52.84	54.11
MenUnet-DA	**49.32**	**45.33**	**43.33**

Table 4. Evaluation of the proposed MenUnet with data augmentation (MenUnet-DA) in the testing phase

Dice_ET (%)	Dice_TC (%)	Dice_WT (%)
83.01	82.01	76.05
Hausdorff_ET (mm)	Hausdorff_TC (mm)	Hausdorff_WT (mm)
46.87	47.68	55.88

5 Conclusions

This study proposes MenUnet, an accurate network for meningioma segmentation. MenUnet adopts a UNet-like architecture that integrates abstract features with precise spatial control. Our method is ranked 5th in the validation set of the BraTS 2023 Meningioma Challenge. The dice scores of Enhancing Tumor (ET), Tumor core (TC), and whole tumor (WT), respectively, are 82.62%, 82.21%, and 83.00%. The Hausdorff Distance (HD) of ET, TC, and WT are, respectively, 49.32, 45.33, and 43.33 mm. On the test set, the dice scores of Enhancing Tumor (ET), Tumor core (TC), and whole tumor (WT), respectively, are 83.01%, 82.01%, and 76.05%. The Hausdorff Distance (HD) of ET, TC, and WT are, respectively, 46.87, 47.68, and 55.88 mm.

One of the limitations is that the main errors are in the Non-enhancing tumor core (NCR). One future work would be focusing on improving the accuracy of the NCR region. Another limitation is that the generalizability of the proposed method is only validated in the BraTS 2023 Meningioma Challenge Dataset. The challenge dataset is limited in numbers, patients, vendors, etc. More experiments could be done to explore the model's generalization ability.

One of the future works would be weighting different modalities in the input channels. Four modalities weigh the same in the current input. One direction is to use channel-wise attention. Another direction is to train only on T1Gd MRI to enhance the accuracy of NCR region segmentation.

References

1. Chen, J., Li, H., Zhang, J., Menze, B.: Adversarial convolutional networks with weak domain-transfer for multi-sequence cardiac mr images segmentation. In: Statistical Atlases and Computational Models of the Heart. Multi-Sequence CMR

Segmentation, CRT-EPiggy and LV Full Quantification Challenges: 10th International Workshop, STACOM 2019, Held in Conjunction with MICCAI 2019, Shenzhen, China, 13 October 2019, Revised Selected Papers 10, pp. 317–325. Springer, Heidelberg (2020)
2. Galdran, A., Carneiro, G., Ballester, M.A.G.: On the optimal combination of cross-entropy and soft dice losses for lesion segmentation with out-of-distribution robustness. In: Diabetic Foot Ulcers Grand Challenge, pp. 40–51. Springer, Heidelberg (2022)
3. Gordillo, N., Montseny, E., Sobrevilla, P.: State of the art survey on mri brain tumor segmentation. Magn. Reson. Imaging **31**(8), 1426–1438 (2013)
4. Isensee, F., Jaeger, P.F., Kohl, S.A., Petersen, J., Maier-Hein, K.H.: nnu-net: a self-configuring method for deep learning-based biomedical image segmentation. Nat. Methods **18**(2), 203–211 (2021)
5. Jadon, S.: A survey of loss functions for semantic segmentation. In: 2020 IEEE Conference on Computational Intelligence in Bioinformatics and Computational Biology (CIBCB), pp. 1–7. IEEE (2020)
6. Kamnitsas, K., et al.: Efficient multi-scale 3d cnn with fully connected crf for accurate brain lesion segmentation. Med. Image Anal. **36**, 61–78 (2017)
7. Karargyris, A., et al.: Federated benchmarking of medical artificial intelligence with medperf. Nat. Mach. Intell. **5**(7), 799–810 (2023)
8. LaBella, D., et al.: The asnr-miccai brain tumor segmentation (brats) challenge 2023: intracranial meningioma. arXiv preprint arXiv:2305.07642 (2023)
9. Lin, H., Li, B., Wang, X., Shu, Y., Niu, S.: Automated defect inspection of led chip using deep convolutional neural network. J. Intell. Manuf. **30**, 2525–2534 (2019)
10. Lin, H., Liu, T., Katsaggelos, A., Kline, A.: Stenunet: automatic stenosis detection from x-ray coronary angiography. arXiv preprint arXiv:2310.14961 (2023)
11. Lin, H., et al.: Usformer: a light neural network for left atrium segmentation of 3d lge mri. In: 2023 31st European Signal Processing Conference (EUSIPCO), pp. 995–999. IEEE (2023)
12. Liu, T., Lin, H., Katsaggelos, A.K., Kline, A.: Yolo-angio: an algorithm for coronary anatomy segmentation. arXiv preprint arXiv:2310.15898 (2023)
13. Mao, Y., et al.: A deep learning framework for layer-wise porosity prediction in metal powder bed fusion using thermal signatures. J. Intell. Manuf. **34**(1), 315–329 (2023)
14. Nanda, A., Javalkar, V., Banerjee, A.D.: Petroclival meningiomas: study on outcomes, complications and recurrence rates. J. Neurosurg. **114**(5), 1268–1277 (2011)
15. Niu, S., Lin, H., Niu, T., Li, B., Wang, X.: Defectgan: weakly-supervised defect detection using generative adversarial network. In: 2019 IEEE 15th International Conference on Automation Science and Engineering (CASE), pp. 127–132. IEEE (2019)
16. Ogasawara, C., Philbrick, B.D., Adamson, D.C.: Meningioma: a review of epidemiology, pathology, diagnosis, treatment, and future directions. Biomedicines **9**(3), 319 (2021)
17. Ronneberger, O., Fischer, P., Brox, T.: U-net: convolutional networks for biomedical image segmentation. In: Navab, N., Hornegger, J., Wells, W.M., Frangi, A.F. (eds.) MICCAI 2015. LNCS, vol. 9351, pp. 234–241. Springer, Cham (2015). https://doi.org/10.1007/978-3-319-24574-4_28
18. Viaene, A.N., et al.: Transcriptome signatures associated with meningioma progression. Acta Neuropathol. Commun. **7**, 1–13 (2019)
19. Wadhwa, A., Bhardwaj, A., Verma, V.S.: A review on brain tumor segmentation of mri images. Magn. Reson. Imaging **61**, 247–259 (2019)

Exploring Compound Loss Functions for Brain Tumor Segmentation

Anita Kriz[1,2(✉)], Raghav Mehta[1,2], Brennan Nichyporuk[1,2], and Tal Arbel[1,2]

[1] McGill University, Montreal, QC, Canada
{anitakriz,arbel}@cim.mcgill.ca
[2] MILA, (Quebec AI Institute), Montreal, Canada
https://www.cim.mcgill.ca/~pvg/

Abstract. In this study, we introduce a modified 3D U-Net framework tailored for the BraTS 2023 Segmentation - Adult Glioma challenge. Alongside conventional techniques such as data augmentation, post-processing, and Monte Carlo dropout, we investigate the efficacy of compound loss functions with a primary focus on mitigating class imbalance. In particular, we investigate various combinations of cross-entropy, boundary, and dice loss functions to identify the most suitable loss for the given data distribution. By engineering the baseline U-Net model with these modifications, we have determined that the combination of dice and cross-entropy loss yields encouraging results, exemplified by lesion-wise dice scores of 0.753, 0.791, and 0.886. Our analysis justifies the use of specially designed loss functions for the underlying data distribution at hand.

Keywords: Tumor Segmentation · Deep Learning · Computer Vision

1 Introduction

Medical imaging serves as a fundamental tool for disease diagnosis, treatment planning, and clinical research. However, the manual identification of anatomical structures in these images by radiologists is error-prone, contributing to approximately 40 million diagnostic errors involving imaging occuring annually worldwide [6,10]. While Computer-Aided Diagnosis (CAD) systems have become the gold standard due to their reduction in cost, time, and human error, they still rely on radiologist interpretation [7]. Given the escalating demands placed on radiologists and the intricacies inherent in interpreting medical images, deep learning is actively being explored to develop automatic, robust, and standardized methods - particularly for tasks such as medical image segmentation [17].

One important characteristic that needs to be considered in medical image segmentation is the number of classes and their prevalence in the data distribution [12,13]. For example, in datasets such as BraTS, there is a class imbalance of the tissue types, with whole tumor (WT) labels greatly exceeding tumor core (TC) or enhanced tumor (ET) labels. This makes classifying minority labels challenging for the deep learning algorithm as there are simply less positive signals to learn from in the training data. Model-centric challenges arise from factors associated with the chosen model architecture, hyperparameter tuning, and optimization techniques. The two aspects are highly interconnected. The quality and characteristics of the data greatly influence which model architecture and hyperparameters will be most effective. Moreover, the model's performance and ability to generalize are heavily dependent on the quality and diversity of the data it is trained on. Thus, addressing challenges in one aspect often requires consideration of the other, emphasizing the importance of a holistic approach to deep learning model development and deployment.

In this work, we use a modified version of the popularized 3D U-Net for the brain tumor segmentation BraTS 2023 challenge. While the U-Net architecture has proven to be successful in various medical image segmentation tasks, the adaptation of specialized loss functions remains crucial for achieving state-of-the-art performance across different datasets, as emphasized by the authors [8]. Tailored loss functions may help to address specific challenges in medical image segmentation, such as class imbalance and boundary location. Thus, along with data augmentation, post-processing, and Monte Carlo dropout, we provide an in-depth analysis of different compound loss functions. With a focus on understanding the fundamental data distribution our model relies on, we explore ways to customize the loss function to enhance performance on underrepresented classes. Compound losses combine the loss functions from the other groups and have proven to be a robust choice for loss functions. They inherit the benefits of the individual loss functions and have been found to achieve high performance across different datasets [15]. Given the advantages and objectives of the different losses, tailoring a compound loss function based on the characteristics of the problem at hand is worth exploring. Along with data augmentation and connected component post-processing, our model using a compound loss of dice and cross-entropy was able to achieve segmentation results on the online validation dataset of 0.753, 0.791, and 0.886 for lesion-wise enhancing tumor, tumor core, and whole tumor, respectively.

2 Methods

2.1 Model Architecture

The architecture of our model is shown in Fig. 1 and is adapted from Ronnenberger et al.'s U-Net architecture with some modification [16]. We set k, the initial number of feature channels, to be 64. Each part of the contracting path consists of a dropout of 30%, two $3 \times 3 \times 3$ convolutions each with a padding of one, instance normalization, and a Leaky ReLU activation function. This is then followed by a $2 \times 2 \times 2$ max pooling, doubling the number of features. In each part of the expansion path of the model, the feature maps from the previous step are upsampled using trilinear interpolation. The corresponding feature map from the contracting path is copied over, and a dropout of 30% is applied to both the upsampled and copied feature maps. Next, a $3 \times 3 \times 3$ convolution is applied to both the feature maps, they are concatenated, and instance normalization and Leaky ReLU activation is then applied to their concatenation. A final $1 \times 1 \times 1$ convolution is used to map the 64 feature channels to the 4 desired classes (i.e. 0, 1, 2, or 3) to yield the segmentation mask.

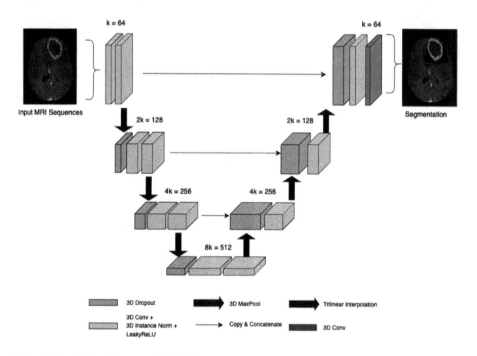

Fig. 1. Model Architecture: 3D U-Net takes as input the 4 MRI sequences and outputs a predicted multi-class segmentation.

2.2 Hyperparameters

Our network structure, processes input channels, indexed by $i = 4$ and initiates with $k = 64$ filters, ultimately producing an output with $o = 4$ filters. The optimizer used was AdamW with a learning rate of 1e–4 and a weight decay of 1e–5. The network was trained for a total number of 120 epochs. To train, various losses were experimented with and are detailed in the following section.

To enhance the model's robustness and generalization capabilities, a combination of data augmentation techniques was employed. These techniques included random flips along any of the three dimensions, rotation by 90° in any direction, random contrast adjustment with gamma correction values sampled from the range (3/4, 4/3), and random affine transformations. The probability of each augmentation varied, with random flips and rotation having a probability of 0.15, contrast adjustment having a probability of 0.4, and affine transformations having a probability of 0.4 as well. The affine transformations involved rotation by $\frac{16\pi}{360}$ radians, a shear range of 0.08, and a scale range of (0.1, 0.1) in each dimension. These augmentation strategies collectively aimed to introduce diverse variations in the input data, thereby improving the model's ability to generalize to different scenarios and enhancing its overall performance.

To optimize memory usage, we employed a strategy of randomly selecting image patches sized 128 × 128 × 128 from each training image. These patches served as input to the U-Net architecture during training. This approach not only conserves memory resources but also aids in accelerating computation, thereby facilitating more efficient model training.

2.3 Loss Functions

Categorical Cross Entropy Loss. is a distribution-based loss used in multi-class classification problems [11]. Given a set of predicted probabilities for each class and the corresponding true labels, the categorical cross-entropy loss measures the dissimilarity between the predicted and true distributions. The equation for the loss function is given below:

$$\mathcal{L}(\hat{\mathbf{y}}, \mathbf{y}) = -\frac{1}{N} \sum_{i=1}^{N} \sum_{j=1}^{C} y_{i,j} \log(\hat{y}_{i,j})$$

where N is the number of samples, C is the number of classes, $\hat{\mathbf{y}}$ is the predicted probabilities following a softmax function, and $\mathbf{y}$ is the one-hot encoded true labels. The softmax function is given by:

$$\hat{y}_{i,j} = \frac{\exp(z_{i,j})}{\sum_{c=1}^{C} \exp(z_{i,c})}$$

where $z_{i,j}$ is the ith samples j^{th} class.

Categorical cross-entropy loss is the most widely-used loss function for classification problems due to its well-behaved gradients. However, cross entropy loss is based on minimizing pixel-wise error, which is demonstrated by the comparison between each voxel in the prediction and ground truth. In class imbalanced datasets such as BraTS, this leads to over-representation of larger objects and results in poorer quality segmentation of smaller objects [15]. For this reason, cross entropy loss is often combined or replaced with other losses in class imbalanced problems [11,15].

Dice Loss. is commonly used in tasks like image segmentation. Its primary objective is to maximize the overlap between the predicted segmentation and the ground truth. This loss function is popular in region-based tasks because it focuses on the agreement between the predicted and ground truth regions rather than pixel-wise classification, as is the case with cross-entropy loss [11].

Dice Loss is based off the Dice Similarity Coefficient (DSC), which is a statisical measure used to quantify the similarity between two sets. It is written as:

$$\text{DSC} = \frac{2 \times |A \cap B|}{|A| + |B|}$$

where $|A|$ is the cardinality of set A, $|B|$ is the cardinality of set B, and $|A \cap B|$ represents the cardinality of the intersection of the two sets. When used in comparing the ground truth from predictions, the dice score requires that the predictions are passed through an argmax function, ensuring that the predictions are one-hot encoded with their most-probable class. For this reason, it is not possible to backpropogate through. Thus, to adapt this as a loss function, the probabilites for each label after the softmax function are used.

The Dice loss is particularly useful in addressing class-imbalanced problems, where certain classes may be underrepresented in the dataset. This is because it evaluates the similarity between two sets (ground truth and predicted segmentation of a particular class) without being heavily influenced by class frequencies. However, it is noted for its inherent instability, mainly due to potentially small denominators in the DSC [11], which could lead to numerical issues during optimization.

Studies have shown that when Dice loss is applied to class-imbalanced tasks, the resulting segmentation tends to have high precision but low recall scores [18]. This implies that while the model may perform well in correctly identifying positive instances, it may miss many relevant instances.

Boundary Loss. is a relatively new type of loss function aimed to minimize the *distance* between ground truth and predicted segmentations [11]. As mentioned above, Dice loss may suffer from unstable optimization. Boundary losses are designed to mitigate these shortcomings of region-based losses, particularly in scenarios where there are significant class imbalances [9].

Boundary losses are computed by performing a voxel-wise multiplication between the softmax predictions generated by the network and a pre-calculated distance map. This distance map is derived from the ground truth segmentation map, wherein the distance to the nearest boundary voxel is determined for each voxel. The resulting loss is obtained by averaging across all voxels associated with a specific sub-tissue type.

It is important to note that boundary losses cannot be used alone. They are typically used in conjunction with region-based losses. This is because boundary losses alone may have limitations, such as getting stuck in local minima or saddle points, especially in cases where there are empty foreground regions [9]. In such situations, the gradients may vanish, leading to difficulties in optimization.

A common approach is to combine boundary loss with region-based losses to leverage the strengths of both types of loss functions. This hybrid approach aims to improve segmentation accuracy by considering both regional and boundary information.

Compound Losses. are designed to inherit benefits from the individual loss functions they combine. Based on the above analysis, we chose to train 6 models, each with different losses, namely Cross-Entropy (CE), Cross-Entropy + Dice (CE + Dice), Cross-Entropy + Boundary (CE + BD), Dice, Dice + Boundary (Dice + BD), and Cross-Entropy + Dice + Boundary loss (CE + Dice + BD). For the Dice and Boundary losses, we implement the loss per sub-region that is considered in evaluation for the BraTS competition rather than the labels themselves. These sub regions are the ET, consisting of label 3, the TC consisting of labels 1 and 3, and the WT consisting of labels 1, 2, and 3.

3 Experimental Setup

3.1 Dataset

The dataset used in this work is the BraTS 2023 Segmentation - Adult Glioma training and validation data [1–5,14]. This includes a total of 5,880 MRI scans from 1,470 brain diffuse glioma patients, with 1251 patients in the training set and 219 patients in the validation set. Each patient file contains native (T1), post-contrast T1 weighted (T1Gd), T2-weighted (T2), and T2 Fluid Attenuated Inversion Recovery (T2-FLAIR) volumes. The mpMRI scans were acquired at multiple different institutions with different clinical protocols and various scanners [5]. The images were annotated by one to four raters following the same annotation protocol and were approved by experienced neuro-radiologists. The segmentation labels given for the annotations are (1) for necrotic parts (NCR) of the tumor, which typically appear hypo-intense in T1Gd when compared to T1, (2) for peritumoral edematous/invaded tissue (ED), which typically appears hyper-intense in FLAIR, (3) for enhancing tumor, which typically appears hyper-intense in T1Gd when compared to both T1 and "healthy" white matter in T1Gd, and (0) for everything else [5]. To do local testing on the dataset, we split the provided training data into 75%, 15%, and 10% for the training, validation, and test split, respectively.

3.2 Preprocessing

The BraTS challenge provides images that have been co-registered to the same anatomical template, interpolated to the same resolution ($1mm^3$) and skull-stripped [5]. We then find the bounding box around the largest brain in the dataset and crop the dimensions of the images to the bounding box's next greatest power of 2. Finally, we standardize the voxel values within the brain to have a 0 mean and standard deviation of 1.

3.3 Inference

This year, the evaluation metrics focus on lesion-wise scoring. To enhance our predictions, we integrated a connected component post-processing step during testing. This process involves removing connected components with fewer than a specified threshold of voxels, set at 1000 voxels. Additionally, to introduce variability in predictions, we maintained a dropout rate of 30% during inference. For robustness, we used Monte Carlo dropout during inference using 20 runs through the test dataset. We used maximum voting for each voxel in each image from these 20 runs to obtain the final prediction.

3.4 Metrics

In the BraTS 2023 Adult Glioma-Segmentation challenge, results were assessed at the lesion-level. In other words, lesion-based Dice scores and Hausdorff distance-95 (HD95) were used rather than entire slice-based scoring. Consequently, the traditional approach of selecting the solution with the highest DSC and/or HD95 may not lead to optimal performance in the BraTS2023 competition. In light of this, we implemented lesion-wise (WT, ET, TC) dice score metrics to be used for evaluation of our models. We then averaged these three scores together to select the best performing model on average.

4 Results and Discussion

4.1 Quantitative Results

To evaluate the effectiveness of compound loss functions, we trained six separate models using different combinations of loss functions: CE, CE + Dice, CE + BD, Dice, Dice + BD, and CE + Dice + BD. We measured performance by calculating the average lesion-wise dice score on the validation split. Based on the average lesion-wise dice score, the top-performing models were those utilizing CE + BD, CE + Dice, and Dice + BD loss functions. The performance of these three models, both with and without augmentation, on the held-out test split is summarized in Table 1 below. Further optimization was carried out by applying the aforementioned data augmentations to these three models. Overall, the model trained with data augmentation and using the combined loss function of CE + Dice performed the best, achieving an average lesion-wise dice score of 0.7647. These scores were calculated before applying connected component post-processing. During inference, we employed majority voting based on 20 Monte Carlo samples for each voxel to ensure the model's predictions' robustness. Given its performance on our held-out test set, we tested the CE + Dice + data augmentation model that was trained on 75% of the training data on the online validation set and obtained dice scores of 0.753, 0.791, and 0.886 for lesion-wise enhancing tumor, tumor core, and whole tumor, respectively.

4.2 Qualitative Results

In Fig. 2, we present 2D slices showing the ground-truth segmentation alongside the output generated by our trained U-Net model using DA, a CCE + Dice

Table 1. Lesion-wise Dice scores on the Test split

	WT Dice	ET Dice	TC Dice	Avg. Lesion-wise Dice
CE + BD	0.7501	0.7366	0.7773	0.7547
CE + BD + DA	**0.7536**	0.6804	0.7668	0.7336
Dice + BD	0.7069	0.738	**0.8304**	0.7584
Dice + BD + DA	0.7473	0.7063	0.801	0.7515
CE + Dice	0.7586	0.7158	0.7819	0.7521
CE + Dice + DA	0.7262	**0.7599**	0.808	**0.7647**

loss function, connected-component post-processing, and Monte Carlo dropout at inference. These overlays are juxtaposed with their corresponding T1c MR images from the held-out test set within our training data. The visual comparison illustrates the model's performance in approximating the ground truth segmentation. Overall, our model demonstrates a high level of accuracy in the example instances. However, a notable exception is observed in patient 00021-001, where the quality of the image appears to be compromised, with artifacts seen throughout the scan. In this case, the model struggles to achieve precise segmentation. Particularly noteworthy is the misclassification observed between necrotic tumor core and enhancing tumor core. This discrepancy underscores the model's weakness to low-quality image data, as such instances are not frequently encountered within the training distribution. In future work, careful data augmentation can alleviate this issue by applying transformations to high quality images that simulate low quality data.

In Fig. 3, we show promising results of our model on the online validation set data. As we did not have access to the validation labels, we only show our predictions next to the T1c image itself.

5 Conclusion

Our comprehensive approach involving the utilization of a U-Net architecture alongside data augmentation, post-processing techniques, Monte Carlo dropout, and compound loss functions tailored to the specific dataset and task has proven to be promising for image segmentation. Through in-depth analysis of various loss combinations, we have determined that the combination of dice and cross-entropy loss yields encouraging results, exemplified by lesion-wise dice scores of 0.753, 0.791, and 0.886 for the enhancing tumor, tumor core, and whole tumor, respectively, on the online validation set.

The incorporation of a boundary loss has shown potential during inference, particularly in enhancing tissue-type scores. This suggests that future approaches should focus on fine-tuning the contribution of each loss component. For instance, reassessing the weighting of individual loss functions within the compound function could further enhance the training process.

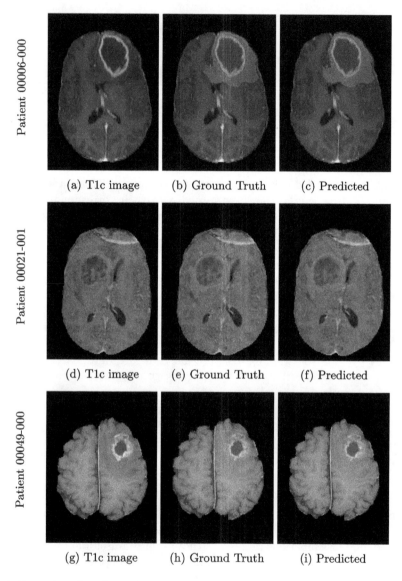

Fig. 2. Examples of results with our trained U-Net model using DA, a CCE + Dice loss function, connected-component post-processing, and Monte Carlo dropout at inference for our held-out test split of the BraTS 2023 Segmentation - Adult Glioma training dataset. The T1c MR volume is on the left, the ground truth overlaid in the center, and the predicted segmentation on the left. The green label corresponds to edema, the red label corresponds to the necrotic tumor core, and the purple label corresponds to the enhancing tumor core. (Color figure online)

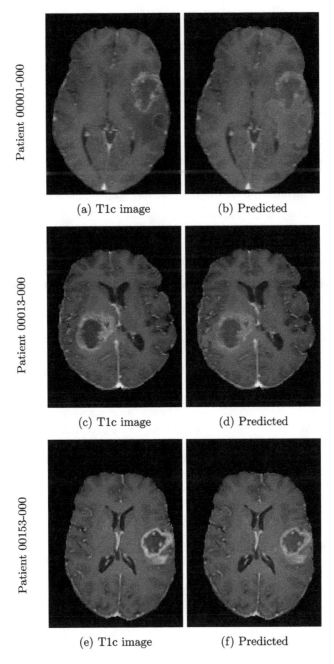

Fig. 3. Examples of Segmentation - Adult-Glioma results with our best performing model for the BraTS 2023 validation dataset. The T1c MR volume is on the left, the ground truth overlaid in the center, and the predicted segmentation on the right. The green label corresponds to edema, the red label corresponds to the necrotic tumor core, and the purple label corresponds to the enhancing tumor core. (Color figure online)

It's crucial to acknowledge the challenges encountered by our model, particularly in its ability to generalize to lower quality images. As evidenced by the performance degradation observed in Patient 00021-001, depicted in Fig. 2, when confronted with such conditions, further efforts may be necessary to address this issue effectively. Specifically, more rigorous data augmentation that simulates low-quality images may significantly improve performance.

In light of this work, continued efforts to develop holistic approaches that align model development with the underlying data distribution hold significant promise for applications such as medical image segmentation. By refining deep learning strategies while remaining mindful of the inherent complexities and nuances of medical imaging datasets, we can strive towards more accurate and reliable segmentation solutions that positively impact patient care and clinical outcomes.

References

1. Baid, U., et al.: The rsna-asnr-miccai brats 2021 benchmark on brain tumor segmentation and radiogenomic classification. arXiv preprint arXiv:2107.02314 (2021)
2. Bakas, S., Akbari, H., Sotiras, A., Bilello, M., Rozycki, M., Kirby, J., et al.: Segmentation labels and radiomic features for the pre-operative scans of the tcga-gbm collection. Cancer Imag. Arch. (2017). https://doi.org/10.7937/K9/TCIA.2017.KLXWJJ1Q
3. Bakas, S., Akbari, H., Sotiras, A., Bilello, M., Rozycki, M., Kirby, J., et al.: Segmentation labels and radiomic features for the pre-operative scans of the tcga-lgg collection. Cancer Imag. Arch. (2017). https://doi.org/10.7937/K9/TCIA.2017.GJQ7R0EF
4. Bakas, S., Akbari, H., Sotiras, A., Bilello, M., Rozycki, M., Kirby, J.S., et al.: Advancing the cancer genome atlas glioma mri collections with expert segmentation labels and radiomic features. Nat. Sci. Data (2017). https://doi.org/10.1038/sdata.2017.117
5. Bakas, S., Baid, U., Meier, Z.: The international brain tumor segmentation (brats) cluster of challenges. In: International Conference on Medical Image Computing and Computer Assisted Intervention (MICCAI) 2023 (MICCAI 2023) (2023)
6. Brady, A.P.: Error and discrepancy in radiology: inevitable or avoidable? Insights Imag. (2017)
7. Doi, K.: Computer-aided diagnosis in medical imaging: historical review, current status and future potential. Comput. Med. Imag. Graph. **31**, 198–211 (2007)
8. Isensee, F., Jäger, P.F., Full, P.M., Vollmuth, P., Maier-Hein, K.H.: nnu-net for brain tumor segmentation. In: Brainlesion: Glioma, Multiple Sclerosis, Stroke and Traumatic Brain Injuries (2021)
9. Kervadec, H., Bouchtiba, J., Desrosiers, C., Granger, E., Dolz, J., Ayed, I.B.: Boundary loss for highly unbalanced segmentation. In: Medical Image Analysis (2021)
10. Itri, J.N., Tappouni, R.R., McEachern, R.O., Pesch, A.J., Patel, S.H.: Fundamentals of diagnostic error in imaging. Radiographics **38**(6), 1845–1865 (2018)
11. Ma, J., et al.: Loss odyssey in medical image segmentation. Med. Image Anal. **71**, 102035 (2021)

12. Johnson, J.M., Khoshgoftaar, T.M.: Survey on deep learning with class imbalance. J. Big Data **6**(1), 1–54 (2019)
13. Gao, L., Zhang, L., Liu, C., Wu, S.: Handling imbalanced medical image data: a deep-learning-based one-class classification approach. Artif. Intell. Med. **108**, 101935 (2020)
14. Menze, B.H., Jakab, A., Bauer, S., Kalpathy-Cramer, J., Farahani, K., Kirby, J., et al.: The multimodal brain tumor image segmentation benchmark (brats). IEEE Trans. Med. Imaging (2015). https://doi.org/10.1109/TMI.2014.2377694
15. Yeung, M., Sala, E., Schonlieb, C.B., Rundo, L.: Unified focal loss: Generalising dice and cross entropy-based losses to handle class imbalanced medical image segmentation. Comput. Med. Imag. Graph. **95**, 102026 (2022)
16. Ronneberger, O., Fischer, P., Brox, T.: U-net: convolutional networks for biomedical image segmentation. In: Navab, N., Hornegger, J., Wells, W.M., Frangi, A.F. (eds.) MICCAI 2015. LNCS, vol. 9351, pp. 234–241. Springer, Cham (2015). https://doi.org/10.1007/978-3-319-24574-4_28
17. Aggarwal, R., et al.: Diagnostic accuracy of deep learning in medical imaging: a systematic review and meta-analysis. NPJ Dig. Med. **4**(1), 65 (2021)
18. Salehi, S.S.M., Erdogmus, D., Gholipour, A.: Tversky loss function for image segmentation using 3D fully convolutional deep networks. In: Wang, Q., Shi, Y., Suk, H.-I., Suzuki, K. (eds.) MLMI 2017. LNCS, vol. 10541, pp. 379–387. Springer, Cham (2017). https://doi.org/10.1007/978-3-319-67389-9_44

Local Synthesis of Healthy Brain Tissue Using an Enhanced 3D Pix2Pix Model for Medical Image Inpainting

M. S. Sadique[✉], M. M. Rahman, W. Farzana, A. Glandon, A. Temtam, and K. M. Iftekharuddin

Old Dominion University, Norfolk, VA 23529, USA
{msadi002,mrahm006,wfarz001,aglan001,atemt001,kiftekha}@odu.edu
https://sites.wp.odu.edu/VisionLab/

Abstract. The restoration of voided regions in three-dimensional (3D) brain Magnetic Resonance Imaging (MRI) data is a critical task in medical image processing. This paper proposes a 3D pix2pix GAN modeling strategy for 3D brain MRI image inpainting, with the goal of improving the quality and diagnostic utility of medical images. The proposed method renders advanced algorithms to accurately predict and reconstruct the voided regions of 3D brain MRI scans. The inpainting outcomes are assessed via online evaluation on BraTS-2023 inpainting challenge data using established metrics, such as the Mean Squared Error (MSE), Peak Signal-to-Noise Ratio (PSNR), and Structural Similarity Index (SSIM). The experimental results demonstrate the effectiveness of the method in achieving a mean SSIM, PSNR, and MSE score of 0.70, 17.52, and 0.049, respectively, indicating spatial coherence and visual accuracy. The improved PSNR and reduced MSE further underscore the quality enhancement achieved by the proposed inpainting method. This work contributes to the field of medical imaging by addressing the crucial challenge of 3D brain MRI image inpainting and demonstrates its potential to enhance medical image analysis, diagnosis, and patient care.

Keywords: Image inpainting · brain tumor · medical imaging · 3D Pix2Pix · segmentation · diagnosis

1 Introduction

Medical imaging, a cornerstone of modern healthcare, has transformed the way medical professionals diagnose and treat various conditions. Among the diverse array of medical imaging techniques, Magnetic Resonance Imaging (MRI) stands out as a powerful tool for non-invasive visualization of intricate structures within the human body. In the realm of brain imaging, the acquisition of three-dimensional (3D) MRI data has revolutionized our understanding of brain anatomy and pathology. However, the acquired MRI images are not always pristine; they often exhibit voided regions due to various factors such as patient motion, limited acquisition time, and technical artifacts. A brain tumor diagnosis heavily relies on accurate medical imaging. The BraTS Image Inpainting Challenge emphasizes the significance of restoring brain tumor images to enhance the accuracy of subsequent analysis.

The application of deep learning to analyze medical images has yielded promising results in several different settings, including tumor detection, segmentation, and classification [1–7]. As the field of medical imaging continues to evolve, the development of advanced techniques for 3D brain MRI image inpainting is essential. Accurate inpainting of missing or corrupted regions enhances the quality of medical images, leading to improved diagnoses and more informed treatment decisions. Different generating models that can create high-quality synthetic data have been introduced since the advent of generative adversarial networks (GANs) [8]. Many of these models produce unlabeled imaging data that could be useful for semi-supervised or self-supervised applications. Some other models can perform conditional generation, which allows for the creation of an image based on a set of criteria drawn from clinical, textual, or imaging data. The latter class of generative models facilitates the generation of labeled synthetic data, which advances machine learning, medical imaging, and clinical practice.

Image inpainting, initially developed for computer vision, has since expanded to encompass various tasks and industries, including medical imaging. Early efforts focused on fixing problems in medical images, such as speckle noise and glossy appearance, to enhance image clarity and diagnostic accuracy. Anomaly detection has also shown its value in this field, as it can remove discrepancies in critical tasks like image registration and segmentation. Inpainting can also improve brain atrophy detection and improve diagnostic procedures. The advent of deep learning has led to a paradigm shift in inpainting techniques, with modern techniques favoring the use of deep neural networks. The adversarial network developed by Armanious et al. [9] is particularly noteworthy for inpainting MR images and a new network designed for medical image modalities. This allows for more complex restorations and faithful feature preservation. The use of neural networks for image restoration has been active research area. In order to train in an unsupervised manner, Pathak et al. [10] proposed the model Context Encoder, which combines encoder decoder and Generative Adversarial Network (GAN) [11]. The adversarial loss is employed to make the inpainted image appear as a real image. However, there are limitations to context encoding, such as the fact that the fully connected layer does not reliably store spatial information and that it occasionally produces blurry textures that do not blend in with the rest of the image. Subsequently, Chao Yang et al. [12] proposed a new approach to inpaint high-resolution images by combining the concepts of style transfer and the context encoder. However, their model is not robust enough to fill the voided region with complex structures. Similar to DCGAN [13], Yeh et al. [14] employ image inpainting for generating and filling in the missing parts of the image. However, the image at the border remains hazy. A new generative model with a single generator and two discriminators is proposed by Satoshi et al. [15]. Results show that this model can improve the details of inpainting. Also proposing a generative model for face completion, Yijun Li et al. [16] use a generator and two discriminators. The image filled with this method appears more realistic and semantically coherent, and the generator is an encoding-decoding architecture. However, this method isn't without its flaws; the model doesn't fully investigate the spatial dependencies between adjacent pixels, and the result isn't great when dealing with some misaligned faces. Many other techniques

[17–19] can also achieve realistic outcomes, enhanced blurring of the inpainted images. Kim et al. demonstrated that it is possible to reconstruct 3D magnetic resonance images of the brain from sparse 2D scans, simplifying imaging without sacrificing data quality or quantity. Kim et al.'s [19] suggestion of using inpainting to generate tumors inside a healthy brain to visualize tumor spreading is an example of the potential for creative application of image inpainting in medicine. A lack of high-level coherence and the difficulty of dealing with the problem of missing large areas or complex structures are still issues that aren't adequately addressed by these methods.

The task of 3D brain MRI image inpainting arises as a critical challenge to address these deficiencies in medical imaging. Inpainting, in this context, involves the restoration of the missing or corrupted portions of 3D brain MRI images, thereby reconstructing a complete and accurate representation of the brain structure. This task holds immense importance as it directly impacts the subsequent analysis, diagnosis, and treatment planning processes conducted by medical professionals. The challenges associated with 3D brain MRI image inpainting are multifaceted. First, the inpainted regions need to be visually coherent and consistent with the surrounding brain anatomy, ensuring that the restored image is diagnostically meaningful. Second, the inpainting process should account for the intricate 3D spatial relationships within the brain, necessitating the development of algorithms that effectively capture such spatial context. Lastly, the inpainted images should be seamlessly integrated with existing medical imaging pipelines, ensuring compatibility with subsequent tasks such as segmentation and feature extraction. This paper introduces a novel approach that leverages a modified 3D Pix2Pix [20] model for inpainting task [21] voided brain tumor images, contributing to the advancement of brain tumor diagnosis and treatment planning.

We present a method for inpainting images in this paper. Our proposed algorithm results in a completion model with generator and discriminator. The discriminator's goal is to determine if the repair result is globally consistent and if the inpainted area is correct after the generator has inpainted it. The generator has an autoencoder structure. The autoencoder has two parts: an encoder that takes an input image and turns it into a latent representation, and a decoder that takes the latent representation and turns it back into the original image. This framework enables the generator to accurately inpaint missing areas by capturing the underlying structure and context of the image.

2 Methodology

Our proposed approach involves the adaptation of the 2D Pix2Pix [20] model to a 3D setting for handling volumetric brain tumor data. This modification enables the network to learn complex spatial relationships within the images. The model is trained to predict the voided regions within brain tumor images by learning from paired examples of voided images and their corresponding ground truth.

2.1 Dataset

We employ the BRATS dataset [22–26], which contains diverse multimodal brain tumor images. The dataset includes various imaging modalities, providing a comprehensive representation of brain tumor cases. The Radiological Society of North America (RSNA), the American Society of Neuroradiology (ASNR), and the Medical Image Computing and Computer Assisted Interventions (MICCAI) society released the Brain Tumor Segmentation Challenge (BraTS) in 2023, from which we used 1251 skull-stripped brain MRI studies. All studies are retrieved using the Neuroimaging Informatics Technology Initiative (NIfTI) format, which consists of a 240 × 240 × 155-pixel 3D imaging array with a pixel dimension of 1 mm along all three axes. At least one high-grade glioma lesion is present in each study, and an NIfTI file is provided for each study with annotated masks for the necrotic tumor core, tumoral edema, and tumoral enhancement (Fig. 1).

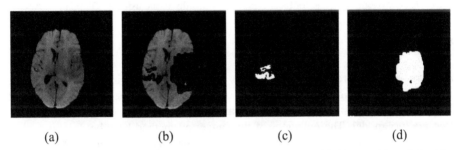

Fig. 1. Examples of a training samples, (a) t1n original image, (b) voided image, (c) mask-healthy, (d) mask-unhealthy

In this competition, only t1n scans from the multi-modal BraTS 2023 glioma segmentation challenge are used as training data. A training set of 1251 cases and a validation set of 219 cases are available for use in training and validating models, respectively. T1n image pairs (including the original and its mask, as well as the void image and its healthy and unhealthy counterparts) make up the training dataset. The following figure shows an example from the training samples.

2.2 Modified 3D Pix2Pix Architecture

Our modified 3D Pix2Pix architecture incorporates a 3D generator and discriminator. The generator learns to map incomplete images to their complete versions while considering the 3D context. The discriminator evaluates the realism of the inpainted images. Skip connections between encoder and decoder facilitate gradient flow, enhancing the network's ability to learn spatial features effectively (Fig. 2).

Generator: The generator network takes the voided image and the mask as inputs and generates a completed image that fills in the masked regions. It's a U-Net architecture with skip connections in encoder and decoder blocks that help preserve high-frequency details. For 3D inpainting, the generator is adapted to handle volumetric data.

Discriminator: The discriminator network evaluates the quality of the generated images by comparing them to the ground truth complete images. It aids in training the generator to produce more realistic inpainted images.

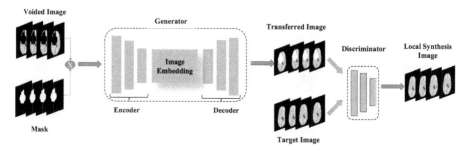

Fig. 2. The overall pipeline for local synthesis of healthy tissue using a 3D pix2pix GAN.

3 Experiments

We carried out comprehensive experiments on the Brain tumor images (BraTS Adult Glioma Dataset) [26] dataset, using a total of 1000 images for the training dataset and 251 images for the testing dataset, to confirm the efficacy and accuracy of the proposed deep pix2pix model. The outcomes of the suggested method have been compared to the results of two base models (Autoencoder and the original pix2pix GAN models). Training parameters: We used the PyTorch open-source framework (v2) and the python programming language (version 3.7) to build the architecture of the suggested model and implement it. When it comes to a hardware system, the model was performed on an NVIDIA V100 HPC platform with a Tesla V100-SXM2-16GB, and CUDA for accelerated training were used in the experiment. There are 300 experimental training iterations. Adam's optimization function is chosen as an optimizer. The batch size was set at 1 and the learning rate is 1e−3.

Network Structure and Implementation Details: All of the models used in the study have $128 \times 128 \times 96$ (Model 1), $128 \times 128 \times 128$ (modified Pix2PixHD Model 2) reshaped images. Train and test data are loaded separately. Then, we create the generator and discriminator models are implemented with PyTorch framework. In addition, we define training parameters learning rate, batch size, epochs and single training step as a step function. The generator of pix2pix model resembles a U-Net architecture and discriminator for both model we keep the same structure. The following section we briefly describe the two different generators.

Model 1: The generator is a U-Net consists of an encoder (downsampler) and decoder (upsampler). The encoder is responsible for downsampling (reducing dimension and increasing channels) of the image whereas the upsampler performs the opposite functionality.

- Each block in the encoder is: Convolution - > Batch normalization - > Leaky ReLU
- Each block in the decoder is: Transposed convolution - > Batch normalization - > Dropout (applied to the first 3 blocks) - > ReLU
- There are skip connections between the encoder and decoder (as in the U-Net).

Model 2: We modify pix2pixHD's [28] generator framework. For better resolution, the Unet divides into a global generator (G1) network and a local enhancer network (G2).

G1 is the core of the generator, and it is surrounded by G2. While the global generator network can only produce images with a resolution of x and y, the local enhancer network can produce images with a resolution four times as large. More local enhancer networks could be used to synthesize images at a higher resolution.

When G1 is fed a semantic label map with a resolution of x × y, it produces an image with the same dimensions. A convolutional front-end, residual block, and a transposed convolutional back-end make up the local enhancer network. The input label map to G2 has a resolution of 2x in every dimension. The input to the residual block differs from that of the global generator network in that it is the element-wise sum of two feature maps: the feature map produced by the convolutional frontend of G2 and the feature map produced by the backend of G1. The integration of global information from G1 to G2 is facilitated by this.

The discriminator's architecture for each model consists of modules following the pattern convolution-BatchNorm-ReLu [29]. Information about the architecture for the discriminator can be found in [20].

Furthermore, we compared the model performance with the baseline model provided by the organizer. In Model 2, we implemented Spatially adaptive normalization with Resnet block, which is derived from [29]. Additionally, we conducted experiments to analyze the impact of different hyperparameters on the discriminator's performance. Our findings suggest that the Spatially adaptive normalization with Resnet block significantly improved the model's ability to learn complex patterns compare to Model 1. Nevertheless, Model 2's performance lags far behind the Baseline model because of input shape. For the Baseline model, an input size of 240 × 240 × 155 was utilized, while Model 2 had to be adjusted to an input shape of 128 × 128 × 128 due to memory constraints.

Evaluation Metrics: We compare our approach to the baselines using three distinct measures of similarity: First, the Peak Signal-to-Noise Ratio (PSNR), second, the Structural Similarity Index Measure (SSIM) [27], and third, the Mean Squared Error (MSE). Metrics are derived exclusively from the region of interest (ROI) where inpainting has occurred. These measures are chosen to comprehensively evaluate the performance of our approach in terms of image quality and fidelity. By focusing on the ROI, we can specifically assess how well our inpainting technique preserves the details and texture of the missing regions.

Results: We evaluated our proposed 3D Pix2Pix model on the BRATS dataset using well-known metrics as peak signal-to-noise ratio (PSNR), structural similarity index (SSIM), and mean squared error (MSE). Our model's ability to successfully restore voided regions produces PSNR and SSIM scores of 0.717 and 16.53, respectively, when compared to the baseline model The baseline model is provided by the organizer. We utilized the trained model and reproduced the results. Model 1 performs better than Model 2 in terms of all three metrics. The inpainted images exhibited a high level of visual coherence and consistency. Additionally, our method was successful in preserving important anatomical structures, as well as the overall integrity of the images that were taken originally. These encouraging results suggest that our proposed 3D Pix2Pix model has the potential to significantly improve the accuracy and reliability of tasks involving the inpainting of medical images.

The 1251 cases for the brain tumor inpainting task are used for training the three model configurations as shown in Table 1. We used the best performing pix2pix models using the training dataset provided by the Brain Tumor Segmentation (BraTS) Challenge 2023 organizer to predict the validation cohort.

Table 1. Online Evaluation on Validation dataset (219 cases).

Model	Statistical Parameter	MSE	PSNR	SSIM
Base	Mean	0.015071001	19.24659077	0.773862472
	Std	0.0097598	3.257652426	0.129973019
	25quantile	0.007440118	17.11192322	0.674699098
	Median	0.013212754	18.79006577	0.778984964
	75quantile	0.019445035	21.28420067	0.869523495
Model 1	Mean	0.032634321	15.71412766	0.6833
	Std	0.020320793	2.917680749	0.182345376
	25quantile	0.01786189	13.96092081	0.591132522
	Median	0.029127529	15.35696316	0.68685919
	75quantile	0.040170558	17.4807539	0.8059403
Model 2 (Ours)	Mean	0.027231	16.53418	0.717443
	Std	0.017125	3.003246	0.141941
	25quantile	0.014881	14.62012	0.608112
	Median	0.023933	16.20998	0.709014
	75quantile	0.034514	18.27369	0.812165

We generated the inpainted images from different variants of pix2pix configurations and submitted for the online evaluation using the validation datasets. The online evaluation results with SSIM, PSNR and MSE DSC are reported in Table 1. The mean SSIM, PSNR and MSE of the proposed model are 0.717, 16.53, and 0.027. The evaluation results show a further improvement of SSIM compared to the model 1.

The inpainting of local healthy tissues is shown for three model configurations in the following Fig. 3: the Baseline Model, Model 1, and Model 2.

The axial, sagittal, and coronal views in the figure provide a comprehensive visualization of the voided image and the corresponding mask. These views allow for a better understanding of how the inpainting process restores the voids in the tissues and ensures that the inpainted areas blend seamlessly with the surrounding tissue. As can be seen in the figure, the Baseline Model restores the voids in the tissues with the highest accuracy, followed by Model 2 and Model 1. The goal of the inpainting process is to make the inpainted areas look consistent with the surrounding tissue. The inpainting process aims to make the inpainted areas look consistent with the surrounding tissue, thereby enhancing the overall visual appearance.

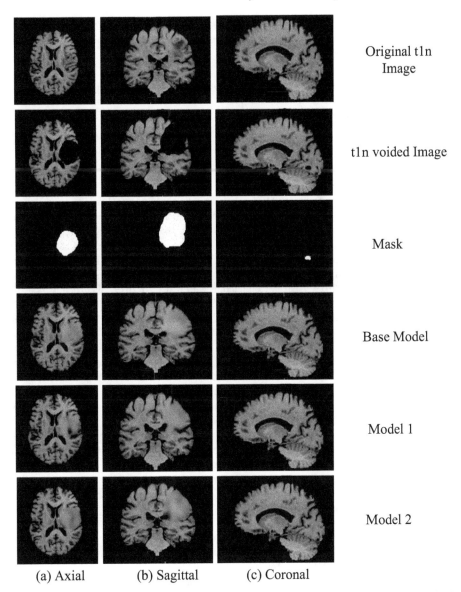

Fig. 3. The visualization of local healthy tissue synthesis on voided images (a) axial, (b) sagittal, and (c) coronal view respectively.

4 Discussion

In this paper, we propose a novel approach for the BRATS Image Inpainting Challenge based on a modified 3D Pix2Pix model for local healthy tissue synthesis. Our findings demonstrate the method's utility for restoring images of brain tumors with high accuracy while preserving the structure of any surrounding healthy tissue. Our method is able to successfully fill in the voided regions with realistic healthy tissue by harnessing the power of the modified 3D Pix2Pix model, resulting in a more complete and accurate representation of the original image.

Acknowledgements. This research was supported in part by an NIH/NIBIB grant with the award number R01EB020683. The authors would like to thank the National Science Foundation for providing partial funding for this work under Grant No. 1828593.

References

1. Pei, L., Vidyaratne, L., Rahman, M.M., Iftekharuddin, K.M.: Deep learning with context encoding for semantic brain tumor segmentation and patient survival prediction. In: Medical Imaging 2020: Computer-Aided Diagnosis, vol. 11314, pp. 102–109. SPIE (2020)
2. Pei, L., Vidyaratne, L., Monibor Rahman, M., Shboul, Z.A., Iftekharuddin, K.M.: Multimodal brain tumor segmentation and survival prediction using hybrid machine learning. In: Brainlesion: Glioma, Multiple Sclerosis, Stroke and Traumatic Brain Injuries: 5th International Workshop, BrainLes 2019, Held in Conjunction with MICCAI 2019, Shenzhen, China, 17 October 2019, Revised Selected Papers, Part II 5, pp. 73–81. Springer, Heidelberg (2020)
3. Pei, L., Vidyaratne, L., Hsu, W.W., Rahman, M.M., Iftekharuddin, K.M.: Brain tumor classification using 3d convolutional neural network. In: Brainlesion: Glioma, Multiple Sclerosis, Stroke and Traumatic Brain Injuries: 5th International Workshop, BrainLes 2019, Held in Conjunction with MICCAI 2019, Shenzhen, China, 17 October 2019, Revised Selected Papers, Part II 5, pp. 335–342. Springer, Heidelberg (2020)
4. Isensee, F., Jaeger, P.F., Kohl, S.A., Petersen, J., Maier-Hein, K.H.: NnU-Net: a self-configuring method for deep learning-based biomedical image segmentation. Nat. Methods **18**(2), 203–211 (2021)
5. Rahman, M.M., Sadique, M.S., Temtam, A.G., Farzana, W., Vidyaratne, L., Iftekharuddin, K.M.: Brain tumor segmentation using UNet-context encoding network. In: International MICCAI Brainlesion Workshop, pp. 463–472. Springer, Cham (2021)
6. Sadique, M.S., Rahman, M.M., Farzana, W., Temtam, A., Iftekharuddin, K.M.: Brain tumor segmentation using neural ordinary differential equations with UNet-context encoding network. In: International MICCAI Brainlesion Workshop, pp. 205–215. Springer, Cham (2022)
7. Sadique, M.S., Farzana, W., Temtam, A., Iftekharuddin, K.M.: Class activation mapping and uncertainty estimation in multi-organ segmentation. In: Medical Imaging 2023: Computer-Aided Diagnosis, vol. 12465, pp. 169–174. SPIE (2023)
8. Efros, A.A., Leung, T.K.: Texture synthesis by non-parametric sampling. In: Proceedings of the Seventh IEEE International Conference on Computer Visio, vol. 2, pp. 1033–1038. IEEE (1999)
9. Armanious, K., Mecky, Y., Gatidis, S., Yang, B.: Adversarial inpainting of medical image modalities. In: ICASSP 2019–2019 IEEE International Conference on Acoustics, Speech and Signal Processing (ICASSP), pp. 3267–3271. IEEE (2019)
10. Pathak, D., Krahenbuhl, P., Donahue, J., Darrell, T., Efros, A.A.: Context encoders: feature learning by inpainting. In: Proceedings of the IEEE Conference on Computer Vision and Pattern Recognition, pp. 2536–2544 (2016)
11. Goodfellow, I., et al.: Generative adversarial nets. Adv. Neural Inf. Process. Syst. **27**, 1–9 (2014)

12. Yang, C., Lu, X., Lin, Z., Shechtman, E., Wang, O., Li, H.: High-resolution image inpainting using multi-scale neural patch synthesis. In: Proceedings of the IEEE Conference on Computer Vision and Pattern Recognition, pp. 6721–6729 (2017)
13. Radford, A., Metz, L., Chintala, S.: Unsupervised representation learning with deep convolutional generative adversarial networks (2015). arXiv preprint arXiv:1511.06434
14. Yeh, R.A., Chen, C., Yian Lim, T., Schwing, A.G., Hasegawa-Johnson, M., Do, M.N.: Semantic image inpainting with deep generative models. In: Proceedings of the IEEE Conference on Computer Vision and Pattern Recognition, pp. 5485–5493 (2017)
15. Iizuka, S., Simo-Serra, E., Ishikawa, H.: Globally and locally consistent image completion. ACM Trans. Graph. (ToG) **36**(4), 1–14 (2017)
16. Li, Y., Liu, S., Yang, J., Yang, M.H.: Generative face completion. In: Proceedings of the IEEE Conference on Computer Vision and Pattern Recognition, pp. 3911–3919 (2017)
17. Demir, U., Unal, G.: Patch-based image inpainting with generative adversarial networks (2018). arXiv preprint arXiv:1803.07422
18. Yu, J., Lin, Z., Yang, J., Shen, X., Lu, X., Huang, T.S.: Generative image inpainting with contextual attention. In: Proceedings of the IEEE Conference on Computer Vision and Pattern Recognition, pp. 5505–5514 (2018)
19. Kim, S., Kim, B., Park, H.: Synthesis of brain tumor multicontrast MR images for improved data augmentation. Med. Phys. **48**(5), 2185–2198 (2021)
20. Isola, P., Zhu, J.Y., Zhou, T., Efros, A.A.: Image-to-image translation with conditional adversarial networks. In: Proceedings of the IEEE Conference on Computer Vision and Pattern Recognition, pp. 1125–1134 (2017)
21. Kofler, F., et al.: The Brain Tumor Segmentation (BraTS) Challenge 2023: Local Synthesis of Healthy Brain Tissue via Inpainting (2023). arXiv preprint arXiv:2305.08992
22. Baid, U., et al.: The rsna-asnr-miccai brats 2021 benchmark on brain tumor segmentation and radiogenomic classification (2021). arXiv preprint arXiv:2107.02314
23. Menze, B.H., et al.: The multimodal brain tumor image segmentation benchmark (BRATS). IEEE Trans. Med. Imaging **34**(10), 1993–2024 (2014)
24. Bakas, S., et al.: Advancing the cancer genome atlas glioma MRI collections with expert segmentation labels and radiomic features. Sci. Data **4**(1), 1–13 (2017)
25. Bakas, S., et al.: Segmentation labels and radiomic features for the pre-operative scans of the TCGA-GBM collection (2017). *10.7937 K, 9*
26. Bakas, S., et al.: Segmentation labels and radiomic features for the pre-operative scans of the TCGA-LGG collection. Cancer Imag. Arch. **286** (2017)
27. Wang, Z., Bovik, A.C., Sheikh, H.R., Simoncelli, E.P.: Image quality assessment: from error visibility to structural similarity. IEEE Trans. Image Process. **13**(4), 600–612 (2004)
28. Wang, T.C., Liu, M.Y., Zhu, J.Y., Tao, A., Kautz, J., Catanzaro, B.: High-resolution image synthesis and semantic manipulation with conditional gans. In: Proceedings of the IEEE Conference on Computer Vision and Pattern Recognition, pp. 8798–8807 (2018)
29. Park, T., Liu, M.Y., Wang, T.C., Zhu, J.Y.: Semantic image synthesis with spatially-adaptive normalization. In: Proceedings of the IEEE/CVF Conference on Computer Vision and Pattern Recognition, pp. 2337–2346 (2019)

Brain Tumor Segmentation: Glioma Segmentation in Sub-Saharan Africa Patients Using nnU-Net

M. S. Sadique^(✉), M. M. Rahman, W. Farzana, A. Glandon, A. Temtam, and K. M. Iftekharuddin

Old Dominion University, Norfolk, VA 23529, USA
{msadi002,mrahm006,wfarz001,aglan001,atemt001,kiftekha}@odu.edu

Abstract. Accurate and automatic segmentation of glioblastoma multiforme (GBM) is crucial for effective treatment planning, disease diagnosis, surgical planning, and brain tumor tracking. MRI and other imaging modalities are used to capture the complex nature of GBM, however the intrinsic heterogeneity in tumor features adds to the difficulty of segmentation. Consequently, advanced computational algorithms and machine learning approaches are being developed to improve the accuracy and efficiency of GBM segmentation. Recently, deep learning-based U-Net architecture has been the state-of-the-art method for segmenting medical images. This work builds on our prior work on U-Net for GBM segmentation and proposes state-of-the-art nnU-Net for adult glioma segmentation in the brain tumor segmentation challenge-2023 (BraTS-Africa Adult Glioma). The nnU-Net allows training of different multiple networks: 2D U-Net, 3D U-Net to perform semantic segmentation of 3D images with high accuracy and performance. We find the best configurations from different variants of nn-UNet and combine an ensemble of these variants to improve segmentation performance. We utilize 3D U-Net to perform segmentation of brain tumor for BraTS Africa dataset. In addition, we compare the result with our 3D UNetcontext encoding model which is pretrained on BraTS Adult glioma data and then fine-tuned on BraTS Africa dataset. The accuracy of our proposed nn-UNet for brain segmentation from multi-modal MRI is evaluated using a 5-fold cross-validation over 15 manually segmented images from the BraTS 2023 challenge. The mean of the lesion-wise Dice Similarity Coefficient (DSC) of the BraTS -Africa validation dataset is 0.7445, 0.7244, and 0.8526 for Enhance Tumor (ET), Tumor Core (TC), and Whole Tumor (WT), respectively. The performance of our model on the BraTS-Africa data set indicates that higher segmentation accuracy may be attained utilizing the latest nn-UNet method.

Keywords: Glioblastoma · Brain Tumor Segmentation · nnU-Net · Neural Ordinary Differential Equations · Deep neural network · U-Net

1 Introduction

GBM is the most common and aggressive primary malignant brain tumor in adults [1, 2]. The prognosis for GBM is generally poor due to its aggressive nature, infiltrative growth pattern, and limited treatment options. Survival rates for GBM are typically low, with most patients surviving for less than two years after diagnosis. Despite advancements in treatment options such as surgery, radiation therapy, and chemotherapy, the tumor's ability to spread rapidly throughout the brain makes it difficult to completely eradicate. The median survival for newly diagnosed GBM is around 12 to 15 months with optimal treatment, which typically includes surgery, radiation therapy, and chemotherapy [3].

Automatic and accurate brain tumor segmentation from multi-modal magnetic resonance imaging (MRI) can support clinical workflows across multiple domains including diagnostic interventions, treatment planning, and treatment delivery. Brain tumor segmentation is a crucially important step for computer-aided diagnosis and biomarker measurement systems [4]. Semantic segmentation of treatment volumes and organs at risk are also essential for radiotherapeutic planning [5]. More generally, semantic segmentation-based patient-specific anatomical models transform raw biomedical image data into meaningful, spatially structured information and can aid in surgical planning and execution through intraoperative image guidance systems [6] or tumor growth monitoring [7]. Manual segmentation of 3D brain tumor images is labor intensive and impractical for most clinical workflows. Brain tumor segmentation can be difficult, because more information must be shared through the network, exacerbating the memory challenges. The weighting of the losses for different abnormal tissue types can have unpredictable effects on convergence and final error. The Dice Similarity Coefficient (DSC) is used to address these problems but remains poorly characterized. Imposing shape and topological constraints between specified abnormal tissue types also remains difficult.

Despite these challenges, recent advances in machine learning, computational power, and data availability have allowed the training of more complex methods, including deep convolutional neural networks (CNN), which promise higher segmentation accuracy [8]. However, these pipelines are often limited in their applicability to specific image analysis problems of the end-user and could not have achieved higher accuracies than the most accurate registration-based methods for most cases. In this work, we present the application of nnU-Net [9] for the segmentation task of BraTS-2023 Challenge on Sub-Sahara-Africa Adult Glioma. The nnUNet is a powerful open-source tool that can be used state-of-the-art segmentation pipeline to help scientific progress in automated method design. The pipeline can be trained and inferred on any medical dataset, providing an end-to-end automated pathway for segmentation. The nnU-Net has outperformed the state-of-the-art architecture in the Medical Decathlon Challenge [10], consisting of 10 different datasets, by using an ensemble of the same U-Net architecture with an automated pipeline consisting of pre-processing, data augmentation, and post-processing. It has set a new standard in the field of medical image segmentation, without having to set a new structure for each dataset individually. The pipeline itself can automatically tune hyper-parameters, so there is no need to make any changes to the network architecture in order to achieve state-of-the-art results. Context encoding [11] with the Neural Ordinary Differential Equations (NODEs) [12, 13], which have shown promise for semantic segmentation of brain tumors due to enhanced representative feature learning, was implemented in the prior BraTS competition [14–20].

We implemented state-of-the-art nnU-Net for adult glioma segmentation. The nnU-Net model is widely recognized for its superior performance in medical image segmentation tasks. By leveraging advanced deep learning techniques, our implementation of nnU-Net has achieved remarkable accuracy and efficiency in segmenting adult gliomas. In addition, we compare the result with our 3D UNet-context encoding (UNCE) model which is pretrained on BraTS Adult glioma data and then fine-tuned on BraTS-Africa dataset. Our comparison shows that the nnU-Net outperforms our 3D UNet-context encoding model in terms of segmentation accuracy and efficiency for adult gliomas. This highlights the effectiveness of leveraging state-of-the-art techniques in medical image segmentation tasks.

2 Methodology

2.1 Dataset

For training data, we use the datasets provided by BraTS2023 challenge. In the BraTS-Africa Challenge 2023 Task, a total of 60 cases with voxel-level annotations of different tumor sub-tissues: necrotic (NC), peritumoral edema (ED), and enhancing tumor (ET) are presented. Standardized brain tumor imaging protocols were used to acquire the multi-parametric magnetic resonance imaging (mpMRI) scans from multiple institutions for this data set. T1-weighted (T1), T1-weighted (T1Gd), T2-weighted (T2), and T2-FLAIR (T2-fluid attenuated inversion recovery) MRI image volumes are used for the mpMRI scans. All imaging data are reviewed by board-certified radiologists with extensive experience in neuro-oncology, pre-processed, and manually annotated using the BraTS pre-processing and annotation protocols. Tumor sub-region ground truth annotations are reviewed and accepted by board-certified neuroradiologists [21–26]. For online evaluation in the validation phase, there are 15 cases provided without any associated ground truth. Figure 1 presents an example from the training data overlaid with a tumor mask.

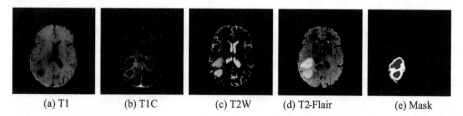

Fig. 1. Example of a training case: four different MRI modalities:(a) T1, (b) T1C, (c) T2, (d) FLAIR with (e) Ground Truth.

2.2 Network Training

The nnU-Net pipeline uses a heuristic rule to determine the data-dependent hyper-parameters, or "data fingerprint", to ingest the training data. The blueprint parameters (loss function, optimizer, architecture) and derived parameters (image resampling, normalization, stack and patch size) along with the data fingerprint create pipeline fingerprints. Pipeline fingerprints generate network training for 2D, 3D, and 3D Cascade

U-Net using the hyperparameters identified so far. The ensemble of different network configurations, along with post-processing, determines the best average Dice coefficient for the training data. The best configuration will then be used to produce the predictions for the test data.

Table 1. Network configurations generated by nnU-Net and UNCE-NODE for the BraTS-Africa 2023 Challenge Dataset

Parameters	2D U-Net	3D full resolution U-Net	UNCE-NODE
Target spacing (mm)	$1 \times 1 \times 1$	$1 \times 1 \times 1$	$1 \times 1 \times 1$
Median image shape at target spacing	175×137.5	$139 \times 175 \times 137.5$	$240 \times 240 \times 155$
Patch size	192×160	$128 \times 160 \times 112$	$192 \times 160 \times 128$
Batch size	105	2	2

Table 1 represents the variants of network configuration generated by nnUNet for the Multi-Modal Brain tumor Segmentation (BraTS) 2023 challenge. In the following sections, we summarized the detailed information for implementation of nnU-Net.

2.3 Dataset Fingerprint

The dataset fingerprint contains a set of heuristic rules to infer data-dependent hyperparameters of the pipeline. The nnU-Net creates this fingerprint based on the cropped training data that captures all the relevant parameters and properties: image size (i.e. number of voxels per spatial dimension) before and after cropping image, image spacing (i.e. physical size of the voxels), modalities (from metadata like CT, MRI), and number of classes for all images and total number of training cases.

2.4 Blueprint Parameters

a. **Network Architecture Template:** The nnU-Net architecture closely follows the original U-Net [13], and recent variations such as residual connection, attention mechanisms, squeeze and excitation, and dilated convolutions have been proposed. Large patch sizes and small batch sizes are used in the nnU-Net. Figure 2 shows the architecture of the 3D U-Net model and its different components. The U-Net architecture consists of a contracting and an expanding path that aims to build a bottleneck in its innermost part through a combination of convolution, instance norm, and leaky ReLU operations. After this bottleneck, the image is reconstructed by combining convolutions and upsampling. Skip connections are added to help the backward flow of gradients, in an effort to improve the training.

b. **Training Schedule:** All configurations of nnU-Net are trained for 1000 epochs with one epoch defined as iteration over 250 mini-batches. For learning the network weights, Stochastic gradient descent with Nesterov momentum and an initial learning

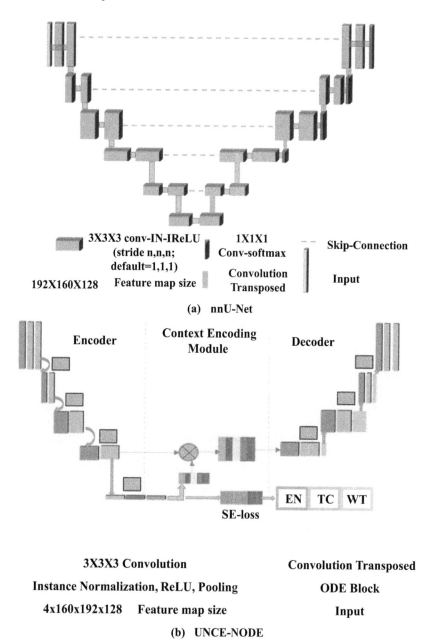

Fig. 2. The (a) nnU-Net and (b) UNCE-NODE processing pipeline (see details implementation [19]). nnU-Net is a fully automatic, end-to-end deep learning pipeline that segments multiple organs from 3D scans across different imaging modalities.

rate of 0.01 is used. All models are trained with an Adam optimizer. The loss function for the nnU-Net is a combination of cross-entropy and dice loss. An oversampling technique is implemented to handle class imbalance. Different data augmentation techniques: rotation, scaling, Gaussian noise, Gaussian blur, brightness, contrast, and simulation of low resolution and gamma resolution have been applied.

c. **Inference:** Images are predicted by using a sliding window approach, where the window size is the same as the patch size used during training. Predictions that are adjacent will overlap by half the size of a patch. To reduce stitching artifacts and reduce the influence of positions close to the borders, a Gaussian importance weighting is applied, increasing the weight of the center voxels in the softmax aggregation.

2.5 Inferred Parameters

Two different image intensity normalization schemes are supported by the nnU-Net. All modalities except CT images use z-scoring as the default setting. For CT, it follows a global normalization scheme, which uses 0.5 and 99.5 percentiles of the foreground voxels for clipping. To justify the heterogeneity of the medical field, all images are resampled to the same target spacing using third-order splines, linear interpolation, or nearest-neighbor interpolation. The network topology for all U-Net configurations is selected based on the median image size after resampling and the target distance at which the images were resampled. The architecture is configured by specifying the number of downsampling operations to be performed until the feature map is reduced to 4 voxels or the feature map space becomes anisotropic. The high-resolution axes are down-sampled separately until their resolution is within a factor of 2 of the lower resolution axes. Each axis is down-sampled individually, until the feature map constraints are activated. The default kernel sizes for aggregates are $3 \times 3 \times 3$ and 3×3 for 3D U-Net and 2D U-Net, respectively.

2.6 Empirical Parameters

a. **Ensembling and selection of U-Net configuration(s):** Models are ensembled by averaging softmax probabilities. Automatically ensembles are implemented based on average foreground Dice coefficient computed via cross validation on training data to use for inference. Variants of the configuration model(s) include single models (2D, 3D_fullres) or an ensemble of any two of these configurations.

b. **Post-processing:** Post-processing is applied based on the connected component used. All foreground classes are treated as a single component, to improve the average foreground Dice coefficient, and if this does not reduce the Dice coefficient for any classes. nnU-Net relies on the outcome of this step and decides whether the same process should be followed for individual classes.

3 Experiments

The 60 multi-modal MRI scans for the segmentation task are used for training each configuration as a five-fold cross-validation. We use 2D, and 3D_fullres models and find the best configurations obtained from the cross-validation on the training cases as an ensemble predict the validation cohort. We generated the segmented mask from different variants of nnU-Net configurations and submitted for the online evaluation using the validation datasets. In addition, we also validated our UNCE-NODE model for comparison. The online evaluation results with Lesion wise DSC and HD95 are reported in Table 2.

Table 2. Online Evaluation on Validation dataset (219 cases).

Model	Statistical Parameter	Lesion wise Dice Score			Lesion wise Hausdroff95		
		ET	TC	WT	ET	TC	WT
nnU-Net	mean	0.7445	0.7244	0.8526	72.32	75.08	16.07
	std	0.3205	0.3386	0.2644	125.9	126.7	47.77
	25quantile	0.6214	0.4475	0.8905	1	1.866	2
	median	0.9146	0.9262	0.9549	2.236	2.236	2.236
	75quantile	0.9444	0.9622	0.9735	96.94	115.0	4.659
UNCE-NODE	mean	0.7005	0.7424	0.8480	54.87	53.67	28.37
	std	0.2326	0.2310	0.1914	93.43	84.62	66.23
	25quantile	0.4905	0.5331	0.8582	2.103	2.342	2.342
	median	0.8647	0.8753	0.9340	3	3.162	3
	75quantile	0.8799	0.9349	0.9540	68.06	104.2	5.381

The dice scores of the UNCE-NODE model are 0.7005, 0.7424, and 0.8480 for en-hancing tumor (ET), tumor core (TC), and whole tumor (WT), respectively. The Hausdorff95 distances of the same model are 54.87 for ET, 53.67 for TC, and 28.37 for WT. The Dice scores of the nnU-Net model are 0.74455, 0.7244, and 0.8526 for enhancing tumor (ET), tumor core (TC), and whole tumor (WT), respectively. The Hausdorff95 distances of the same model are 72.32 for ET, 75.08 for TC, and 16.07 for WT. The evaluation results show an overall improvement of Hausdroff95 scores compared to the nnU-Net model for enhance tumor and tumor core and in terms of dice score nnU-Net outperforms than UNCE-NODE model for whole tumor and enhance tumor Nevertheless, there has been no substantial enhancement in the performance of nnU-Net, attributed to the limited number of training cases.

The UNCE-NODE model demonstrated lower performance on lesion-wise DSC compared to the nnU-Net. Nevertheless, the dice score of the enhance tumor (ET) is notably low for the DIPG dataset, indicating a potential domain shift in the data distribution from the source (BraTS) to the target dataset (DIPG). Figure 3 shows the T2 image overlaid with predicted segmentation mask in the first (nnUNet) and second row (UNCE-NODE) respectively for the same case.

During the Testing phase, we submitted MLCubes to assess the performance of our model on data that had not been previously seen. The MLCubes that have been submitted will be executed and assessed on the challenge platform utilizing MedPerf [27] a benchmarking platform designed for medical artificial intelligence.

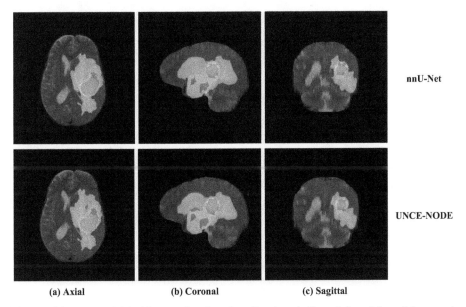

(a) Axial	(b) Coronal	(c) Sagittal

Fig. 3. T2 image overlaid with ground truth and predicted mask. From left to right: axial, coronal, and sagittal view respectively.

4 Discussion

The purpose of this paper is to demonstrate the comparative application of nn-UNET and UNCE-NODE models for the Multi-Modal Brain Tumor Segmentation (BraTS) Challenge 2023. The nnU-Net framework is customized to fit the specifications of the BraTS Challenge 2023 dataset. Using a transfer learning approach, we also evaluate the generalizability of the UNCE-NODE model. Our UNCE-NODE model exhibits comparative performance, demonstrating its potential for broader applications in medical imaging.

Acknowledgements. This work was partially funded through NIH/NIBIB grant under award number R01EB020683. The authos would like to acknowledge partial support of this work by the National Science Foundation Grant No. 1828593.

References

1. Louis, D.N., et al.: The 2016 World Health Organization classification of tumors of the central nervous system: a summary. Acta Neuropathol. **131**, 803–820 (2016)
2. Ostrom, Q.T., Gittleman, H., Truitt, G., Boscia, A., Kruchko, C., Barnholtz-Sloan, J.S.: CBTRUS statistical report: primary brain and other central nervous system tumors diagnosed in the United States in 2011–2015. Neuro-oncology **20**(suppl_4), pp.iv1–v86 (2018)
3. Krex, D., et al.: Long-term survival with glioblastoma multiforme. Brain **130**(10), 2596–2606 (2007)

4. Van Ginneken, B., Schaefer-Prokop, C.M., Prokop, M.: Computer-aided diagnosis: how to move from the laboratory to the clinic. Radiology **261**(3), 719–732 (2011)
5. Sykes, J.: Reflections on the current status of commercial automated segmentation systems in clinical practice. J. Med. Radiat. Sci. **61**(3), 131–134 (2014)
6. Howe, R.D., Matsuoka, Y.: Robotics for surgery. Ann. Rev. Biomed. Eng. **1**(1), 211–240 (1999)
7. Weber, W.A., Figlin, R.: Monitoring cancer treatment with PET/CT: does it make a difference? J. Nucl. Med. **48**(1 suppl), 36S-44S (2007)
8. Litjens, G., et al.: A survey on deep learning in medical image analysis. Med. Image Anal. **42**, 60–88 (2017)
9. Isensee, F., Jäger, P.F., Kohl, S.A., Petersen, J., Maier-Hein, K.H.: Automated design of deep learning methods for biomedical image segmentation. arXiv preprint arXiv:1904.08128 (2019)
10. Antonelli, M., et al.: The medical segmentation decathlon. Nat. Commun. **13**(1), 4128 (2022)
11. Zhang, H., et al.: Context encoding for semantic segmentation. In: Proceedings of the IEEE Conference on Computer Vision and Pattern Recognition, pp. 7151–7160 (2018)
12. Pinckaers, H., Litjens, G.: Neural ordinary differential equations for semantic segmentation of individual colon glands. arXiv preprint arXiv:1910.10470 (2019)
13. Chen, R.T., Rubanova, Y., Bettencourt, J., Duvenaud, D.K.: Neural ordinary differential equations. Adv. Neural. Inf. Process. Syst. **31**, 1–13 (2018)
14. Pei, L., Vidyaratne, L., Rahman, M.M., Iftekharuddin, K.M.: Deep learning with context encoding for semantic brain tumor segmentation and patient survival prediction. In: Medical Imaging 2020: Computer-Aided Diagnosis, vol. 11314, pp. 102–109. SPIE (2020)
15. Pei, L., Vidyaratne, L., Monibor Rahman, M., Shboul, Z.A., Iftekharuddin, K.M.: Multimodal brain tumor segmentation and survival prediction using hybrid machine learning. In: Brainlesion: Glioma, Multiple Sclerosis, Stroke and Traumatic Brain Injuries: 5th International Workshop, BrainLes 2019, Held in Conjunction with MICCAI 2019, Shenzhen, China, 17 October 2019, Revised Selected Papers, Part II 5, pp. 73–81. Springer, Heidelberg (2020)
16. Pei, L., Vidyaratne, L., Hsu, W.W., Rahman, M.M., Iftekharuddin, K.M.: Brain tumor classification using 3d convolutional neural network. In: Brainlesion: Glioma, Multiple Sclerosis, Stroke and Traumatic Brain Injuries: 5th International Workshop, BrainLes 2019, Held in Conjunction with MICCAI 2019, Shenzhen, China, 17 October 2019, Revised Selected Papers, Part II 5, pp. 335–342. Springer, Heidelberg (2020)
17. Isensee, F., Jaeger, P.F., Kohl, S.A., Petersen, J., Maier-Hein, K.H.: NnU-Net: a self-configuring method for deep learning-based biomedical image segmentation. Nat. Methods **18**(2), 203–211 (2021)
18. Rahman, M.M., Sadique, M.S., Temtam, A.G., Farzana, W., Vidyaratne, L., Iftekharuddin, K.M.: Brain tumor segmentation using UNet-context encoding network. In: International MICCAI Brainlesion Workshop, pp. 463–472. Springer, Cham (2021)
19. Sadique, M.S., Rahman, M.M., Farzana, W., Temtam, A., Iftekharuddin, K.M.: Brain tumor segmentation using neural ordinary differential equations with UNet-context encoding network. In: International MICCAI Brainlesion Workshop, pp. 205–215. Springer, Cham (2022)
20. Sadique, M.S., Farzana, W., Temtam, A., Iftekharuddin, K.M.: Class activation mapping and uncertainty estimation in multi-organ segmentation. In: Medical Imaging 2023: Computer-Aided Diagnosis, vol. 12465, pp. 169–174. SPIE (2023)
21. Adewole, M., et al.: The brain tumor segmentation (BraTS) challenge 2023: glioma segmentation in Sub-Saharan Africa patient population (BraTS-Africa). arXiv preprint arXiv:2305.19369 (2023)
22. Baid, U., et al.: The rsna-asnr-miccai brats 2021 benchmark on brain tumor segmentation and radiogenomic classification. arXiv preprint arXiv:2107.02314 (2021)

23. Menze, B.H., et al.: The multimodal brain tumor image segmentation benchmark (BRATS). IEEE Trans. Med. Imaging **34**(10), 1993–2024 (2014)
24. Bakas, S., et al.: Advancing the cancer genome atlas glioma MRI collections with expert segmentation labels and radiomic features. Sci. Data **4**(1), 1–13 (2017)
25. Bakas, S., et al.: Segmentation labels and radiomic features for the pre-operative scans of the TCGA-GBM collection (2017). 10.7937 K, 9
26. Bakas, S., et al.: Segmentation labels and radiomic features for the pre-operative scans of the TCGA-LGG collection. Canc. Imaging Arch. **286** (2017)
27. Karargyris, A., et al.: Federated benchmarking of medical artificial intelligence with MedPerf. Nat. Mach. Intell. **5**(7), 799–810 (2023)

Pediatric Brain Tumor Segmentation Using Multiresolution Fractal Deep Neural Network

A. Temtam[✉], M. S. Sadique, M. M. Rahman, W. Farzana, and K. M. Iftekharuddin

Old Dominion University, Norfolk, VA 23529, USA
{atemt001,msadi002,mrahm006,wfarz001,kiftekha}@odu.edu
https://sites.wp.odu.edu/VisionLab/

Abstract. Pediatric (PED) central nervous system tumors are the leading cause of cancer-related deaths in children, with highgrade gliomas having a dismal five-year survival rate below 20%. The rarity of these tumors often leads to delayed diagnosis, difficult treatment regimens, and necessitates multi-institutional collaborations for clinical trials. Automated and precise volumetric measurements can offer a more standardized way to determine the extent of disease and monitor the effectiveness of treatments. Multiresolution Fractal Deep Neural Network (MFDNN) has been proposed earlier for multiscale deep learning fractal-based tissue segmentation. In this work, we hypothesize that a MFDNN can automatically extract intricate multiresolution texture features when analyzing data from pediatric patients with high-grade glioma. We employ MFDNN on a data set of pediatric MRI scans that include diverse tumor subtypes. The training data set consists of multi-parametric MRI (mpMRI) scans from BraTS-PEDs 2023 challenge. The model segmentation efficacy is assessed against separate validation and unseen mpMRI data of high-grade pediatric glioma. The MFDNN model excels in pediatric brain tumor segmentation. It achieves the highest Lesion Wise Dice scores of 0.444 (ET), 0.634 (TC), and 0.783 (WT), with corresponding dice scores of 0.356, 0.672, and 0.830, respectively. The Dice score-based evaluation and uncertainty analysis within MFDNN offer improved brain tumor segmentation compared to the state-of-the-art methods in the literature.

Keywords: Deep learning · pediatric brain tumor · MRI · segmentation · BraTS-PEDs 2023 · Multiresolution Fractal Deep Neural Network (MFDNN)

1 Introduction

Brain tumors rank among the most lethal forms of cancer. The brain tumor segmentation (BraTS) Challenge has played a pivotal role in generating resources to analyze and segment glioblastoma multiforme (GBM), one of the most aggressive and prevalent primary tumors found in adults' central nervous systems. For children, while brain and central nervous system tumors are relatively rare, they tragically stand as the leading disease-related cause of death. These pediatric tumors, though sharing some similarities with those found in adults, often manifest differently both clinically and on imaging scans.

GBMs and pediatric diffuse midline gliomas (DMGs) both belong to the category of high-grade gliomas.

On average, patients with these tumors have a life expectancy of around 11–13 months' post-diagnosis [1]. In terms of frequency, GBMs are diagnosed in 3 out of every 100,000 individuals. DMGs, on the other hand, are around three times less prevalent. [2]. In terms of location and age of diagnosis: GBMs typically manifest in the frontal or temporal lobes and are commonly diagnosed around the age of 64. DMGs, on the other hand, are mostly found in the pons and are typically diagnosed in children between the ages of 5 and 10. As for imaging characteristics, GBMs often show enhanced tumor regions in post-gadolinium T1 weighted MRI scans and have identifiable necrotic areas. DMGs, however, don't exhibit these imaging traits as distinctly. Given the distinct differences in imaging and clinical presentation between pediatric and adult brain tumors, there's a pressing need for specialized imaging tools. Such tools would not only assist in differentiating these tumors but also play a significant role in improving diagnosis and prognosis predictions for pediatric brain tumors.

In comparison with the adult brain tumor literature, machine learning applications [3, 4] for pediatric brain remain poorly characterized. Unique pathological differences and limited data make developing machine learning tools for children particularly challenging. Since machine learning models need specific training and validation for each intended use, [5–7] concentrated research initiatives for the pediatric demographic are essential to determine machine learning's role in treating pediatric brain tumors. While there's a growing interest in applying machine learning to pediatric brain tumor imaging, significant hurdles remain in incorporating it into clinical procedures. Many machine learning methods suffer from a lack of transparency, often referred to as a "black box", which can cause apprehension among clinicians and patients [7–10]. The continuous advancements in machine learning techniques necessitate ongoing efficacy assessments to ensure patient safety.

In this work, we apply our previously proposed Multiresolution Fractal Deep Neural Network (MFDNN), that combines Wavelet Convolutional Neural Network and Multiresolution modeling, to segment pediatric brain tumors. Using the BraTS-PEDs 2023 challenge dataset, the MFDNN model offers better tumor segmentation performance when compared to U-Net in tumor segmentation accuracy and reliability.

2 Dataset Overview

The BraTS-PEDs 2023 dataset [11–14] comprises conventional or structural MRI scans from 228 pediatric patients with high-grade glioma. These scans include pre- and post-gadolinium T1-weighted images (referred to as T1 and T1CE), T2-weighted images (T2), and T2-weighted fluid attenuated inversion recovery images (T2-FLAIR). Such multiparametric MRI (mpMRI) scans are standard in clinical imaging for brain tumors. However, a notable challenge is the variation in image acquisition protocols and MRI equipment across institutions. This has resulted in discrepancies in image quality within the dataset. For inclusion in the dataset, pediatric patients needed to:

1. Have a confirmed diagnosis of high-grade glioma, specifically high-grade astrocytoma or DMG. This includes those with either radiological or histological evidence of diffuse intrinsic pontine glioma (DIPG).
2. Have all four of the mpMRI sequences from imaging sessions before any treatment from the dataset are:
   1. MRI images that are of poor quality or had artifacts compromising reliable tumor segmentation.
   2. Infants under one month old.

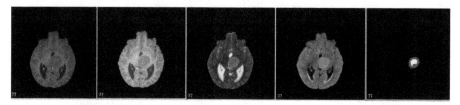

Fig. 1. Four (MRI) sequences used in BraTS-PEDs 2023 Exclusions.

The data sources included: Children's Brain Tumor Network (CBTN) (138 patients), Boston's Children Hospital (61 patients), and Yale University (29 patients).

The BraTS-PEDs 2023 challenge dataset is divided into training (99 cases), validation (45 cases), and testing subsets. Participants receive the mpMRI scans along with the corresponding ground truth labels for the training subset and the mpMRI sequences for the validation subset, but without the associated ground truth.

3 Method

3.1 Training and Optimization of the MFDNN Algorithm

The MFDNN computational modeling is illustrated in Fig. 2. The structure integrates a multiresolution encoding module, a fractal dimension (FD) context encoding module, and a multiresolution decoding module. The framework is split into two paths: contracting and expansive. The contracting pathway processes the data by successively applying convolution and pooling, followed by a rectified linear unit (ReLU) activation, thereby condensing the data and amplifying feature information. Conversely, the expansive path fuses both feature and spatial data via up-convolutions and concatenation processes.

The image that serves as input for the proposed MFDNN algorithm is structured to break down an image into multiple frequency sub bands., The network's training is facilitated by the Adam optimizer, which minimizes this loss and updates the relevant parameters, where N is the total number of pixels in the image. We utilize the Multimodal Brain Tumor Segmentation BraTS-PEDs 2023 dataset with the MFDNN. This dataset contains 99 cases for training and 45 for validation. Each case encompasses all 4 MRI sequences. These mMRIs undergo preprocessing by the challenge coordinators, including co-registration, noise reduction, and skull stripping, resulting in a preprocessed image size of 240 × 240 × 155. Ground truth is coded as 1 for nonenhancing component (NC - a combination of nonenhancing tumor, cystic component, and necrosis), 2 for peritumoral edematous area (ED), 4 for enhancing tumor (ET), and 0 for all other categories. It's essential to note that the public only has access to the ground truth for the training phase.

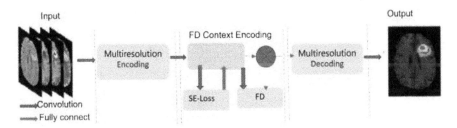

Fig. 2. Proposed computational model for MFDNN.

Each modality in the original dataset has dimensions of 240 × 240 × 155. To make the computational process more memory-efficient and cost-effective, the image sizes were modified. Specifically, they were cropped to a more manageable size of 192 × 160 × 128. The resultant image dimensions after the cropping process are illustrated in Fig. 3.

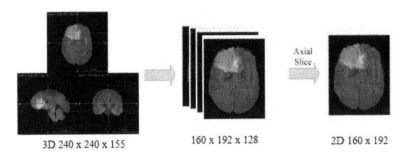

Fig. 3. Image Size preprocessing.

Evaluation metrics center on three tumor subregions: the whole tumor (WT), tumor core (TC), and enhancing tumor (ET). The WT aggregates all tumor subtypes; the TC comprises both NC and ET, whereas the ET specifically addresses the enhancing tumor. We first develop a model using the training data via the proposed MFDNN. we apply our trained model to the validation dataset and subsequently forward our segmentation results to the official Challenge portal for real-time assessment.

4 Performance Assessment

The efficacy of the models presented for the BraTS-PEDs 2023 challenge is assessed using Lesion Wise Dice, Dice score and the 95th percentile of the symmetric Hausdorff distance (HD95). These metrics are applied across the whole tumor (WT), core tumor

(TC), and enhancing tumor (ET) subdivisions. The Dice score, represented by Eq. (1), gauges the accuracy of automated segmentation, highlighting both the size and location alignment in relation to the provided ground truth:

$$\text{Dice} = \frac{2\text{TP}}{\text{FP} + 2\text{TP} + \text{FN}}. \tag{1}$$

Equation (1) effectively illustrates the alignment in both size and position compared to the actual data. For the segmentation task, the BraTS 2023 Challenge also factors in the HD95 metric, which offers insight into the accuracy of segmentation calculations, denoted as:

$$\text{HD95} = 95\% \left(d(Y, \hat{Y}) || d(Y, \hat{Y})\right) \tag{2}$$

where d is the element-wise distance of every voxel Y to the closest voxel of the same label in the second, $\hat{Y}$ are the segmented of each voxel, Y are the GT of each voxel, and || is the concatenation operator.

5 Uncertainty Analysis

Uncertainty measures in deep learning [3] are essential for understanding the reliability of a model's predictions and assigning a level of confidence to model predictions. There are several methods available for estimating the uncertainty of a deep learning model. We conduct two different techniques for quantifying uncertainty as discussed in the next section.

i. Monte Carlo Dropout Monte Carlo Dropout (MCDO) leverages dropout layers within deep neural network (DNN) structures to introduce variability in model predictions, which helps assess the uncertainty of these predictions. For our MFDNN, we've incorporated this approach by enabling dropout layers within the network. During testing, each sample, denoted as y, is iteratively processed N-times with the dropout layers activated during the evaluation phase, leading to N varied predictions, represented as $P_N(y)$. To ascertain the epistemic uncertainty in our predictions, we implement test-time augmentation (TTA) on inputs and compute the average prediction score.

$$P_N(y) = \frac{1}{N} \sum_{n=1}^{N} P_n(y) \tag{3}$$

ii. Deep Ensembles In Deep Ensembles, primarily we randomized initial weights and obtain multiple MFDNN models trained on the same training data then construct multiple best performing MFDNN models, each with their own set of parameters, denoted as $\{\theta_1, \theta_2, \ldots \theta_n\}$. Each model in the ensemble makes a prediction, denoted as $\{y_1(x; \theta_1), y_2(x; \theta_2), \ldots, y_n(x; \theta_n),\}$[16], where x is the image input data and θ_i is the set of parameters for the i-th model.

$$y(x) = \frac{1}{N} \sum_{i=1}^{N} y_i(x, \theta_i) \tag{4}$$

The final prediction made by the ensemble is then computed by averaging the predictions of all the models in the ensemble. This can be represented as:

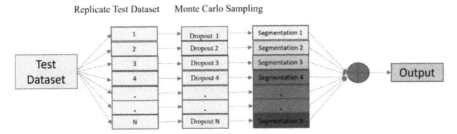

Fig. 4. Monte Carlo Dropout computation framework for Uncertainty Estimation.

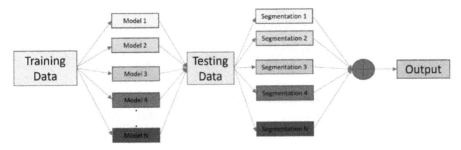

Fig. 5. Deep Ensemble computation framework for Uncertainty Estimation.

6 Results and Discussion

We employ our MFDNN model alongside both the Monte Carlo and deep ensemble methods to evaluate Lesion Wise Dice, dice score, and HD95 metrics. A comparison is made between these three techniques.

Table 1. Presents the online evaluation performance of the three models when tested on the BraTS-PEDs 2023 challenge validation dataset for brain tumor segmentation using dice score.

MFDNN Model	Dice			Dice HD95		
	ET	TC	WT	ET	TC	WT
MFDNN	0.3555	0.6727	0.8302	241.02	24.91	13.20
MFDNN MCDO	0.3555	0.7585	0.8165	241.02	14.28	12.64
MFDNN Ensemble	0.3555	0.7651	0.8265	241.02	14.28	12.66

Table 1 illustrates the online evaluation performance of the MFDNN Ensemble model upon testing with the BraTS-PEDs 2023 challenge validation dataset for brain tumor segmentation. The Dice scores for enhancing tumor (ET), tumor core (TC), and whole tumor (WT) are reported as 0.3555, 0.7651, and 0.8265, respectively. These metrics highlight the model's capability to accurately delineate tumor regions (Table 2).

Table 2. Presents the online evaluation performance of the three models when tested on the BraTS-PEDs 2023 challenge validation dataset for brain tumor segmentation using lesion wise Dice.

MFDNN Model	Mean ± std	Lesion Wise Dice			Lesion Wise Dice HD95		
		ET	TC	WT	ET	TC	WT
MFDNN	mean	0.44444	0.63478	0.78322	207.777	47.3027	35.0750
	std	0.50251	0.27580	0.23027	187.942	89.759	75.584
MFDNN MCDO	mean	0.44444	0.73628	0.78741	207.777	30.4721	31.6588
	std	0.50251	0.21752	0.21673	187.942	63.1905	71.6336
MFDNN Ensemble	mean	0.44444	0.73639	0.80238	207.777	29.1705	23.6030
	std	0.5025	0.2172	0.1935	187.94	58.877	54.0872

Figure 6 provides a visual representation of the results obtained using our proposed model on pediatric brain tumor segmentation. Essentially, it showcases how our model performs when tasked with delineating tumors in pediatric brain images.

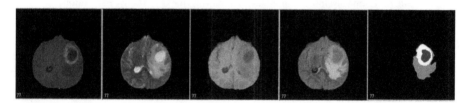

Fig. 6. Example of our proposed model for pediatric brain tumors segmentation.

The results in Table 3 demonstrate the online evaluation performance of the MFDNN Ensemble model on the BraTS-PEDs 2023 challenge testing dataset for brain tumor segmentation. Notably, the lesion-wise Dice scores for the tumor core (TC) and whole tumor (WT) are reported as 0.71117 and 0.72874, respectively. These metrics showcase the model's effectiveness in accurately delineating tumor boundaries and highlight its potential for clinical application in pediatric brain tumor diagnosis and treatment planning.

Table 4 displays the Sensitivity and Specificity metrics for the online evaluation performance of the MFDNN Ensemble model when assessed on the BraTS-PEDs 2023 challenge testing dataset for brain tumor segmentation. Notably, the lesion-wise Dice scores for the tumor core (TC) and whole tumor (WT) are reported as 0.7111 and 0.6758, respectively. These results underscore the model's capacity to accurately identify tumor regions and its potential clinical utility in pediatric brain tumor diagnosis and treatment planning.

Table 3. Presents the online evaluation performance of the MFDNN Ensemble model when tested on the BraTS-PEDs 2023 challenge testing dataset for brain tumor segmentation using lesion wise Dice.

MFDNN Model	Mean ± std	Lesion Wise Dice			Lesion Wise Dice HD95		
		ET	TC	WT	ET	TC	WT
MFDNN	mean	0.1666	0.7111	0.6758	311.666	38.402	68.181
	std	0.3806	0.2483	0.2594	142.3793	71.0132	89.5636

Table 4. Presents the Sensitivity and Specificity for the online evaluation performance of the MFDNN Ensemble model when tested on the BraTS-PEDs 2023 challenge testing dataset for brain tumor segmentation.

MFDNN Model	Mean ± std	Lesion Wise Sensitivity			Lesion Wise Specificity		
		ET	TC	WT	ET	TC	WT
MFDNN	mean	0.16666	0.69595	0.72874	1	0.99939	0.99960
	std	0.38069	0.22759	0.21150	0	0.00112	0.00043

7 Conclusion

In this study, we apply the MFDNN, a model for pediatric brain tumor segmentation using BraTS-PEDs 2023 challenge dataset. The data comprises over 45 patient cases. Moreover, uncertainty analysis is used to demonstrate the model's consistency and dependability. Dice score-based evaluation and uncertainty assessments, indicate that MFDNN surpasses contemporary techniques in PED brain tumor volume segmentation. This study underscores the potential of our proposed method to enhance the precision and dependability of automated abnormal brain tissue segmentation. Such advancements may aid in earlier diagnoses and more strategic treatment planning for PED brain tumors. Looking forward, the MFDNN's performance can be further scrutinized using datasets that blend adult and PED samples. In the future, the proposed MFDNN model can be adapted for various abnormal tissue segmentation tasks.

Acknowledgements. This work was partially funded through NIH/NIBIB grant under award number R01EB020683. The authos would like to acknowledge partial support of this work by the National Science Foundation Grant No. 1828593.

References

1. Findlay, I.J., De Iuliis, G.N., Duchatel, R.J., Jackson, E.R., Vitanza, N.A., Cain, J.E., Waszak, S.M., Dun, M.D.: Pharmacoproteogenomic profiling of pediatric diffuse midline glioma to inform future treatment strategies. Oncogene. **41**(4), 461–475 (2022)

2. Serrallach BL, Tran BH, Bauer DF, Mohila CA, Adesina AM, McGovern SL, Lindsay HB, Huisman TA.
3. Pediatric spinal cord diffuse midline glioma, H3 K27-altered with intracranial and spinal leptomeningeal spread: a case report. Neuroradiol. J. **35**(5):634–639 (2022)
4. Rahman, M.M., Sadique, M.S., Temtam, A.G., Farzana, W., Vidyaratne, L., Iftekharuddin, K.M.: Brain tumor segmentation using UNet-context encoding network. In: International MICCAI Brainlesion Workshop, pp. 463–472. Springer International Publishing, Cham (2021). https://doi.org/10.1007/978-3-031-08999-2_40
5. Sadique, M.S., Rahman, M.M., Farzana, W., Temtam, A., Iftekharuddin, K.M.: Brain tumor segmentation using neural ordinary differential equations with UNet-context encoding network. In: International MICCAI Brainlesion Workshop, pp. 205–215. Springer Nature Switzerland, Cham (2022). https://doi.org/10.1007/978-3-031-33842-7_18
6. Kim, S.H., et al.: Deep learning reconstruction in pediatric brain MRI: comparison of image quality with conventional T2-weighted MRI. Neuroradiology **65**(1), 207–214 (2023)
7. Maspero, M., et al.: Deep learning-based synthetic CT generation for paediatric brain MR-only photon and proton radiotherapy. Radiotherapy Oncol. **1**(153), 197–204 (2020)
8. Curtin, S.C., Miniño, A.M., Anderson, R.N.: Declines in cancer death rates among children and adolescents in the United States, 1999–2014. US Department of Health & Human Services, Centers for Disease Control and Prevention, National Center for Health Statistics (2016)
9. Pollack, I.F., Agnihotri, S., Broniscer, A.: Childhood brain tumors: current management, biological insights, and future directions. J. Neurosurgery: Pediatrics **23**(3), 261–273 (2019)
10. Li, M., Shang, Z., Yang, Z., Zhang, Y., Wan, H.: Machine learning methods for MRI biomarkers analysis of pediatric posterior fossa tumors. Biocybern. Biomed. Eng. **39**(3), 765–774 (2019)
11. Fathi Kazerooni, A., et al.: Automated tumor segmentation and brain tissue extraction from multiparametric MRI of pediatric brain tumors: a multi-institutional study. Neuro-Oncol. Adv. **5**(1), vdad027 (2023)
12. Baid, U., et al.: The RSNA-ASNR-MICCAI brats 2021 benchmark on brain tumor segmentation and radiogenomic classification. arXiv preprint arXiv:2107.02314 (2021)
13. Menze, B.H., Jakab, A., Bauer, S., Kalpathy-Cramer, J., Farahani, K., Kirby, J., Burren, Y., Porz, N., Slotboom, J., Wiest, R., Lanczi, L.: The multimodal brain tumor image segmentation benchmark (BRATS). IEEE Trans. Med. Imaging **34**(10), 1993–2024 (2014)
14. Bakas, S., et al.: Advancing the cancer genome atlas glioma MRI collections with expert segmentation labels and radiomic features. Sci. Data **4**(1), 1–13 (2017)
15. Bakas S., et al.: Segmentation labels and radiomic features for the pre-operative scans of the TCGA-LGG collection. The Cancer Imaging Archive, 286 (2017)
16. Roy, S., et al.: MedNeXt: transformer-driven scaling of ConvNets for medical image segmentation. arXiv preprint arXiv:2303.09975 (2023)

BPML, MLops and 3D-UNet Network Integration in End-to-End Application Design Applied to the Segmentation of Human Brain Tumors in Clinic Cases

José Armando Hernández[✉]

Université Paris-Saclay, ENS Paris-Saclay, CNRS, Centre Borelli,
91190 Gif-sur-Yvette, France
ja.hernandez906@uniandes.edu.co

Abstract. This work aims to facilitate the integration of the scientific findings obtained from the BraTS challenge with business processes and applicable in real clinical cases. We describe the 3D-UNet neural network originally proposed by Ronneberger et al. in 2015 for biomedical image segmentation. We evaluate its performance for segmenting human brain tumors from real MRI-scan images data BraTS 2023 challenge. We very briefly explain the details of how these MRI scans are interpreted and the neural network architecture of the model obtained. Finally, we present the entire end-to-end BPM business integration through MLops for a clinical case of segmentation of brain tumors. We conclude that the proposed methodology allows the creation of an end-to-end operational proof of concept app in a business logic agilely based on a segmentation model to value the research results.

1 Introduction

There is currently a general shortage of specialist radiologists due to many factors that depend on each country. Population growth, the increase in the elderly population, and aging. The BraTS2023 competition is the top reference for segmentation algorithms.

It has been suggested [1] that artificial intelligence could perform many functions, to the point that one study raises the question of whether radiologists could be replaceable. However, in previous editions of BraTS, the results of which are mentioned in the MICCAI conference show significant advances in this field of artificial intelligence. In this sense, the automatic segmentation of tumors through machine learning represents a promising alternative solution to

---

This research was made possible by support from the French National Research Agency, the SESAME's OVD-SaaS project from Région Île de France and BPI France, and Ministry of Science, Technology and Innovation of Colombia (Minciencias), call 885 of 2020. and BraTS Challenge 2023.

this growing problem for timely and efficient diagnosis. In Centre Borelli, there is a particular interest in creating medical applications in an agile way.

Given that the IPOL demo system allows quick creation of online demos, we proposed a simple demo that permits radiologists, the general public, and other interested parties to carry out experiments with their images and compare results. In this way, test images of healthy patients and patients with tumors will be constantly obtained in the online demo. However, it is still necessary to develop methodologies to integrate more complex processes and models.

Considering the above, this paper studies the segmentation of human brain tumors with the 3D-UNet network within the framework of the BraTS challenge to develop and integrate advanced segmentation models in MLops development cycles. 3D-Unet is chosen, because it is a widely studied architecture with a good response, and its complexity is adequate proof of concept for end-to-end application development.

According to [2], the performance of different architectures, including U-Net concerning the Dice loss function for application of brain extraction is expected to be 0.97 ± 0.01 with U-Net, ResUNet 0.98 ± 0.01, and FCN (Fully Convolutional Network) 0.97 ± 0.01. For brain tumor sub-region segmentation U-Net 0.65 ± 0.05, ResUNet 0.71 ± 0.05, FCN 0.62 ± 0.05, and UInc 0.64 ± 0.05.

The document is organized as follows. First, a brief review of state-of-the-art 3D-UNet for biomedical image segmentation The Methodology MLops and BPML with 3D-UNet architecture model is described in Sect. 2. The end-to-end BraTS APP functionalities, such as data preparation, training and validation of the used model is described in Sect. 3. Finally, Sect. 4 concludes the paper and presents ideas for future work.

2 Method

The purpose is the creation of the entire business workflow of an application through MLops. In this case, the dataset is BraTS Glioma (BraTS-GLI) [3–6], and the neural network architecture is 3D-Unet, see Fig. 2 from previous work on IPOL[1] we have a graphical online interface demonstration and a basic Unet model, but it is constrained. In such a way, an End-to-End application of Segmentation of brain glioma can be created from storytelling in a business logic Fig. 1, interacting role 1 (patient), role 2 (Radiologist), role 3 (MLengineer) in a AAA(Authentication, Authorization, Accounting) environment. Through the orchestration of microservices (REST APIS connectors) with business processes BPML (business process language) Fig. 5 we can achieve reproducibility and interactive visualization frontend with low code tools like Streamlit[2]. There are important more complex initiatives such as [7] that are compatible with MLcubes. However, our approach is more oriented to simplify business logic, quickly value research results, and develop agilely.

User story:

---

[1] https://ipolcore.ipol.im/demo/clientApp/demo.html?id=77777000461.
[2] https://streamlit.io/.

"As a radiologist, I wish to have updated and increasingly accurate neural network models available in emergency rooms to assist in interpreting brain magnetic resonance images. So, a diagnosis of the patient's severity and treatment authorization is required very quickly"

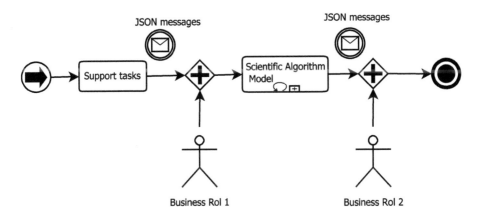

Fig. 1. Model Inserted in a replicable Business Logic

the topology is a basic 3D-Unet, Fig. 2

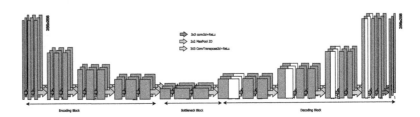

Fig. 2. The 3D-UNet architecture is characterized by its U-shaped structure, consisting of a contraction section (encoder) and an expansion section (decoder). Here, we should see the U shape with its Encoding, Decoding Blocks, and Bridging (Bottleneck) blocks.

2.1 MLops

For Model versioning, traceability, and replicability of artifacts we use the MLflow tool, Fig. 3.

Besides MLcube obtained to be evaluated against the test unseen dataset of the BraTS challenge, we create a containerized API with the final model, Fig. 4.

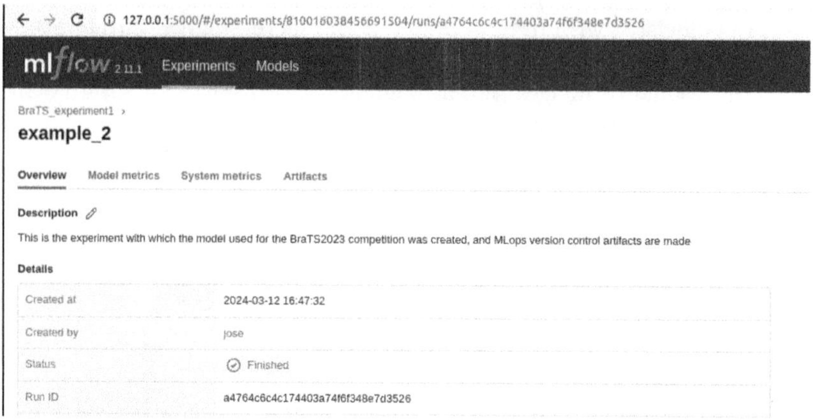

Fig. 3. MLflow dashboard for BraTS Model tracking and versioning.

2.2 BPML

In the context of a hospital's business process, BPML Fig. 5 allows orchestrating the backend APIs of the model, as well as the frontend of the roles that participate, such as the radiologist, Fig. 6 who, after diagnosing, authorizes treatments or new procedures.

Figure 2 describes the architecture trained with the BraTS2023 dataset, specifying the different layers and their interaction at the code level

Figure 7 describes the 3 channels T1CE, FLAIR, T2, and the three-color mask representing each class as input for the training process.

BraTS Dataset Annotations(Labels). Figure 7:

- Label 0: Unlabeled Volume (black color)
- Label 1: Necrotic and non-enhancing tumor core (NCR/NET) (dark green color)
- Label 2: Peritumoral edema (ED) (yellow color)
- Label 3: GD-enhancing tumor (ET) (green color)

3 Results

The network continues to train at 100 epochs with loss function based on dice score, for which a partial result is presented Tabla 1 as part of the Mlops methodology's first iterative cycle. As can be seen, the model can make good inferences, Fig. 7, but to reach its optimal point, several MLops tuning improvement cycles are required. Figure 8.

$$\text{DICE\_SCORE} = \frac{2 \sum_{i=1}^{N} x_i y_i}{\sum_{i=1}^{N} x_i^2 + \sum_{i=1}^{N} y_i^2}$$

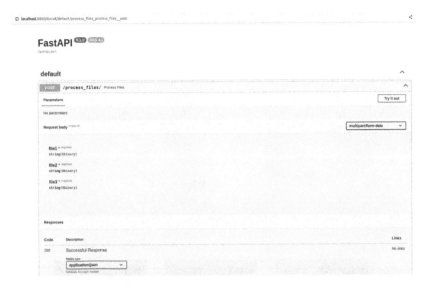

Fig. 4. Model Backend REST API. Receives 3 MRI image files (.nii.gz format) and returns segmentation result (.nii.gz format)

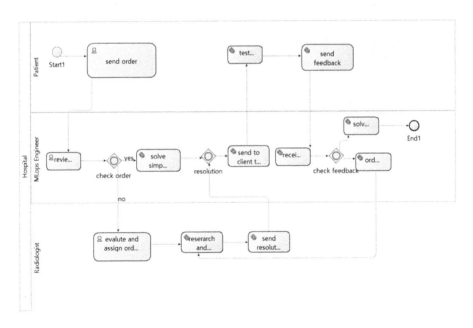

Fig. 5. The figure describes the entire process BPM, from when the Patient requests an exam and the Radiologist makes validations, with a technology intermediary such as the MLops engineer.

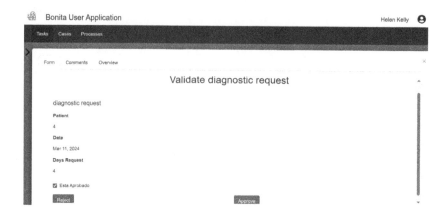

Fig. 6. BPML diagnosis and authorization form for radiologist role (authenticated user Helen Kelly)

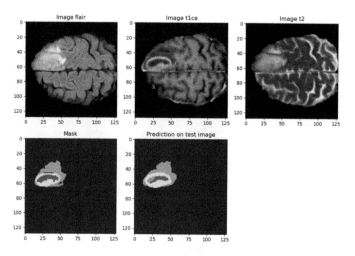

Fig. 7. Input validation image and prediction image obtained from the model.

where:

- DICE_SCORE represents the Dice coefficient used as a similarity metric in image segmentation tasks. It measures the overlap between two sets.
- N is the total number of pixels in the images.
- x_i represents the value of the i-th pixel in the predicted segmentation image.
- y_i represents the value of the i-th pixel in the ground truth segmentation image.
- The summations $\sum_{i=1}^{N} x_i y_i$, $\sum_{i=1}^{N} x_i^2$, and $\sum_{i=1}^{N} y_i^2$ denote the sum of the cross products and sums of the squares of pixel values in both images.

Finally, we have an end-to-end BraTS APP Fig. 9a, 9b, very useful in health care (Hospital) domain context and their business process needs. In this sim-

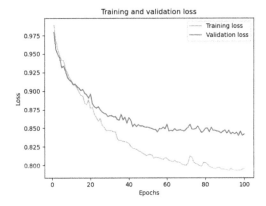

Fig. 8. The 3D-UNet architecture training result.

ple flow, the patient requests diagnosis and treatment from the radiologist, the radiologist attaches the 3 images in nii.gz format, sends them to the inference model API, and returns a segmentation file. The radiologist can choose the slide and view the tumor's possible location in 3D, generate a diagnosis, and issue a treatment authorization.

As a sample, the IPOL graphical interface is presented, an online Demo example Fig. 11 with a simple model.

3.1 Blockchain API for Medical Records

Optionally, Although it is not directly related to segmentation, it can be located within the BPM business logic, an API can be included within the business process, where the treatment authorization can be digitally signed. This order can be recorded in a blockchain API for authenticity verification, Fig. 10). However, only a small API prototype is proposed and is subject to future improvements.

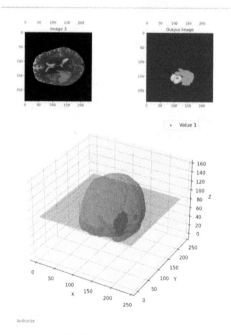

(a) BraTS APP. The radiologist can choose slide image of interest, write a diagnosis and authorize treatment.

(b) The 3D BraTS APP.

Fig. 9. BraTS APP Functionalities

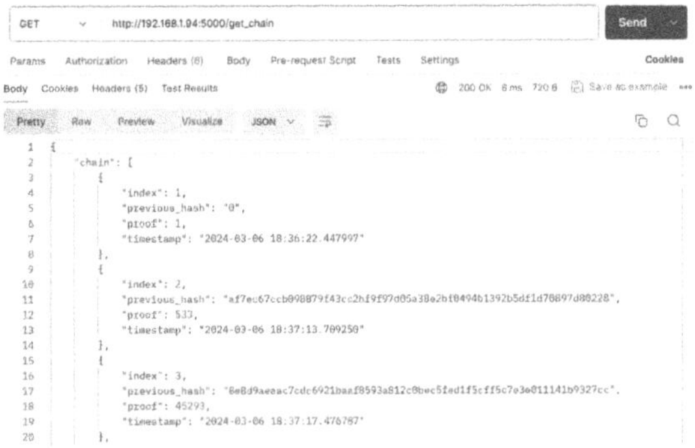

Brain Segmentation 349

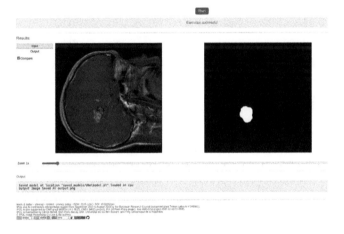

Fig. 10. Authorization Blockchain API. Postman client consuming the API

Fig. 11. First User Interface Output, basic Unet model, Online Demo IPOL

Table 1. Model performance on BraTS2023 Challenge

scan_id	LesionWise_Score_Dice	LesionWise_Score_HD95	Sensitivity	Specificity
ET (Edema Tissue)				
mean	0.43	176.99	0.77	0.9995
std	0.32	136.07	0.26	0.0005
25quantile	0.15	3.00	0.75	0.9994
median	0.36	188.80	0.87	0.9997
75quantile	0.79	299.57	0.93	0.9999
TC (Tumor Core)				
mean	0.48	168.20	0.81	0.9996
std	0.34	134.99	0.27	0.0008
25quantile	0.18	3.32	0.80	0.9996
median	0.44	188.66	0.92	0.9998
75quantile	0.90	283.59	0.96	0.9999
WT (Whole Tumor)				
mean	0.36	225.36	0.92	0.9996
std	0.32	127.58	0.11	0.0018
25quantile	0.10	187.71	0.90	0.9996
median	0.23	281.25	0.96	0.9998
75quantile	0.48	327.62	0.98	0.9999

4 Conclusion

The methodology is described as end-to-end implementation, but optimizing the model and its integration into the MLops continuous improvement cycles is necessary.

The model had some false positives, suggesting that radiologists should use medical criteria to validate the results. The tool can significantly help but in no way replaces doctors. For this reason, the radiologist's participation is mandatory in the hospital's BPM business process.

We hope that, together with the work developed in IPOL and the Brats2023 competition, it will be of help to radiologists, researchers, industry, and students who wish to obtain an agile method for putting into production, reproducibility, verification, and optimization of brain tumor segmentation models. The IPOL online demonstration for one channel and end-to-end medical application BraTS APP based on BPM and MLops methodologies, are proofs of concept for future, more advanced implementations.

References

1. Langlotz, C.P.: Will artificial intelligence replace radiologists? Radiol. Artif. Intell. **1**(3), e190058 (2019)
2. Işın, A., Direkoğlu, C., Şah, M.: Review of MRI-based brain tumor image segmentation using deep learning methods. Procedia Comput. Sci. **102**, 317–324 (2016)
3. Bakas, S., et al.: Advancing the cancer genome atlas glioma MRI collections with expert segmentation labels and radiomic features. Sci. Data **4**(1), 170117 (2017)
4. Menze, B.H., et al.: The multimodal brain tumor image segmentation benchmark (BRATS). IEEE Trans. Med. Imaging **34**(10), 1993–2024 (2015)
5. Baid, U., et al.: The RSNA-ASNR-MICCAI BraTS 2021 benchmark on brain tumor segmentation and radiogenomic classification. arXiv:2107.02314 [cs] (2021)
6. Karargyris, A., et al.: Federated benchmarking of medical artificial intelligence with MedPerf. Nat. Mach. Intell. **5**(7), 799–810 (2023)
7. Pati, S., et al.: GaNDLF: the generally nuanced deep learning framework for scalable end-to-end clinical workflows. Commun. Eng. **2**(1), 23 (2023)

CrossMoDA

An Efficient Cross-Modal Segmentation Method for Vestibular Schwannoma and Cochlea on MRI Images

Cancan Chen[1], Dawei Wang[2], and Rongguo Zhang[3](✉)

[1] School of Computer Engineering, Jiangsu Ocean University, Lianyungang, China
[2] Infervision Advanced Research Institute, Beijing, China
[3] Academy for Multidisciplinary Studies, Capital Normal University, Beijing, China
zrongguo@cnu.edu.cn

Abstract. To obtain the segmentation results of vestibular schwannoma (VS) and cochlea on high-resolution T2 (hrT2) MR images according to the annotated contrast-enhanced T1 (ceT1) MR images, we propose an efficient cross-modal segmentation framework in this study. An image-to-image model is first applied to transfer ceT1 scans to hrT2 modality to alleviate the domain shift between them. In the model training phase, we adopted data augmentation for both original images and segmentation target regions to adapt to the diversity and heterogeneity of multi-center imaging data. Furthermore, random cropping along the z-axis and random flipping at all axial directions representing the different observation perspectives were implemented. We also utilized a 2.5D ResUnet model as the segmentation backbone. These strategies collectively contribute to improved segmentation output. Eventually, a post-processing method based on image contrast is applied to improve the quality of the pseudo-labels on the hrT2 modality. Our experimental results address the effectiveness of the proposed framework for the crossMoDA23 segmentation task of the vestibular schwannoma and cochlea on hrT2 modality, with average Dice scores of 0.8358 and 0.828 for VS and average Dice scores of 0.8355 and 0.844 for cochlea, respectively on validation and test data.

Keywords: Unsupervised domain adaptation · Cross-modality · Image translation · Heterogeneity · Magnetic resonance imaging (MRI)

1 Introduction

Vestibular schwannoma (VS) is the most common tumor of the cerebellar angular cisterna and the internal auditory canal, and contrast-enhanced T1 (ceT1) MR images are commonly used for the diagnosis and surveillance of patients with VS. Given the risk of gadolinium-containing contrast agents used in scanning ceT1 MR images [1], high-resolution T2 (hrT2) MR image has raised the interest of researchers as a replacement modality given its lower risk and more efficient cost. However, gadolinium-enhanced MR images are required for certain scenarios and equivocal findings. The goal of CrossMoDA challenge 2021–2023 [4,6,13,15] is to segment VS and cochlea on contrast-enhanced T1(ceT1) and high-resolution T2 (hrT2) MR images for monitoring tumor growth in consecutive follow-ups and even for treatment planning. In this challenge, the aim is to obtain the segmentation results of VS and cochlea on hrT2 MR images with the ceT1 MR images as the gold standard. Besides, the additional segmentation task on the intra- and extra-meatal regions of the tumor from the multi-center heterogeneous scans makes the work more challenging and clinically significant.

Based on the previous excellent work and studies [3,4,14], we propose a simple and efficient cross-modal segmentation framework to tackle the unsupervised domain adaptation segmentation task on unseen data. Firstly, the labeled images on the ceT1 sequence need to be transferred to the hrT2 domain by the image-to-image translation model, such as CycleGAN or CUT [4,10,16]. In this work, we apply CUT as the image-to-image translation model. Secondly, the initial segmentation model for hrT2 sequence is trained on the translated pseudo-hrT2 images and the gold standard annotations on ceT1 sequence, and the pseudo-labels for training target data are obtained. Furthermore, the segmentation model is updated on real hrT2 scans and pseudo-labels by self-training, which could find a better decision boundary on the hrT2 domain [3]. The better experiments on the validation set demonstrate that our approach is effective.

The main contributions of this paper are summarized as follows:

- We propose an efficient cross-modal segmentation method, which could effectively and efficiently perform the segmentation of VS and Cochlea on cross-modality MRI images.
- We first calculate the spacing resolution distribution of all MRI images, especially the thickness on the z-axis, which sparks the helpful ideas or details about patch size, augmentation and 2.5D ResUnet backbone [2,5] at the segmentation stage.
- The strong data augmentation is used in the model training process, such as random crop, random flip, etc., and a post-processing method of the pseudo-labels on hrT2 modality to improve the final output results.
- The experiments demonstrate the effectiveness of our proposed method.

2 Methods

The proposed cross-modal segmentation framework mainly consists of unsupervised domain adaption module for translating MR images from ceT1 to hrT2 modality, and semantic segmentation module for the VS and cochlea based on hrT2 scans and pseudo-labels of target domain. Domain Adaptation (DA) has recently raised strong interest in the medical imaging community. By encouraging algorithms to be robust to unseen situations or different data domains, domain adaptation has improved the applicability of deep learning approaches to various clinical scenes. In this challenge, we adopt CUT model [10] to realize the image-to-image translation. For the second stage, the semantic segmentation of organs or lesions is a common task in the field of medical image analysis.

There are already a large number of excellent and efficient algorithms available for medical image segmentation, such as U-Net [11], ResU-Net [2], nnU-Net [5], and others. Based on the strong baseline [4] and the strong heterogeneity of MRI images resolution, the optimal 2.5D ResUnet model is used as the segmentation workflow backbone to avoid the up/down-sample along z axis.

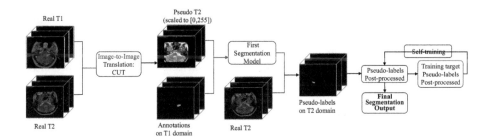

Fig. 1. An overview of our proposed cross-modal segmentation framework

2.1 Preprocessing

The preprocessing steps are listed as follows:

- Cropping strategy:
  Since the segmentation targets (the VS and cochlea) are located in the center of the brain MR image, we crop the center area as the regions of interest (ROIs), i.e., the inputs of our framework. According to the cropping method in reference [3], the 2D ROI images in the image-to-image translation stage are cropped with a range $[\frac{3W}{16} : \frac{13W}{16}, \frac{3H}{16} : \frac{13H}{16}]$ from the original range $[0 : W, 0 : H]$, and the 3D ROI images in the segmentation stage are cropped with a range $[0 : D, \frac{3W}{16} : \frac{13W}{16}, \frac{3H}{16} : \frac{13H}{16}]$ from the original range $[0 : D, 0 : W, 0 : H]$. Especially for the incomplete MRI images such as missing partial areas and irregular shape along x/y axis, the original images without any cropping are used as ROIs.
- Resampling method for anisotropic data:
  The 2D ROI images at the image-to-image translation stage are resampled to 256×256. The 3D ROI images at the segmentation stage are resampled to $D \times 384 \times 384$, the cube is randomly cropped along the z-axis, and the cube size is $40 \times 384 \times 384$.
- Intensity normalization method:
  All 2/3D ROI images are normalized to the range $[-1, 1]$ by the min-max scaler.
- Others:
  To improve the efficiency of the model training and inference, the mixed precision approach is used in the entire process of our framework.

2.2 Proposed Method

Our proposed framework is shown in Fig. 1, which mainly consists of the image-to-image translation and semantic segmentation of tumor and cochlea. The details of two stages are addressed as follows.

The Image-to-Image Translation. We apply the CUT model [10] to learn the mapping from the source domain ceT1 scans to the target domain hrT2 scans, which is similarly composed of the generator and discriminator. It is noteworthy that the discriminator has a stronger learning ability than the generator on this translation task, which implies the lower initial learning rate of the discriminator than generator could be more appropriate. After multiple repeated experiments, the CUT model could well implement the style transfer from the ceT1 scans to hrT2 scans with the following hyper-parameters setting: instance normalization, batch size equals to 10, the images range from -1 to 1, the initial learning late of generator is 0.0002, the initial learning rate of discriminator is 0.1×0.0002, and the proper stopping epoch. Additionally, we did not explore more details about the structure optimization of the CUT model due to the urgent time constraint. The visualization examples are shown in Fig. 2.

Semantic Segmentation. In the semantic segmentation stage, self-training is applied to further improve the segmentation results of the unseen real hrT2 scans. We adopt 2.5D ResUnet as the segmentation backbone, and network architecture has 3 down-sample layers, 3 up-sample layers, and no down-sample at z direction for the high performance and high efficiency of our method, which is shown in Fig. 3. The self-training process consists of the following steps.

- Step 1: The initial segmentation model is trained on the translated hrT2 scans and annotations of the ceT1 scans;
- Step 2: Generate pseudo-labels of real hrT2 scans by the segmentation model;
- Step 3: Select pseudo-labels by the max probability threshold p, and perform post-processing for the pseudo-labels to improve the segmentation quality of intra-meatal VS and cochlea;
- Step 4: Retrain the segmentation model on the selected real hrT2 scans and pseudo-labels;
- Step 5: Repeating Step 2–4, output the segmentation result, and evaluate it on the validation set.

Post-processing method for the pseudo-labels: we follow [12] to improve pseudo-labels of cochlea and intra-meatal VS based on the contrast of real hrT2 scans, and the examples are shown in Fig. 4.

Loss function: we use the summation between Dice loss and Cross-Entropy loss because compound loss functions have been proven to be robust in various medical image segmentation tasks [8].

Other tricks: 1) hard example mining is used in the loss function, and the hard samples are obtained by eroding or dilating the target masks; 2) to tackle

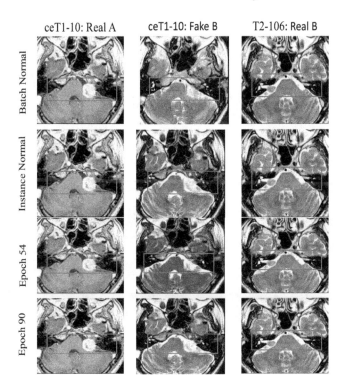

Fig. 2. Visualization for the transferred ceT1 scans and real ceT1/hrT2 scans of different hyper-parameters

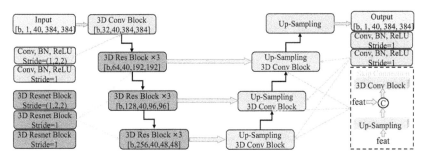

Fig. 3. The proposed network architecture

the structure heterogeneity of multi-center data set, such as the incomplete MRI cases with missing partital areas, the normal images are randomly replaced by the fixed ratio along x/y axis with the value −1, and the incomplete abnormal cases are randomly expanded to balance size x/y.

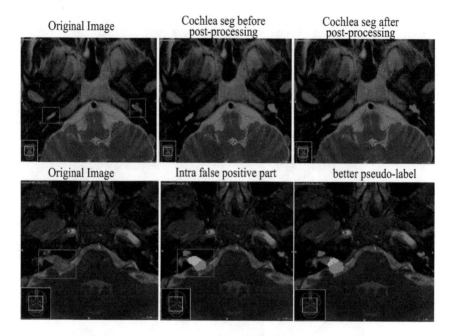

Fig. 4. Visualization for the pseudo-labels after post-processing

3 Results

3.1 Dataset and Evaluation Measures

The crossMoDA challenge 2023 organizer has publicly released 618 MRI scans, consisting of 227 ceT1 scans on the training source domain, 295 hrT2 scans on training target domain and 96 hrT2 scans for validation. The volumetric Dice coefficient, Average Symmetric Surface Distance (ASSD) and boundary ASSD [15] are used to evaluate algorithms.

3.2 Implementation Details

Environment Settings. The development environments and requirements are presented in Table 1.

Table 1. Development environments and requirements

Windows/Ubuntu version	Ubuntu 18.04.06 LTS
CPU	Intel(R) Xeon(R) Silver 4210R CPU @ 2.40 GHz
RAM	128 GB
GPU (number and type)	Two NVIDIA RTX A6000 48G
CUDA version	11.4
The programming language	Python 3.7
Deep learning framework	PyTorch (Torch 1.7.1+cu110, torchvision 0.8.2)
(Optional) Link to code	https://github.com/chencancan1018/crossMoDA

Data Augmentation. At the segmentation stage, random cropping ([0.8, 1.2]), flipping (z, y, z axis), elastic transforms (project MONAI [9]), contrast ([0,6, 1.5]), brightness ([0,6, 1.5]), and gamma augmentation ([0,6, 1.5]) are all applied to images, and contrast ([0,6, 1.5]), brightness ([0,6, 1.5]), and gamma augmentation ([0,6, 1.5]) are applied again to targets in the training process.

Training Protocols. Details of our training protocols are shown in Table 2 and Table 3.

Table 2. Training protocols for image-to-image translation

Network initialization	"he" normal initialization
Batch size	10
Patch size	256 × 256
Total epochs	200
Optimizer	ADAM ($weightdecay = 1e-4$)
Initial learning rate (lr)	2 × 1e−4, 0.2 × 1e−4
Lr decay schedule	plateau

Table 3. Training protocols for semantic segmentation

Network initialization	"he" normal initialization
Batch size	10
Patch size	40 × 384 × 384
Total epochs	200
Optimizer	ADAMW [7] ($weightdecay = 1e-4$)
Initial learning rate (lr)	1e−4
Lr decay schedule	CosineAnnealing

3.3 Results on the Validation and Test Set

The final scores on the validation and test set are listed in Table 4. Besides, the average inference time of the validation set is 27 s, and the max GPU occupancy is 5413M.

Table 4. Results of the proposed cross-modal segmentation framework on the validation set

Set	Intra Dice	extra Dice	VS Dice	Cochlea Dice	
Val	0.7057 ± 0.0959	0.8363 ± 0.108	0.8358 ± 0.1025	0.8355 ± 0.0441	
Test	0.699	0.808	0.828	0.844	
Set	Intra ASSD	extra ASSD	VS ASSD	boundary ASSD	Cochlea ASSD
Val	0.5928 ± 0.6929	0.5023 ± 0.2054	0.5648 ± 0.64	4.7632 ± 37.23	0.2259 ± 0.1449
Test	0.581	0.593	0.562	1.985	0.207

4 Conclusion

Based on 2.5D ResUnet, we propose an efficient cross-modal segmentation framework for the segmentation of VS and cochlea on cross-modality MRI images. The experimental results indicate that our framework is effective, but the lack of structure optimization and innovation of the image-to-image translation model expanded the gap between pseudo images and target domain (hrT2 modality). Moreover, the disadvantage yielded by the image-to-image translation could not be compensated at the segmentation stage, and we will focus on the designing and optimization of the translation model such as the exploration of 3D structure or the supervision of segmentation head.

References

1. Coelho, D.H., Tang, Y., Suddarth, B., Mamdani, M.: MRI surveillance of vestibular schwannomas without contrast enhancement: clinical and economic evaluation. Laryngoscope (2018)
2. Diakogiannis, F.I., Waldner, F., Caccetta, P., Wu, C.: ResUNet-a: a deep learning framework for semantic segmentation of remotely sensed data. ISPRS J. Photogramm. Remote. Sens. **162**, 94–114 (2020)
3. Dong, H., Yu, F., Zhao, J., et al.: Unsupervised domain adaptation in semantic segmentation based on pixel alignment and self-training. arXiv preprint arXiv:2109.14219 (2021)
4. Dorent, R., Kujawa, A., Ivory, M., Bakas, S., et al.: Crossmoda 2021 challenge: benchmark of cross-modality domain adaptation techniques for vestibular schwannoma and cochlea segmentation. Med. Image Anal. (2023)
5. Isensee, F., Jaeger, P.F., Kohl, S.A., Petersen, J., Maier-Hein, K.H.: nnU-net: a self-configuring method for deep learning-based biomedical image segmentation. Nat. Methods **18**(2), 203–211 (2021)

6. Kujawa, A., Dorent, R., Connor, S., Thomson, S., et al.: Deep learning for automatic segmentation of vestibular schwannoma: Dstudy from multi-centre routine mri. MedRxiv (2023)
7. Loshchilov, I., Hutter, F.: Decoupled weight decay regularization. arXiv preprint arXiv:1711.05101 (2017)
8. Ma, J., Chen, J., Ng, M., Huang, R., Li, Y., et al.: Loss odyssey in medical image segmentation. Med. Image Anal. **71**, 102035 (2021)
9. Nic, M., Wenqi, L., Richard, B., Yiheng, W., Behrooz, H.: MONAI. https://github.com/Project-MONAI/MONAI. [Version 0.8.1]
10. Park, T., Efros, Alexei, A., Zhang, R., Zhu, J.Y.: Contrastive learning for unpaired image-to-image translation (2020)
11. Ronneberger, O., Fischer, P., Brox, T.: U-net: convolutional networks for biomedical image segmentation. In: International Conference on Medical Image Computing and Computer-Assisted Intervention, pp. 234–241 (2015)
12. Sallé, G., Conze, P.H., Bert, J., et al.: Tumor blending augmentation using one-shot generative learning for crossmodal MRI segmentation (2022). https://crossmoda-challenge.ml/media/papers-2022/latim.pdf
13. Shapey, J., Kujawa, A., Dorent, R., Wang, G., Dimitriadis, A., et al.: Segmentation of vestibular schwannoma from MRI an open annotated dataset and baseline algorithm. medRxiv (2021)
14. Shin, H., Kim, H., Kim, S., et al.: COSMOS: cross-modality unsupervised domain adaptation for 3D medical image segmentation based on target-aware domain translation and iterative self-training. arXiv preprint arXiv:2203.16557 (2022)
15. Wijethilake, N., Kujawa, A., Dorent, R., Asad, M., et al.: Boundary distance loss for intra-/extra-meatal segmentation of vestibular schwannoma. In: International Workshop on Machine Learning in Clinical Neuroimaging (2022)
16. Zhu, J.Y., Park, T., Isola, P., Efros, Alexei, A.: Unpaired image-to-image translation using cycle-consistent adversarial networks, pp. 2223–2232 (2017)

Fine-Grained Unsupervised Cross-Modality Domain Adaptation for Vestibular Schwannoma Segmentation

Luyi Han[1,2], Tao Tan[3,2(✉)], and Ritse Mann[1,2]

[1] Department of Radiology and Nuclear Medicine, Radboud University Medical Center, Geert Grooteplein 10, 6525 GA Nijmegen, The Netherlands
[2] Department of Radiology, The Netherlands Cancer Institute, Plesmanlaan 121, 1066 CX Amsterdam, The Netherlands
taotanjs@gmail.com
[3] Faculty of Applied Sciences, Macao Polytechnic University, Macao 999078, China

Abstract. The domain adaptation approach has gained significant acceptance in transferring styles across various vendors and centers, along with filling the gaps in modalities. However, multi-center application faces the challenge of the difficulty of domain adaptation due to their intra-domain differences. We focus on introducing a fine-grained unsupervised framework for domain adaptation to facilitate cross-modality segmentation of vestibular schwannoma (VS) and cochlea. We propose to use a vector to control the generator to synthesize a fake image with given features. And then, we can apply various augmentations to the dataset by searching the feature dictionary. The diversity augmentation can increase the performance and robustness of the segmentation model. On the CrossMoDA2023 test phase leaderboard, our method received a mean Dice score of 0.773 and 0.843 on VS and cochlea, respectively.

Keywords: Domain Adaptation · Segmentation · Vestibular Schwannoma

1 Introduction

The use of domain adaptation in clinical settings has become increasingly popular to enhance the effectiveness of deep learning methods. The objective of the Cross-Modality Domain Adaptation (CrossMoDA) challenge [5] is to accurately segment two brain structures: the vestibular schwannoma (VS) and cochlea. Although contrast-enhanced T1 (ceT1) MR imaging is a common diagnostic and surveillance tool for patients with VS, the research on non-contrast imaging, such as T2-weighted imaging (T2), is increasing due to its lower risk and cost-effectiveness. To prevent the need for extra annotation, CrossMoDA works towards transferring acquired knowledge from ceT1 images to T2 images through the creation of domain adaptation between unpaired ceT1 and T2. The use of multi-center data from London SC-GK (ldn), Tilburg SC-GK (etz), and UK MC-RC (ukm) poses a challenge in domain adaptation due to intra-domain bias. Simply transferring images from the ceT1 domain to the T2 domain using a single model results in a loss of diversity in the multi-center T2 images. Thus, we propose a fine-grained domain adaptation model controlled with more specific features to synthesize T2 images. Our primary contributions are as follows: (1) The proposed domain adaptation model can control the appearance of the output image through the characteristic conditions of the input target sequence. (2) The proposed HyperDiscriminator can simplify adversarial training for multiple image styles. (3) We improve model segmentation performance by generating images with different appearances for augmentation.

2 Related Work

Extensive validation of unsupervised domain adaptation for the vestibular system and cochlea segmentation has been conducted through the CrossMoDA challenge [5]. In present studies, an image-to-image translation technique, such as CycleGAN [16], is utilized to produce pseudo-target domain images from source domain images. These generated images and their corresponding manual annotations are subsequently employed to train the segmentation models. Several recent studies have utilized varying versions of CycleGAN to convert ceT1 images into hrT2 images for brain tumor segmentation. The main objective of these studies is to maintain the structural integrity of the low-intensity regions in real hrT2 scans, such as the VS and cochleas. Specifically, Dong et al. [4] utilize Nice-GAN [2], which employs discriminators for encoding, while Choi et al. [3] use CUT [11] and post-processing techniques. Furthermore, Shin et al. [14] implement an additional decoder and an iterable self-training strategy. Kang et al. [9] utilize two image translation models in parallel, each incorporating a pixel-level consistent constraint and a patch-level contrastive constraint, respectively. Sallé et al. [12] propose tumor blending augmentation combined with CycleGAN, which diversifies target regions of interest during training, improving the segmentation generalization of the model during testing. Han et al. [6] acquire a shared representation from both ceT1 and hrT2 images alongside the successful recovery of another modality from the latent representation. In addition, they utilized proxy tasks of VS segmentation and brain parcellation to regulate the consistency of image structures in domain adaptation effectively.

3 Method

3.1 Framework Overview

Figure 1 illustrates the proposed fine-grained unsupervised domain adaptation segmentation framework. We first employ a conditional generator (Seq2Seq) [7] to synthesize the corresponding T2 image from a given ceT1 image. The T2 image can be augmented by changing the feature codes used to control the Seq2Seq generator. Using the fake T2 dataset after augmentation, we can train a robust segmentation network – the nnU-Net [8] model.

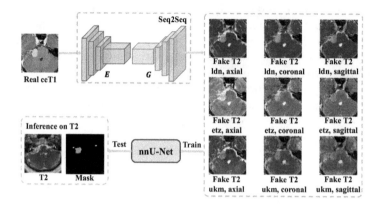

Fig. 1. Overview of the proposed fine-grained unsupervised domain adaptation segmentation framework. The plane (axial, coronal, and sagital) presents the plane of 2D slices for the input image to the Seq2Seq model. The plane (axial, coronal, and sagittal) presents the plane of 2D slices for the image to input to the Seq2Seq model. The SeqSeq model can only process 2D slices and re-stack these slices into 3D images. For better comparison, we only show the axial plane of these images.

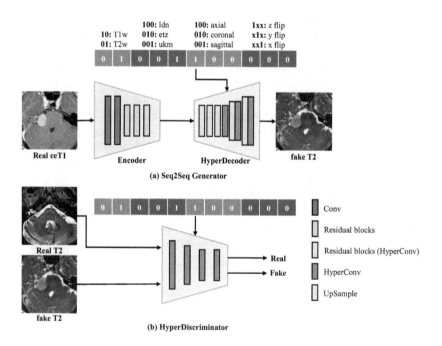

Fig. 2. The architecture of (a) Seq2Seq generator and (b) HyperDiscriminator. The given conditional zero-one code can control the synthesized image of the generator. The conditional code is the combination of target modality (T1w or T2w), center (ldn, etz, ukm), plane (axial, coronal, sagittal), and flip augmentation (z-axis, y-axis, x-axis).

3.2 Fine-Grained Domain Adaptation

Figure 2 illustrates the architecture of the Seq2Seq generator [7] and Hyper-Discriminator. The seq2Seq generator is a conditional autoencoder-like model, inputting with a real ceT1 image and a conditional zero-one code and outputting with the fake T2 image. The conditional code combines the target modality, center, plane, and flip augmentation code. Note that, the plane in the conditional code presents the plane of 2D slices for the input image because the proposed model can only handle 2D slices. Adversarial learning involves differentiating between real and generated images. However, due to the varying appearances of data from different centers even within the same modality, the discriminator needs to distinguish between a much larger number of domains than just the ceT1 and T2 categories. Having a separate discriminator for each case would result in a very tedious and challenging training process, and would fail to capture the shared information between these images. Therefore, we propose the use of a HyperDiscriminator, which, like the generator, has two inputs: image and conditional encoding. Under different conditional codes, the discriminator can differentiate between true and false images. We train our models by following the training process and loss function in [6], and keep all the hyper-parameters the same.

3.3 Segmentation with Domain Augmentation

With the proposed Seq2Seq, we can control the intra-domain diversity of the fake T2 images. Specifically, we augment each real ceT1 image into nine fake images with the combination of the image center and plane view as shown in Fig. 1. Finally, we train the nnU-Net [8] model feeding with the augmented dataset.

4 Experimental Results

4.1 Materials and Implementation Details

Dataset. The dataset for the CrossMoDA challenge is an extension of the publicly available Vestibular-Schwannoma-SEG collection [10,13,15], which is divided into the training dataset (227 subjects with ceT1 images and other unpaired 295 subjects with T2 images) and the validation dataset (96 subjects with T2 images). All imaging datasets were manually segmented for cochlea and VS, and the VS segmentation was split into the intra- and extra-meatal regions.

Data Preprocessing. The pipeline of image preprocessing is modified from MSF-Net [6]. All the images are first resampled to the spacing of $0.4102 \times 0.4102 \times 0.4102$ mm due to various spacing of images from different centers, and normalized image size to $256 \times 256 \times 256$ by central cropping or zero padding. Then we normalize images to $[0, 1]$ by setting the intensity range from 0 to 99.5 percentile. We select an identical ceT1 image (ldn_1_ceT1) as the atlas (atlas should have a complete brain structure so that other incomplete images can be easily matched) to improve domain adaptation performance and employ intra- and inter-modality affine transformation on all the ceT1 and T2 images, respectively. Here, the affine registration is implemented by Advanced Normalization Tools (ANTs) [1], and we utilize mutual information (MI) loss for T2 images and normalized cross-correlation (NCC) loss for ceT1 images. Finally, based on the distribution of tumor areas in the training set, we crop the images to the size of $256 \times 256 \times 256$ by setting a fixed region. Finally, 2D slices selected from axial, coronal, and sagittal planes are used to train the models.

Implementation Details. We implemented our method[1] using PyTorch with NVIDIA 3090 RTX. The encoder architecture of Seq2Seq is comprised of three convolutional layers and six residual blocks. The first convolutional layer is responsible for encoding the intensities into features, while the second and third convolutional layers conduct four-time downsampling of images. The high-level representation is then extracted by the residual blocks, whose channels are of sizes 64, 128, 256, and 256, respectively. The HyperDecoder of Seq2Seq is an inverse architecture of the encoder, which has all the convolutional layers replaced with HyperConv [7]. HyperConv is a convolutional layer whose kernel is generated from the input conditional code. The HyperDiscriminator is implemented with four HyperConv layers with a kernel size of 4, stride of 2, and output channel of 64, 128, 256, and 512, respectively, followed by a convolutional layer with a kernel size of 1 and an output channel of 1. The Seq2Seq generator is trained with Adam optimizer, a learning rate of 2×10^{-4}, a default of 1,000 epochs, and a batch size of 1. nnU-Net is trained with its default 3D full-resolution settings.

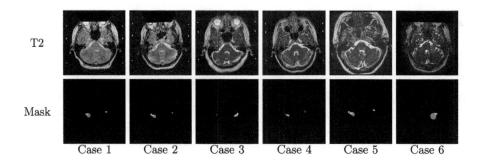

Fig. 3. Examples of vestibular schwannoma (VS) and cochlea segmentation.

---

[1] https://github.com/fiy2W/cmda2022.superpolymerization.

4.2 Results

Figure 3 shows the performance of VS and cochlea segmentation. With fine-grained modality augmentation, the segmentation model can correctly segment images from different centers. We compare our proposed method with MSF-Net [6] on ceT1 and T2 domain adaptation to evaluate the influence of different generation performances for further segmentation. Table 1 and Table 2 show the segmentation results for the nnU-Net models training with fake T2 images generated by different methods and whether augmented with varying styles of planes and centers. The proposed method achieves better results than MSF-Net and Seq2Seq on the validation set, and the ablation study shows that more augmentation can increase the generalization ability of the segmentation model.

Table 1. Segmentation results of VS and cochlea for nnU-Net utilizing generated T2 images with different domain adaptation methods. The best result is in bold.

Methods	VS		Cochlea	
	Dice ↑	ASSD ↓	Dice ↑	ASSD ↓
MSF-Net [6]	0.671 ± 0.304	10.6 ± 38.4	0.820 ± 0.039	0.300 ± 0.371
Seq2Seq [7]	0.702 ± 0.282	9.29 ± 38.3	0.804 ± 0.040	0.275 ± 0.136
Seq2Seq+Plane	0.710 ± 0.275	8.74 ± 37.9	0.833 ± 0.034	0.229 ± 0.128
Seq2Seq+Plane+Center	**0.765 ± 0.255**	**7.49 ± 37.4**	**0.836 ± 0.031**	**0.218 ± 0.127**

Table 2. Segmentation results of intra- and extra-meatal region of VS for nnU-Net utilizing generated T2 images with different domain adaptation methods. The best result is in bold.

Methods	Intra-Meatal		Extra-Meatal	
	Dice ↑	ASSD ↓	Dice ↑	ASSD ↓
MSF-Net [6]	0.542 ± 0.277	11.1 ± 38.7	0.706 ± 0.273	14.6 ± 64.0
Seq2Seq [7]	0.561 ± 0.264	9.77 ± 38.6	0.750 ± 0.222	**5.98 ± 37.7**
Seq2Seq+Plane	0.550 ± 0.267	16.1 ± 61.7	0.757 ± 0.227	12.7 ± 63.7
Seq2Seq+Plane+Center	**0.598 ± 0.242**	**7.67 ± 37.4**	**0.813 ± 0.174**	8.56 ± 52.4

5 Discussion

According to the findings depicted in Fig. 3, despite noticeable differences in the visual appearance of T2 images from different centers due to variations in scanning devices and parameters, our segmentation model has accomplished the task of accurately segmenting VS and cochlea. This outcome highlights the efficacy of data augmentation through fine-granted domain adaptation in enhancing the generalization of subsequent segmentation models. In addition, as indicated by the results presented in Table 1 and Table 2, generating images from diverse planes of view and multiple centers through augmentation can enhance the segmentation precision of VS and cochlear. Nevertheless, due to the model being able only to process 2D slices and the absence of spatial 3D information extraction, the resulting fake T2 images inadequately display the morphology of certain minute tumors, ultimately failing to segment these smaller tumors accurately.

6 Conclusion

In this study, we propose a method for fine-grained unsupervised cross-modality domain adaptation. Our approach enables the synthesis of T2 images from different centers, thereby increasing the generalization of the segmentation model. Our proposed method achieves a third rank during the test phase for cross-modal VS (intra- and extra-meatal region) and cochlear segmentation in the CrossMoDA 2023 challenge.

Acknowledgement. Luyi Han was funded by Chinese Scholarship Council (CSC) scholarship. This work is supported by Macao Polytechnic University Grant (RP/FCA-05/2022).

References

1. Avants, B.B., Tustison, N., Song, G., et al.: Advanced normalization tools (ANTs). Insight J. **2**(365), 1–35 (2009)
2. Chen, R., Huang, W., Huang, B., Sun, F., Fang, B.: Reusing discriminators for encoding: towards unsupervised image-to-image translation. In: Proceedings of the IEEE/CVF Conference on Computer Vision and Pattern Recognition, pp. 8168–8177 (2020)
3. Choi, J.W.: Using out-of-the-box frameworks for contrastive unpaired image translation for vestibular schwannoma and cochlea segmentation: an approach for the crossMoDA challenge. In: International MICCAI Brainlesion Workshop, pp. 509–517. Springer (2021)
4. Dong, H., Yu, F., Zhao, J., Dong, B., Zhang, L.: Unsupervised domain adaptation in semantic segmentation based on pixel alignment and self-training. arXiv preprint arXiv:2109.14219 (2021)
5. Dorent, R., et al.: CrossMoDA 2021 challenge: benchmark of cross-modality domain adaptation techniques for vestibular schwannoma and cochlea segmentation. Med. Image Anal. **83**, 102628 (2023)
6. Han, L., Huang, Y., Tan, T., Mann, R.: Unsupervised cross-modality domain adaptation for vestibular schwannoma segmentation and koos grade prediction based on semi-supervised contrastive learning. arXiv preprint arXiv:2210.04255 (2022)
7. Han, L., et al.: Synthesis-based imaging-differentiation representation learning for multi-sequence 3D/4D MRI. Med. Image Anal. **92**, 103044 (2024)

8. Isensee, F., Jaeger, P.F., Kohl, S.A., Petersen, J., Maier-Hein, K.H.: nnU-net: a self-configuring method for deep learning-based biomedical image segmentation. Nat. Methods **18**(2), 203–211 (2021)
9. Kang, B., Nam, H., Han, J.W., Heo, K.S., Kam, T.E.: Multi-view cross-modality MR image translation for vestibular schwannoma and cochlea segmentation. arXiv preprint arXiv:2303.14998 (2023)
10. Kujawa, A., et al.: Deep learning for automatic segmentation of vestibular schwannoma: a retrospective study from multi-centre routine MRI. medRxiv, pp. 2022–08 (2022)
11. Park, T., Efros, A.A., Zhang, R., Zhu, J.Y.: Contrastive learning for unpaired image-to-image translation. In: Computer Vision–ECCV 2020: 16th European Conference, Glasgow, UK, 23–28 August 2020, Part IX, pp. 319–345. Springer (2020)
12. Sallé, G., Conze, P.H., Bert, J., Boussion, N., Visvikis, D., Jaouen, V.: Cross-modal tumor segmentation using generative blending augmentation and self training. arXiv preprint arXiv:2304.01705 (2023)
13. Shapey, J., et al.: Segmentation of vestibular schwannoma from MRI, an open annotated dataset and baseline algorithm. Sci. Data **8**(1), 286 (2021)
14. Shin, H., Kim, H., Kim, S., Jun, Y., Eo, T., Hwang, D.: COSMOS: cross-modality unsupervised domain adaptation for 3D medical image segmentation based on target-aware domain translation and iterative self-training. arXiv preprint arXiv:2203.16557 (2022)
15. Wijethilake, N., et al.: Boundary distance loss for intra-/extra-meatal segmentation of vestibular schwannoma. In: International Workshop on Machine Learning in Clinical Neuroimaging, pp. 73–82. Springer (2022)
16. Zhu, J.Y., Park, T., Isola, P., Efros, A.A.: Unpaired image-to-image translation using cycle-consistent adversarial networks. In: Proceedings of the IEEE International Conference on Computer Vision, pp. 2223–2232 (2017)

Learning Site-Specific Styles for Multi-institutional Unsupervised Cross-Modality Domain Adaptation

Han Liu[1](✉), Yubo Fan[1], Zhoubing Xu[2], Benoit M. Dawant[1], and Ipek Oguz[1]

[1] Vanderbilt University, Nashville, TN, USA
han.liu@vanderbilt.edu
[2] Siemens Healthineers, Princeton, NJ, USA

Abstract. Unsupervised cross-modality domain adaptation is a challenging task in medical image analysis, and it becomes more challenging when source and target domain data are collected from multiple institutions. In this paper, we present our solution to tackle the multi-institutional unsupervised domain adaptation for the crossMoDA 2023 challenge. First, we perform unpaired image translation to translate the source domain images to the target domain, where we design a dynamic network to generate synthetic target domain images with controllable, site-specific styles. Afterwards, we train a segmentation model using the synthetic images and further reduce the domain gap by self-training. Our solution achieved the 1st place during both the validation and testing phases of the challenge. The code repository is publicly available at https://github.com/MedICL-VU/crossmoda2023.

Keywords: MRI · Vestibular schwannoma · Cochlea · Multi-institutional · Unsupervised domain adaptation · Style transfer · Dynamic network

1 Introduction

The crossMoDA challenges[1] [6] aim to tackle the unsupervised cross-modality segmentation of vestibular schwannoma (VS) and cochleae on MRI scans. Specifically, participants are provided with the labeled source domain data, i.e., contrast-enhanced T1-weighted (ceT1) images, and the unlabeled target domain data, i.e., high-resolution T2-weighted (hrT2) images. The goal of this challenge is to train a segmentation model for the target domain hrT2 images. The crossMoDA 2023 extends the previous editions by introducing (1) a sub-segmentation task for the VS (intra- and extra-meatal components) [28] and (2) more heterogeneous data collected from multiple institutions. The schematic problem description of the crossMoDA 2023 is illustrated in Fig. 1. Specifically, the organizers partition the multi-institutional images into 3 sub-datasets, namely ETZ,

---

[1] https://crossmoda-challenge.ml/.

LDN, and UKM. It can be observed that the hrT2 images from different sub-datasets have significantly different appearances and thus it is critical to ensure the robustness of our segmentation model on the multi-institutional data.

As the images within the same sub-dataset have relatively consistent styles, we assume that the images within each sub-dataset are collected from the same **site**. Note that this assumption is not accurate for the UKM sub-dataset as it includes images collected from multiple sites. However, by considering the UKM images as collected from the same site, we will show that our generative model can learn a UKM-specific style that can be used to diversify the styles of our synthetic images. In this paper, our contributions are summarized as follows:

- We revisit the top-performing solutions of the previous crossMoDA challenges and analyze the factors contributing to their success.
- To addresses the intra-domain variability in multi-institutional UDA, we propose a dynamic network to generate synthetic images with controllable, site-specific styles, which are used to train the downstream segmentation model for improved robustness and generalizability.
- Our proposed method achieves the 1st place during both the validation and testing phases of the crossMoDA 2023 challenge.

2 Related Works

2.1 CrossMoDA Challenges: 2021–2023

While numerous domain adaptation techniques have been proposed for image segmentation, most of these techniques have only been validated either on private datasets or on small public datasets, and mostly addressed single-class segmentation tasks. The crossMoDA challenge [6] introduced the first large and multi-class dataset for cross-modality domain adaptation for medical image segmentation. In the 2021 edition, source and target domain data were collected from a single scanner and the participants were asked to segment the cochleae and the whole VS in hrT2 images, i.e., a 2-class segmentation task. With the same task, the 2022 edition included additional data from another scanner for both source and target domain datasets, making the domain adaptation task more challenging by introducing intra-domain variability. The 2023 edition further enlarged the datasets by including multi-institutional, heterogeneous data for both domains and introduced a sub-segmentation for the VS (intra- and extra-meatal components), leading to a 3-class segmentation task with significant intra-domain variability.

2.2 Top Solutions in CrossMoDA 2021 and 2022

The top solutions in the 2021 and 2022 editions are mainly based on the ***image-level domain alignment*** approach. As illustrated in Fig. 2, it typically consists of three steps. In step 1, unpaired image translation is used to translate ceT1 images to synthetic hrT2 images. The most commonly used techniques include

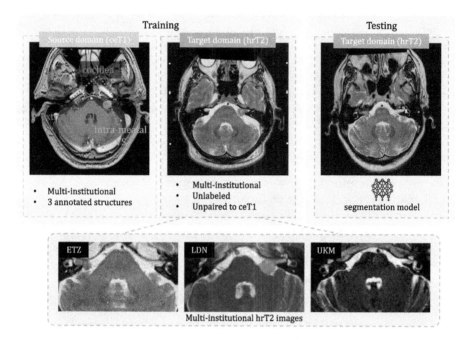

Fig. 1. Schematic problem description of the crossMoDA 2023 challenge. The task of this challenge is cross-modality unsupervised domain adaptation (UDA), where source domain and target domain are contrast-enhanced T1 (ceT1) and high-resolution T2 (hrT2), respectively. Note that both source and target domain data are collected from multiple institutions, leading to additional challenges to the UDA tasks, which primarily focus on the inter-domain gap rather than the intra-domain variability.

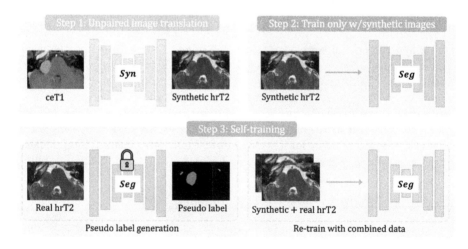

Fig. 2. The training strategy of the image-level domain alignment approaches for UDA.

cycleGAN [32], CUT [24], QS-Attn [11] with either 2D or 3D backbones. In step 2, the synthetic hrT2 images and the associated ceT1 labels are used to train a segmentation model. In step 3, to further reduce the domain gap between synthetic and real hrT2, the unlabeled real hrT2 are used to train the segmentation model via self-training. Specifically, the network trained in step 2 is used to firstly generate the pseudo labels on the real hrT2 images. Then the synthetic and real hrT2 images are combined to re-train a segmentation network. This self-training process can be repeated iteratively by using the most updated pseudo labels generated by the network trained at the previous iteration.

Based on the image-level domain alignment strategy, the top teams have proposed a variety of techniques to further improve the performance. In the 2021 edition, the 1st place team [27] proposed to add segmentation decoders to the generators of the 2D cycleGAN to better synthesize the VS and the cochlea. Additionally, they visually inspected the pseudo labels to select the most reliable ones for self-training. The 2nd place team proposed PAST [5], where 2D NICE-GAN [3] was used for image synthesis and self-training with pixel-level pseudo label filtering was used for segmentation. The 3rd place team [4] used the CUT model for image synthesis and proposed an offline data augmentation technique to simulate the heterogeneous signal intensity of VS. In the 2022 edition, the 1st place team built upon the PAST algorithm and added extra segmentation heads for NICE-GAN. Moreover, to address the intra-domain variability, they trained separate segmentation models for different sites and structures. The 2nd place team [15] proposed to improve the image synthesis via multi-view image translation, where the cycleGAN and the QS-Attn were used in parallel. The 3rd place team [25] proposed to improve the generalizability of the segmentation model by generating diverse appearances of VS via SinGAN [26].

In summary, the top solutions in 2021 and 2022 editions demonstrated three promising directions to improve the image-level domain alignment: (1) better synthetic hrT2 images in step 1, (2) higher-quality pseudo labels for self-training in step 3, and (3) local intensity augmentation for VS in step 2 and 3.

3 Methods

Motivated by the previous works [5,9,18,19,27,31], we propose to tackle the UDA problem by reducing the domain gap at the image-level, and follow the 3-step strategy presented in Sect. 2.2. Since the quality of synthetic hrT2 images is critical to the performance of the downstream segmentation task, our key innovations are mainly focused on the step 1, i.e., unpaired image translation. To address the intra-domain variability, we propose to generate synthetic hrT2 images with **site-specific styles**, which are then used to train the segmentation model for improved robustness to various hrT2 styles. The details of our novel techniques for image translation are provided as follows.

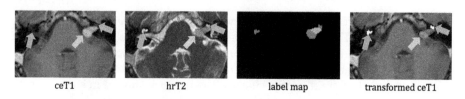

Fig. 3. Illustration of our proposed label-assisted intensity transformation. The VS (yellow arrow) and cochleae (blue arrows) have opposite intensity profiles in ceT1 and hrT2 images. (Color figure online)

3.1 Label-Assisted Intensity Transformation

The VS and the cochleae have significantly different intensity profiles in ceT1 and hrT2. As shown in Fig. 3, the cochleae have weak signals and the VS has strong signals in ceT1 images, but the opposite is true in hrT2. Our preliminary experiment shows that the synthesis network with the original ceT1 as input may fail to capture the appearance difference of these structures between the two modalities. To address this problem, we propose to transform the intensity profiles of VS and cochlea in ceT1 images before feeding them to the synthesis network. After we perform regular preprocessing steps, which include rescaling to $[-1, 1]$ range (see Sect. 3.5), we replace the intensity values of the cochleae by 1.0, i.e., the maximum value of the preprocessed image. In addition, we decrease the intensity values of the VS by $\mu_{VS} + 0.5$, where μ_{VS} is the mean intensity of the VS. With the transformed ceT1, we reduce the appearance difference of the VS and cochleae across two modalities before performing the synthesis task.

3.2 Anatomy-Aware Image Synthesis

We adopt the QS-Attn [11] and extend it to 3D for volumetric unpaired image translation. 3D QS-Attn is used because (1) compared to 2D networks, 3D networks can generate synthetic images with better slice-to-slice continuity by exploiting the inter-slice information, and (2) compared to CycleGAN [32], QS-Attn is less memory-intensive and thus more suitable for 3D networks.

As shown in Fig. 4, we propose to improve the image synthesis by making the generator focus more on the anatomical structures in the downstream segmentation task, i.e., the VS and the cochleae. To this end, we add an extra segmentation decoder D_{seg} to the generator such that our generator learns to synthesize hrT2 images and segment these structures jointly. As demonstrated in [27], this multi-task learning paradigm can help better preserve the shape of the structures-of-interest (SOI) in the synthetic images. Moreover, we employ another segmentation network S to segment SOI from the synthetic hrT2 images, further encouraging the generated SOI to have semantically meaningful boundaries.

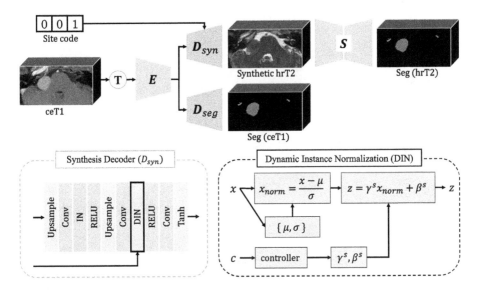

Fig. 4. Illustration of our dynamic generator used for the unpaired image translation. T is the label-assisted intensity transformation. Given a site code (a one-hot vector), our dynamic network is trained to generate site-specific affine parameters for the last instance normalization layer, which is then used to control the output hrT2 styles.

3.3 Site-Specific Styles

To ensure the robustness to different hrT2 styles, we propose to generate the synthetic hrT2 images with site-specific styles to train the segmentation model. Inspired by [20], we propose to modify the synthesis decoder to a dynamic network, where the style of the output hrT2 image is conditioned on a given site prior. Specifically, we replace the last instance normalization (IN) layer of the synthesis decoder by a dynamic instance normalization (DIN) layer. This is motivated by previous studies [7,12,16] where the IN layers are shown to effectively control the **styles** of images. We encode the site condition as a one-hot vector c, which is passed to a controller (a 3D convolutional layer with a kernel size of $1 \times 1 \times 1$) to generate site-specific affine parameters γ^s and β^s for IN. Therefore, we can train a single unified synthesis network on all hrT2 images with a controllable output style, as shown in Fig. 5.

3.4 Oversampling Hard Samples by Style Interpolation

Based on the segmentation results from the validation set, we observe that the VS with either (1) tiny/no extra-meatal components, or (2) large extra-meatal components with heterogeneous appearance, are more challenging to segment. We refer to these cases as *hard samples*. We find that such hard samples are indeed under-represented in the source domain dataset and their associated synthetic hrT2 may need to be oversampled for balanced training. In practice, we

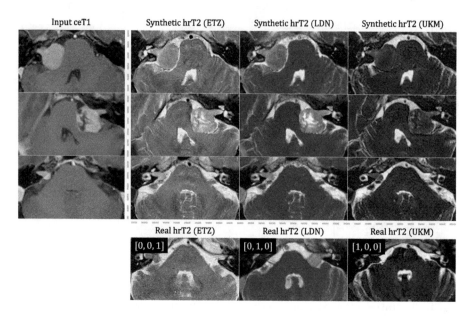

Fig. 5. Synthetic hrT2 images with site-specific styles. In top three rows, each row displays a representative ceT1 image being transformed to hrT2 with different site-specific styles. The bottom row displays real hrT2 images from three different sites, which are used as references for style comparison. Each column corresponds to the same site-specific style and the associated site code is shown on the top left corner at the bottom row.

select the hard samples based on the aforementioned two rules with the help of source domain labels. Inspired by style interpolation [7,10,12], we propose to generate more diverse hrT2 styles for oversampling by feeding the controller with unseen site codes. As shown in Fig. 6, we oversample each hard sample by translating the same ceT1 image into a variety of unseen hrT2 styles, further enriching the diversity of our synthetic dataset. Specifically, out of 226 ceT1 images, we manually identify 32 images with tiny extra-meatal VS and 21 images with large heterogeneous extra-meatal VS, which are oversampled 10 times and added to our training set.

3.5 Implementation Details

Preprocessing. All MR scans are set to the RAI orientation, resampled to the median voxel size of the dataset, i.e., $0.41 \times 0.41 \times 1$ mm^3, and further cropped into $256 \times 144 \times 32$ based on the positions of the cochleae, which are computed by a cochleae localization network. The cropped volumes are used for all the synthesis and segmentation tasks. The cochlea localization network is trained as follows. We firstly train a 2D QS-Attn model to translate the axial slices of whole brain images from ceT1 to hrT2. We stack the generated slices into 3D volumes and train an nnU-Net to segment cochleae. Empirically, we find this model is

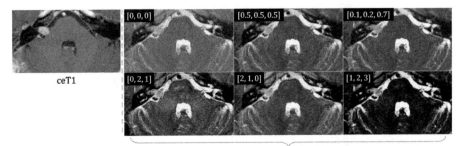

Fig. 6. Examples of hrT2 styles generated by style interpolation. During inference, arbitrary site codes can be used as the site condition to generate unseen hrT2 styles. In each example, the site code is shown at the top left corner.

robust enough to localize cochleae for cropping purposes. To further improve the robustness, we use self-training to retrain the localization model with real hrT2 images and pseudo labels of cochleae.

Synthesis. For image synthesis, we normalize both ceT1 and hrT2 images using Z-score normalization, clip the intensity values to the $[0, 99.9^{th}]$ percentile, and rescale the values to $[-1, 1]$. The backbone of our dynamic generator is a 3D 9-block ResNet. Due to the limit of GPU memory, the input is a 3D patch with a size of $256 \times 144 \times 8$ randomly cropped from the preprocessed image. We use overlapping sliding windows for inference. During training, we apply on-the-fly data augmentation including random contrast adjustment ($p = 0.4$ for ceT1 and $p = 0.1$ for hrT2; smaller p for hrT2 to preserve the site-specific style) and randomly flipping on the LR direction ($p = 0.5$). The loss function for image synthesis is expressed as: $L_G = L_{QS} + \lambda_1 L_{seg}^{ceT1} + \lambda_2 L_{seg}^{hrT2} + \lambda_3 L_{edge}$, where $L_{QS} = L_{adv} + L_{con}^{ceT1} + L_{con}^{hrT2}$ is the default loss function of QS-Attn. L_{seg}^{ceT1} and L_{seg}^{hrT2} are the segmentation losses for D_{seg} and S, respectively. We also adopt an edge loss L_{edge} [8,22,30] to encourage the edge consistency between the input and the output so that the texture within the VS and the cochlea boundary can be well preserved. We use $\lambda_1 = 0.5$, $\lambda_2 = 0.5$ and $\lambda_3 = 1$. We train the network for 400 epochs with a learning rate of $2e-4$ and another 400 epochs with linear decay policy. For our discriminator, we do not condition it on site information and use a single discriminator for all sites. For other hyperparameters, we use the default settings of the QS-Attn.

Segmentation. We use the nnU-Net V2 [14] with 3D fullres configuration for all our segmentation tasks. We build upon the default nnUNetTrainer and make the following modifications. First, we only enable random flipping along LR direction. Second, we introduce two local intensity augmentation functions to only augment the intensity values of the VS and the cochlea. Specifically, we randomly multiply the VS intensity with $u \sim U(1.2, 2)$. In addition, we randomly reduce the cochleae intensity by $v \sim U(0.5, 1)$, since previous study indicates that the cochleae ipsilateral to VS may have weaker signals in hrT2 [2]. We follow [21] to train segmentation models and perform two rounds of self-training. Previous studies suggest that image-level pseudo label filtering can be incorporated into self-training to avoid performance degradation caused by unreliable pseudo labels [13,23,29]. Therefore, we remove the real hrT2 images with unreliable pseudo labels from our training set throughout the self-training process, where the pseudo labels with no tumor prediction or with multiple tumor components on both sides are considered unreliable. Note that the reliability of pseudo labels can be determined by connected component analysis and thus the entire process is fully automatic. Lastly, we use model ensemble by averaging the predictions from 11 models to further boost the performance. These models include 3 standard nnU-Net models trained with different seeds and 8 customized nnU-Net models with the following configurations: 2 different backbone architectures (U-Net or ResU-Net) × 2 different augmentation strategies (strong or weak local intensity augmentation for VS and cochleae) × 2 different sets of unseen site codes for style interpolation.

4 Experiments and Results

We use the dataset[2] provided by the crossMoDA 2023 challenge [17,28]. Dice score and average symmetric surface distance (ASSD) for extra-meatal VS, intra-meatal VS, and cochleae, as well as the boundary ASSD (denoted as 'bound') are used for quantitative evaluation.

Table 1. Quantitative results during the validation phase (96 cases). **Bold** represents the best scores. The three rows at the bottom are our ablation studies. ST: self-training. Tr: modified nnUNetTrainer. OS: oversampling

Method	Dice↑ (%)			ASSD↓ (mm)			
	extra	intra	cochlea	extra	intra	cochlea	bound
Ours (ensemble)	**85.75**	**74.36**	84.07	**0.45**	**0.44**	0.20	**0.51**
Ours (single)	85.08	73.34	84.44	0.48	0.45	0.20	0.53
Team A	83.63	70.57	83.55	0.50	0.59	0.23	4.76
Team B	72.75	56.94	**86.66**	17.62	16.80	**0.18**	32.79
Team C	81.32	59.79	83.56	8.57	7.67	0.22	20.78
w/o ST	84.06	71.42	82.78	0.50	0.59	0.21	0.54
w/o (ST, Tr)	81.74	68.92	82.81	8.58	7.93	0.53	8.69
w/o (ST, Tr, OS)	79.09	64.15	81.94	8.68	11.80	0.56	12.86

[2] https://www.synapse.org/#!Synapse:syn51317912.

Table 2. Quantitative results during the testing phase (341 cases).

Method	Dice↑ (%)			ASSD↓ (mm)			
	extra	intra	cochlea	extra	intra	cochlea	bound
Ours	**84.9**	**72.8**	83.6	**0.452**	**0.496**	**0.201**	**0.675**
Team A	80.8	69.9	**84.4**	0.593	0.581	0.207	1.985
Team B	78.6	60.7	84.3	6.552	9.711	0.246	18.575
Team C	78.4	64.6	81.4	1.625	4.036	1.316	9.953
Team D	63.7	55.8	75.0	20.806	27.814	12.776	24.089
Team E	67.6	56.3	76.7	13.874	18.607	11.026	35.848

4.1 Quantitative Results

In Table 1, we report the evaluation metrics on the validation leaderboard. Our method (a single model) achieves the 1st place on validation leaderboard and model ensembling can slightly improve the performance. Moreover, we perform ablation studies on the validation set to investigate the effectiveness of self-training, our modified nnUNetTrainer, and the oversampling strategy. The results show that each component can effectively improve the segmentation performance. As shown in Table 2, during the testing phase, our method outperforms other methods in all evaluation metrics except the Dice score of cochleae. We note that during both validation and testing phases our method achieves significantly smaller boundary ASSD, i.e., the distance between the intra-meatal and extra-meatal boundary. This demonstrates its superiority in identifying the anatomical separation between the two tumor components.

4.2 Qualitative Results

Representative examples of results obtained with images in the validation set are shown in Fig. 7. In Fig. 7(a), we can observe that even with our oversampling technique (Sect. 3.4), the segmentation results on some hard cases remain unsatisfactory. For example, UKM_150 and LDN_185 include VS with tiny/no extra-meatal components and VS with large extra-meatal components and heterogeneous textures, respectively. Moreover, the field of view and the image quality may also have a negative impact on the segmentation performance, e.g., UKM_174. In Fig. 7(b), even though the hrT2 images may have very different styles, our model can produce good segmentation results for the VS whose shapes are common in the training set, indicating that generating site-specific styles is a promising way to improve model robustness for multi-institutional data.

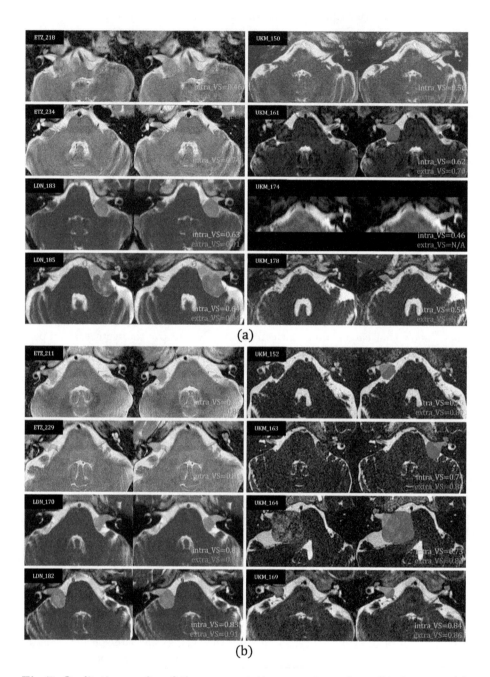

Fig. 7. Qualitative results of the representative cases from the validation sets. (a) Unsatisfactory segmentation results. (b) Satisfactory segmentation results. Dice scores of the intra- and extra-meatal VS are displayed.

5 Discussion and Conclusion

In this paper, we have presented our solution for the crossMoDA 2023 challenge to tackle the multi-institutional UDA problem. Specifically, we have generated synthetic hrT2 images with site-specific styles to improve the robustness of the segmentation model. The results obtained during both the validation and testing phases show that our method has achieved superior performance against other competitors. Notably, the boundary ASSD achieved by our method is much smaller than the ones achieved by other methods. This suggests that our method is more reliable than other approaches for the follow-up clinical analyses, for which the clear separation between intra- and extra-components is crucial. For instance, the size and volume features extracted from the extra-meatal VS are considered as the most sensitive radiomic features for the evaluation of VS growth [1].

Though our solution has achieved promising performance, we believe there are several interesting directions to further improve our method. First, by generating site-specific styles, we assume that the images in each sub-dataset are collected from the same site and have relatively consistent appearances. However, this assumption is not strictly accurate for the UKM sub-dataset, where the images are collected from multiple sites and scanners. Indeed, we find that the images in the UKM sub-dataset may have significantly different appearances, which cannot be simply represented by a single site-specific style. Therefore, an interesting direction for future studies is to transform the **site**-specific style to the **image**-specific style, i.e., the generated style is conditioned on a reference real hrT2 image. Second, though we can produce some synthetic styles by feeding the dynamic generator with unseen site codes (Sect. 3.4), the generated styles and the associated codes do not have strong correspondence and thus our style interpolation process is not explainable. The underlying reason may be that the dynamic generator is optimized to learn only 3 discrete site-specific styles, leading to a discontinuous latent space of styles. In the future, we will explore some regularization techniques to make the latent space more continuous. This would permit to not only generate site-specific styles, but also more diverse and explainable synthetic styles via style interpolation.

Acknowledgement. This work was supported in part by the National Science Foundation grant 2220401 and the National Institutes of Health grant T32EB021937.

References

1. Baccianella, S., Esuli, A., Sebastiani, F.: Evaluation measures for ordinal regression. In: 2009 Ninth International Conference on Intelligent Systems Design and Applications, pp. 283–287. IEEE (2009)
2. Cass, N.D., Fan, Y., Lindquist, N.R., Dawant, B.M., Tawfik, K.O.: Automated whole cochlear T2 signal demonstrates weak correlation with hearing loss in observed vestibular schwannoma. Audiol. Neuro-otol. 1–11 (2023)

3. Chen, R., Huang, W., Huang, B., Sun, F., Fang, B.: Reusing discriminators for encoding: towards unsupervised image-to-image translation. In: Proceedings of the IEEE/CVF Conference on Computer Vision and Pattern Recognition, pp. 8168–8177 (2020)
4. Choi, J.: Using out-of-the-box frameworks for unpaired image translation and image segmentation for the CrossMoDA challenge. arXiv preprint arXiv:2110.01607 (2021)
5. Dong, H., Yu, F., Zhao, J., Dong, B., Zhang, L.: Unsupervised domain adaptation in semantic segmentation based on pixel alignment and self-training. arXiv preprint arXiv:2109.14219 (2021)
6. Dorent, R., et al.: CrossMoDA 2021 challenge: benchmark of cross-modality domain adaptation techniques for vestibular schwannoma and cochlea segmentation. Med. Image Anal. **83**, 102628 (2023)
7. Dumoulin, V., Shlens, J., Kudlur, M.: A learned representation for artistic style. In: International Conference on Learning Representations (2017). https://openreview.net/forum?id=BJO-BuT1g
8. Fan, Y., Khan, M.M., Liu, H., Noble, J.H., Labadie, R.F., Dawant, B.M.: Temporal bone CT synthesis for MR-only cochlear implant preoperative planning. In: Medical Imaging 2023: Image-Guided Procedures, Robotic Interventions, and Modeling, vol. 12466, pp. 358–363. SPIE (2023)
9. Han, L., Huang, Y., Tan, T., Mann, R.: Unsupervised cross-modality domain adaptation for vestibular schwannoma segmentation and koos grade prediction based on semi-supervised contrastive learning. arXiv preprint arXiv:2210.04255 (2022)
10. Hu, D., Li, H., Liu, H., Yao, X., Wang, J., Oguz, I.: Map: domain generalization via meta-learning on anatomy-consistent pseudo-modalities. arXiv preprint arXiv:2309.01286 (2023)
11. Hu, X., Zhou, X., Huang, Q., Shi, Z., Sun, L., Li, Q.: QS-attn: query-selected attention for contrastive learning in I2I translation. In: Proceedings of the IEEE/CVF Conference on Computer Vision and Pattern Recognition, pp. 18291–18300 (2022)
12. Huang, X., Belongie, S.: Arbitrary style transfer in real-time with adaptive instance normalization. In: Proceedings of the IEEE International Conference on Computer Vision, pp. 1501–1510 (2017)
13. Huang, Z., et al.: Revisiting nnU-net for iterative pseudo labeling and efficient sliding window inference. In: Fast and Low-Resource Semi-supervised Abdominal Organ Segmentation: MICCAI 2022 Challenge, FLARE 2022, Held in Conjunction with MICCAI 2022, Singapore, 22 September 2022, pp. 178–189. Springer (2023)
14. Isensee, F., Jaeger, P.F., Kohl, S.A., Petersen, J., Maier-Hein, K.H.: nnU-net: a self-configuring method for deep learning-based biomedical image segmentation. Nat. Methods **18**(2), 203–211 (2021)
15. Kang, B., Nam, H., Han, J.W., Heo, K.S., Kam, T.E.: Multi-view cross-modality MR image translation for vestibular schwannoma and cochlea segmentation. arXiv preprint arXiv:2303.14998 (2023)
16. Karras, T., Laine, S., Aila, T.: A style-based generator architecture for generative adversarial networks. In: Proceedings of the IEEE/CVF Conference on Computer Vision and Pattern Recognition, pp. 4401–4410 (2019)
17. Kujawa, A., et al.: Deep learning for automatic segmentation of vestibular schwannoma: a retrospective study from multi-centre routine MRI. medRxiv pp. 2022–08 (2022)
18. Li, H., Hu, D., Zhu, Q., Larson, K.E., Zhang, H., Oguz, I.: Unsupervised cross-modality domain adaptation for segmenting vestibular schwannoma and cochlea

with data augmentation and model ensemble. In: International MICCAI Brainlesion Workshop, pp. 518–528. Springer (2021)
19. Liu, H., Fan, Y., Cui, C., Su, D., McNeil, A., Dawant, B.M.: Unsupervised domain adaptation for vestibular schwannoma and cochlea segmentation via semi-supervised learning and label fusion. In: International MICCAI Brainlesion Workshop, pp. 529–539. Springer (2021)
20. Liu, H., et al.: ModDrop++: a dynamic filter network with intra-subject co-training for multiple sclerosis lesion segmentation with missing modalities. In: International Conference on Medical Image Computing and Computer-Assisted Intervention, pp. 444–453. Springer (2022)
21. Liu, H., Fan, Y., Oguz, I., Dawant, B.M.: Enhancing data diversity for self-training based unsupervised cross-modality vestibular schwannoma and cochlea segmentation. arXiv preprint arXiv:2209.11879 (2022)
22. Liu, H., Sigona, M.K., Manuel, T.J., Chen, L.M., Dawant, B.M., Caskey, C.F.: Evaluation of synthetically generated computed tomography for use in transcranial focused ultrasound procedures. J. Med. Imaging **10**(5), 055001–055001 (2023)
23. Liu, H., et al.: COSST: multi-organ segmentation with partially labeled datasets using comprehensive supervisions and self-training. arXiv preprint arXiv:2304.14030 (2023)
24. Park, T., Efros, A.A., Zhang, R., Zhu, J.Y.: Contrastive learning for unpaired image-to-image translation. In: Computer Vision–ECCV 2020: 16th European Conference, Glasgow, UK, 23–28 August 2020, Part IX, pp. 319–345. Springer (2020)
25. Sallé, G., Conze, P.H., Bert, J., Boussion, N., Visvikis, D., Jaouen, V.: Cross-modal tumor segmentation using generative blending augmentation and self training. arXiv preprint arXiv:2304.01705 (2023)
26. Shaham, T.R., Dekel, T., Michaeli, T.: SinGAN: learning a generative model from a single natural image. In: Proceedings of the IEEE/CVF International Conference on Computer Vision, pp. 4570–4580 (2019)
27. Shin, H., Kim, H., Kim, S., Jun, Y., Eo, T., Hwang, D.: COSMOS: cross-modality unsupervised domain adaptation for 3D medical image segmentation based on target-aware domain translation and iterative self-training. arXiv preprint arXiv:2203.16557 (2022)
28. Wijethilake, N., et al.: Boundary distance loss for intra-/extra-meatal segmentation of vestibular schwannoma. In: International Workshop on Machine Learning in Clinical Neuroimaging, pp. 73–82. Springer (2022)
29. Yang, L., Zhuo, W., Qi, L., Shi, Y., Gao, Y.: ST++: make self-training work better for semi-supervised semantic segmentation. In: Proceedings of the IEEE/CVF Conference on Computer Vision and Pattern Recognition, pp. 4268–4277 (2022)
30. Yu, B., Zhou, L., Wang, L., Shi, Y., Fripp, J., Bourgeat, P.: Ea-GANs: edge-aware generative adversarial networks for cross-modality MR image synthesis. IEEE Trans. Med. Imaging **38**(7), 1750–1762 (2019)
31. Zhao, Z., Xu, K., Yeo, H.Z., Yang, X., Guan, C.: MS-MT: multi-scale mean teacher with contrastive unpaired translation for cross-modality vestibular schwannoma and cochlea segmentation. arXiv preprint arXiv:2303.15826 (2023)
32. Zhu, J.Y., Park, T., Isola, P., Efros, A.A.: Unpaired image-to-image translation using cycle-consistent adversarial networks. In: Proceedings of the IEEE International Conference on Computer Vision, pp. 2223–2232 (2017)

MS-MT++: Enhanced Multi-scale Mean Teacher for Cross-Modality Vestibular Schwannoma and Cochlea Segmentation

Ziyuan Zhao[✉], Ruikai Lin, Kaixin Xu, Xulei Yang, and Cuntai Guan

Institute for Infocomm Research (I2R), A*STAR, Singapore, Singapore
zhaoz@i2r.a-star.edu.sg

Abstract. Domain shift has been a long-standing issue for medical image segmentation. Unsupervised domain adaptation (UDA) methods have recently achieved promising cross-modality segmentation performance by distilling knowledge from a label-rich source domain to a target domain without labels. Different from CrossMoDA 2022, the challenge of 2023 includes highly heterogeneous MRI scans from more institutions and various scanners and subdivides the segmentation object into three key brain structures (intra/extra-vestibular schwannoma and cochlea), increasing the difficulty of domain adaptation. In this work, we improve our previous method and propose an enhanced multi-scale self-ensembling-based UDA framework for automatic segmentation of Vestibular Schwannoma and Cochlea on high-resolution T2 images. Our method demonstrates a mean Dice score of 0.669 and 0.766 for the extra/intra-VS joint area and Cochlea respectively, securing a top 5 finish in the CrossMoDA 2023 challenge.

Keywords: Medical image segmentation · Unsupervised domain adaptation · Vestibular Schwannoma · Cochlea

1 Introduction

Medical image segmentation plays a pivotal role in medical image analysis, providing crucial information for diagnostic analysis and treatment planning [6]. Accurate segmentation and measurement of Vestibular Schwannoma (VS) and Cochlea from MRI are instrumental in assisting VS treatment planning and streamlining clinical workflows [26]. Recently, machine learning and deep learning [11] have demonstrated remarkable success across various domains [3,9,19, 23,24,32–34]. Consequently, researchers have increasingly employed deep learning techniques for autonomously segmenting VS and Cochlea [5,14,15]. In the case of Vestibular Schwannoma, the tumor area is anatomically classified into intra- and extra-meatal regions based on their location inside or outside the inner ear canal. Reporting guidelines underscore the importance of differentiating between intra- and extra-meatal regions when presenting results [25]. Notably, the largest extra-meatal diameter serves as a key metric for indicating tumor size.

In addition, metrics such as size and volume derived from the extra-meatal region are crucial radiomic features for evaluating Vestibular Schwannoma (VS) growth. In this regard, the CrossMoDA 2023 dataset introduces more detailed annotations of intra- and extra-meatal VS to facilitate more accurate VS segmentation compared to the previous challenge [5]. While Contrast-enhanced T1 (ceT1) MR imaging is commonly used, there is a growing interest in non-contrast sequences, such as high-resolution T2 (hrT2) imaging. Recent findings suggest that high-resolution T2 (hrT2) MRI could be a safer and more cost-efficient alternative to contrast-enhanced T1 (ceT1) MRI. However, the significant domain shift between MRI images with different contrasts, along with the expensive and laborious process of re-annotating medical image scans in another modality, makes it challenging for deep learning models to generalize effectively across both domains. In this regard, unsupervised domain adaptation (UDA) [1,7,37] has emerged as a promising approach in medical imaging to enhance the robustness of deep learning algorithms on complex scenarios from multiple perspectives, such as image adaptation [7,18,42], feature adaptation [16,30,36] and their mixtures [2,40,41], enabling them to adapt to diverse input data domains and extend their utility in various clinical settings. Therefore, we are encouraged to perform unsupervised domain adaptation (UDA) and conduct intra-VS, extra-VS, and Cochlea segmentation in the hrT2 domain by leveraging both labeled ceT1 scans and unlabeled hrT2 scans.

In this work, we improve our previous method [38] and propose an effective cross-modality unsupervised domain adaptation (UDA) framework, called MS-MT++. In our framework, we first translate contrast-enhanced T1 (ceT1) scans to high-resolution T2 (hrT2) modality via a Segmentation-Enhanced Contrastive Unpaired Translation (SE-CUT) network [22]. Subsequently, three CycleGAN networks are employed for pixel-level intensity fine-tuning. We also perform intensity augmentation on the annotated regions of generated images. To generate pseudo labels for unlabeled real hrT2 scans, we apply a 3D full-resolution nnU-Net [8]. Finally, we build a multi-scale mean-teacher (MS-MT) network [12,28] for improving the cross-modality segmentation performance. The experimental results demonstrate the effectiveness of the proposed UDA method in reducing the domain gap between different modalities, achieving promising segmentation performance on ceT2 scans.

2 Methods

Given an unpaired dataset of two modalities, *i.e.*, annotated contrast-enhanced T1 (ceT1) MRI images $\mathcal{D}_s = \{(\mathbf{x}_i^s, y_i^s)\}_{i=1}^{N}$ and non-annotated high-resolution T2 (hrT2) MRI scans $\mathcal{D}_t = \{(\mathbf{x}_i^t)\}_{i=1}^{M}$, both sharing the same classes (intra- and extra-meatal VS, and Cochlea), we aim to exploit $\mathcal{D}_s$ and $\mathcal{D}_t$ for unsupervised domain adaptation, aiming to enhance the cross-modality segmentation performance of the VS and Cochlea on hrT2 MRI images. The overview of our UDA framework is illustrated in Fig. 1.

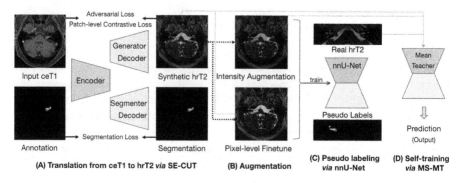

Fig. 1. The workflow of our proposed method. First, the SE-CUT network is proposed to translate ceT1 to hrT2. Then, the target areas are augmented with intensity, and multiple CycleGANs are used for pixel-level enhancement. After that, all synthetic and augmented scans are used for training a 3D nnU-Net, which can generate pseudo labels for all unlabeled real hrT2 images. Finally, an MS-MT network is employed for multi-scale self-ensemble learning.

2.1 Segmentation-Enhanced Translation

To mitigate the domain gap across modalities, we conduct image-level domain adaptation to generate synthetic target samples. This involves training a model on synthetic target images for VS and Cochlea segmentation in real high-resolution T2 (hrT2) scans. For effective image-to-image translation, we leverage the Contrastive Unpaired Translation (CUT) [22] method for time efficiency. To preserve structural information during translation (see Fig. 1(A)), we enhance the 2D CUT with an additional segmentation decoder. The ResNet-based generator (generation decoder) transforms source domain images to the target domain, while a PatchGAN discriminator distinguishes real from generated images [22]. Inspired by the SIFA architecture design [2], we connect two layers of the encoder with the segmenter decoder to produce multi-level segmentation predictions. This segmentation loss guides the encoder to focus on relevant areas, thereby preserving the structure details of Vestibular Schwannoma (VS) and Cochlea in the translated images.

2.2 Intensity Augmentation and Pseudo Labeling

Considering the heterogeneous signal intensity of tumors [20] and the hyperintense signal intensity of cochleas [13] in T2-weighted imaging, we perform intensity augmentation and generate augmented data for diversifying the training distributions. Using the generated hrT2 images and corresponding ground truth annotations, the signal intensities of annotated regions in each scan are randomly adjusted by a factor of 50% or 25% for mute and intensify respectively, effectively doubling the training data. Simultaneously, we employ multiple CycleGANs [42] on different sources of data for further fine-tuning at the pixel level of synthetic hrT2, improving the data utilization and training efficiency, which also augments

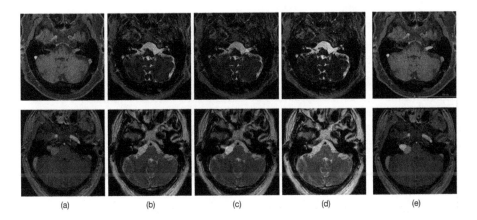

Fig. 2. Visual comparison for (a) Original ceT1, (b) Generated hrT2 using SE-CUT, (c) Generated hrT2 after intensity augmentation, (d) Generated hrT2 after pixel-level fine-tuning via CycleGAN, and (e) Ground truth of VS and cochlea.

the data by another copy. On the other hand, to enhance the segmentation performance on real hrT2 images, we utilize a Pseudo-Labeling (PL) strategy to leverage unlabeled hrT2 images by generating pseudo hrT2 annotations. We train a 3D full-resolution nnU-Net [8] using synthetic hrT2 images and augmented images. These trained models are then used to generate pseudo-labels for the unlabeled hrT2 images, further improving segmentation accuracy.

2.3 Multi-scale Self-ensembling Learning

To maximize the utilization of available data, we propose using the self-ensembling network, mean teacher (MT) [28], where a teacher model is constructed with the same architecture as the student model and updated using an exponential moving average (EMA) of the student's parameters during training. We ensure consistency between student and teacher outputs by minimizing their difference with the mean square error (MSE) loss. Additionally, we leverage the success of multi-scale learning in medical image analysis [12,35,39] and other fields [21,29], and introduce a multi-scale mean teacher (MS-MT) network following [12]. This approach utilizes multi-scale predictions for deep supervision and consistency regularization. Both the teacher and student networks utilize the 3D full-resolution nnU-Net [8] as the backbone, with auxiliary layers connected to each block of the last five blocks to obtain multi-scale predictions. This combination allows us to make the most use of available data, leading to enhanced cross-modality segmentation performance.

3 Experiments and Results

3.1 Dataset

The CrossMoDA 2023 challenge provides a highly heterogeneous dataset, sourced from multiple centers, comprising 227 annotated contrast-enhanced T1 (ceT1) scans and 391 unlabeled high-resolution T2 (hrT2) scans (295 scans are used for training and 96 scans are used as the validation set) [5,10,31]. The London (LDN) and Tilburg SC-GK (ETZ) data are obtained using different scanners and imaging sequences, encompassing both T1-weighted and high-resolution T2-weighted imaging. The UK MC-RC (UKM) data are obtained from various scanners with different magnetic field strengths and slice thickness, in which, voxel volume and intensities vary significantly across all ceT1 weighted and T2 weighted imaging. Besides, 341 unpublished hrT2 scans are used as the external test set during the testing phase.

3.2 Data Preprocessing

Due to variations in voxel spacing in the raw scans, all images were resampled into a common spacing of $0.6 \times 0.6 \times 1.0$ mm and the intensity was normalized to the range [0, 1] using Min-Max scaling. To delineate the regions of interest (ROI) and remove the noises, the images were cropped into 256×256 pixels in the xy-plane using a 75-percentile binary threshold [4], resulting in $256 \times 256 \times N$ image volumes for 3D nnU-Net training. These processed 3D volumes were also sliced along the z-axis to create N 2D images for SE-CUT and CycleGAN training. The Dice Score (DSC [%]) [27] and the Average Symmetric Surface Distance(ASSD [mm]) [17] are used to assess the model performance on VS and Cochlea segmentation.

3.3 Implementation Details

We used a single NVIDIA A40 GPU with 48GB of memory for model training. Figure 2 shows the effects of using SE-CUT to translate (a) original ceT1 into (b) synthetic hrT2 after training for 120 epochs. In the SE-CUT, We followed [22] and [2] to keep the same weights for adversarial loss, contrastive loss, and segmentation loss; the loss weights for additional segmentation were set to 1 and 0.1 for the last layer and the second last downsampling layer, respectively. The segmentation-enhanced architecture effectively retained structural information for Vestibular Schwannoma (VS) and cochlea in the original ceT1 scans, as demonstrated in Figs. 2(c) and (d). These images represent synthetic hrT2 results after intensity augmentation and pixel-level fine-tuning, respectively. To improve pixel intensity similarity to real hrT2 scans, three CycleGANs were individually trained for 50 epochs on scans from different sources (ETZ, LDN, and UKM). The resulting datasets were collectively used to train a 3D full-resolution nnU-Net with generalization ability for hrT2. After 400 epochs of training and 5-fold cross-validation, the nnU-Net generated pseudo labels for all unlabeled

Table 1. Performance of our model during validation and testing phases.

	Cochlea		VS		extra-VS		intra-VS	
	Dice	ASSD	Dice	ASSD	Dice	ASSD	Dice	ASSD
Validation Phase	0.729	19.836	0.568	32.409	0.620	40.384	0.457	40.364
Testing Phase	0.766	11.026	0.669	10.378	0.676	13.874	0.563	18.607

real hrT2 scans. Subsequently, a self-training process using synthetic hrT2 with real labels and real hrT2 with pseudo labels was conducted. The multi-scale mean teacher (MS-MT) network, with a backbone of two 3D nnU-Nets, was trained using stochastic gradient descent for 300 epochs. The initial learning rate was set to 0.01, and the objective function employed a combination of Dice and cross-entropy losses. The deep supervision scheme in nnU-Net [8] was enabled. In the MS-MT network, the exponential moving average (EMA) update α was set to 0.9, and the loss weights for consistency regularization were assigned as $\{0.05, 0.05, 0.05, 0.4, 0.5\}$ in ascending order of feature map size.

3.4 Experimental Results

Following the preprocessing step, the validation set was evaluated using the 5-fold ensemble MS-MT model, as depicted in Fig. 3 and summarized in Table 1. Notably, the Dice scores for Vestibular Schwannoma (VS) and cochlea in the validation phase leaderboard were 0.729 and 0.568, respectively. Finally, the largest connected component (LCC) was calculated, and the segmentation results were post-processed (*i.e.*, the first LCC was preserved for the connected intra and extra VS while the first and second LCCs were preserved for the cochlea) for the final submission during the testing phase. The segmentation performance of the final model on 341 cases of unpublished real high-resolution T2 (hrT2) scans during the testing phase is detailed in Table 1. In the region segmentation of Cochlea, extra-VS, and intra-VS, our method obtained dice scores of 0.766,

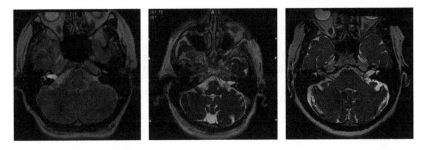

Fig. 3. Segmentation results of the validation set produced by our workflow. The intra-VS, extra-VS, and cochlea are indicated in red, green, and blue color, respectively. (Color figure online)

0.676, and 0.563 respectively, securing the fifth place. The superior performance during the testing phase further confirms the effectiveness of the proposed framework. Figure 3 provides some qualitative results produced by our method.

4 Conclusion

In this study, we propose a comprehensive four-stage cross-modality unsupervised domain adaptation workflow, designed to seamlessly bridge the gap between annotated ceT1 and unlabeled hrT2 MRI scans. Our approach comprises unpaired image translation, intensity augmentation, and pixel-level fine-tuning, followed by pseudo labeling and multi-scale self-training. By leveraging only annotated ceT1 scans, we successfully trained a final model capable of segmenting intra-meatal Vestibular Schwannoma (VS), extra-meatal VS, and cochlea in hrT2 scans. Our proposed method demonstrates its efficacy by achieving a top-5 finish in the testing phase of the CrossMoDA 2023 challenge, highlighting the model's ability to effectively bridge the gap between ceT1 and hrT2 MRI modalities and showcasing its potential in enhancing the segmentation of intra-meatal VS, extra-meatal VS, and cochlea.

References

1. Chen, C., Dou, Q., Chen, H., Qin, J., Heng, P.A.: Synergistic image and feature adaptation: towards cross-modality domain adaptation for medical image segmentation. In: Proceedings of the AAAI Conference on Artificial Intelligence, vol. 33, pp. 865–872 (2019)
2. Chen, C., Dou, Q., Chen, H., Qin, J., Heng, P.A.: Unsupervised bidirectional cross-modality adaptation via deeply synergistic image and feature alignment for medical image segmentation. IEEE Trans. Med. Imaging **39**(7), 2494–2505 (2020)
3. Chen, L., et al.: Data-driven detection of subtype-specific differentially expressed genes. Sci. Rep. **11**(1), 332 (2021)
4. Choi, J.W.: Using out-of-the-box frameworks for unpaired image translation and image segmentation for the crossmoda challenge. arXiv e-prints, pp. arXiv–2110 (2021)
5. Dorent, R., et al.: CrossMoDA 2021 challenge: benchmark of cross-modality domain adaptation techniques for vestibular schwnannoma and cochlea segmentation. arXiv preprint arXiv:2201.02831 (2022)
6. Hesamian, M.H., Jia, W., He, X., Kennedy, P.: Deep learning techniques for medical image segmentation: achievements and challenges. J. Digit. Imaging **32**(4), 582–596 (2019)
7. Huo, Y., Xu, Z., Bao, S., Assad, A., Abramson, R.G., Landman, B.A.: Adversarial synthesis learning enables segmentation without target modality ground truth. In: 2018 IEEE 15th International Symposium on Biomedical Imaging (ISBI 2018), pp. 1217–1220. IEEE (2018)
8. Isensee, F., Jaeger, P.F., Kohl, S.A., Petersen, J., Maier-Hein, K.H.: nnU-net: a self-configuring method for deep learning-based biomedical image segmentation. Nat. Methods **18**(2), 203–211 (2021)

9. Jiang, C., Hui, B., Liu, B., Yan, D.: Successfully applying lottery ticket hypothesis to diffusion model. arXiv preprint arXiv:2310.18823 (2023)
10. Kujawa, A., et al.: Deep learning for automatic segmentation of vestibular schwannoma: A retrospective study from multi-centre routine MRI. In: medRxiv (2022)
11. LeCun, Y., Bengio, Y., Hinton, G.: Deep learning. Nature **521**(7553), 436–444 (2015)
12. Li, S., Zhao, Z., Xu, K., Zeng, Z., Guan, C.: Hierarchical consistency regularized mean teacher for semi-supervised 3D left atrium segmentation. In: 2021 43rd Annual International Conference of the IEEE Engineering in Medicine & Biology Society (EMBC), pp. 3395–3398. IEEE (2021)
13. Lin, E., Crane, B.: The management and imaging of vestibular schwannomas. Am. J. Neuroradiol. **38**(11), 2034–2043 (2017)
14. Liu, H., Fan, Y., Cui, C., Su, D., McNeil, A., Dawant, B.M.: Unsupervised domain adaptation for vestibular schwannoma and cochlea segmentation via semi-supervised learning and label fusion. In: International MICCAI Brainlesion Workshop, pp. 529–539. Springer (2021)
15. Liu, H., Fan, Y., Oguz, I., Dawant, B.M.: Enhancing data diversity for self-training based unsupervised cross-modality vestibular schwannoma and cochlea segmentation. arXiv preprint arXiv:2209.11879 (2022)
16. Long, M., Cao, Y., Wang, J., Jordan, M.: Learning transferable features with deep adaptation networks. In: International Conference on Machine Learning, pp. 97–105. PMLR (2015)
17. Lu, F., Wu, F., Hu, P., Peng, Z., Kong, D.: Automatic 3D liver location and segmentation via convolutional neural network and graph cut. Int. J. Comput. Assist. Radiol. Surg. **12**(2), 171–182 (2017)
18. Lu, Y., Wang, H., Wei, W.: Machine learning for synthetic data generation: a review. arXiv preprint arXiv:2302.04062 (2023)
19. Murungi, N.K., Pham, M.V., Dai, X., Qu, X.: Trends in machine learning and electroencephalogram (EEG): a review for undergraduate researchers. arXiv preprint arXiv:2307.02819 (2023)
20. Nguyen, D., de Kanztow, L.: Vestibular schwannomas: a review. Appl. Radiol. **48**(3), 22–27 (2019)
21. Pahwa, R.S., et al.: 3D defect detection and metrology of HBMS using semi-supervised deep learning. In: 2023 IEEE 73rd Electronic Components and Technology Conference (ECTC), pp. 943–950. IEEE (2023)
22. Park, T., Efros, A.A., Zhang, R., Zhu, J.Y.: Contrastive learning for unpaired image-to-image translation. In: European Conference on Computer Vision, pp. 319–345. Springer (2020)
23. Qiu, Y., Zhao, Z., Yao, H., Chen, D., Wang, Z.: Modal-aware visual prompting for incomplete multi-modal brain tumor segmentation. In: Proceedings of the 31st ACM International Conference on Multimedia, pp. 3228–3239 (2023)
24. Qu, X., Liu, P., Li, Z., Hickey, T.: Multi-class time continuity voting for EEG classification. In: Brain Function Assessment in Learning: Second International Conference, BFAL 2020, Heraklion, Crete, Greece, 9–11 October 2020, pp. 24–33. Springer (2020)
25. Shapey, J., et al.: A standardised pathway for the surveillance of stable vestibular schwannoma. Ann. Roy. Coll. Surgeons England **100**(3), 216–220 (2018)
26. Shapey, J., et al.: An artificial intelligence framework for automatic segmentation and volumetry of vestibular schwannomas from contrast-enhanced T1-weighted and high-resolution T2-weighted MRI. J. Neurosurg. **134**(1), 171–179 (2019)

27. Sudre, C.H., Li, W., Vercauteren, T., Ourselin, S., Cardoso, M.J.: Generalised dice overlap as a deep learning loss function for highly unbalanced segmentations. In: Deep Learning in Medical Image Analysis and Multimodal Learning for Clinical Decision Support, pp. 240–248. Springer (2017)
28. Tarvainen, A., Valpola, H.: Mean teachers are better role models: weight-averaged consistency targets improve semi-supervised deep learning results. arXiv preprint arXiv:1703.01780 (2017)
29. Wang, J., Chang, R., Zhao, Z., Pahwa, R.S.: Robust detection, segmentation, and metrology of high bandwidth memory 3D scans using an improved semi-supervised deep learning approach. Sensors **23**(12), 5470 (2023)
30. Wang, L., Wang, M., Zhang, D., Fu, H.: Unsupervised domain adaptation via style-aware self-intermediate domain. arXiv preprint arXiv:2209.01870 (2022)
31. Wijethilake, N., et al.: Boundary distance loss for intra-/extra-meatal segmentation of vestibular schwannoma. In: MLCN@MICCAI (2022)
32. Wu, J., Ye, X., Mou, C., Dai, W.: FineEHR: refine clinical note representations to improve mortality prediction. In: 2023 11th International Symposium on Digital Forensics and Security (ISDFS), pp. 1–6. IEEE (2023)
33. Zeng, Z., et al.: Robust traffic prediction from spatial-temporal data based on conditional distribution learning. IEEE Trans. Cybern. **52**(12), 13458–13471 (2021)
34. Zhang, Z., Tian, R., Ding, Z.: TrEP: transformer-based evidential prediction for pedestrian intention with uncertainty. In: Proceedings of the AAAI Conference on Artificial Intelligence, vol. 37 (2023)
35. Zhao, Z., et al.: MMGL: multi-scale multi-view global-local contrastive learning for semi-supervised cardiac image segmentation. arXiv preprint arXiv:2207.01883 (2022)
36. Zhao, Z., et al.: SemiGNN-PPI: Self-ensembling multi-graph neural network for efficient and generalizable protein-protein interaction prediction. In: Elkind, E. (ed.) Proceedings of the Thirty-Second International Joint Conference on Artificial Intelligence, IJCAI-23, pp. 4984–4992. International Joint Conferences on Artificial Intelligence Organization (2023). https://doi.org/10.24963/ijcai.2023/554
37. Zhao, Z., Xu, K., Li, S., Zeng, Z., Guan, C.: MT-UDA: towards unsupervised cross-modality medical image segmentation with limited source labels. In: Medical Image Computing and Computer Assisted Intervention–MICCAI 2021: 24th International Conference, Strasbourg, France, 27 September–1 October 2021, Part I, pp. 293–303. Springer (2021)
38. Zhao, Z., Xu, K., Yeo, H.Z., Yang, X., Guan, C.: MS-MT: multi-scale mean teacher with contrastive unpaired translation for cross-modality vestibular schwannoma and cochlea segmentation. arXiv preprint arXiv:2303.15826 (2023)
39. Zhao, Z., Zeng, Z., Xu, K., Chen, C., Guan, C.: DSAL: deeply supervised active learning from strong and weak labelers for biomedical image segmentation. IEEE J. Biomed. Health Inform. **25**(10), 3744–3751 (2021)
40. Zhao, Z., Zhou, F., Xu, K., Zeng, Z., Guan, C., Zhou, S.K.: LE-UDA: label-efficient unsupervised domain adaptation for medical image segmentation. IEEE Trans. Med. Imaging **42**(3), 633–646 (2022)
41. Zhao, Z., Zhou, F., Zeng, Z., Guan, C., Zhou, S.K.: Meta-hallucinator: towards few-shot cross-modality cardiac image segmentation. In: International Conference on Medical Image Computing and Computer-Assisted Intervention, pp. 128–139. Springer (2022)
42. Zhu, J.Y., Park, T., Isola, P., Efros, A.A.: Unpaired image-to-image translation using cycle-consistent adversarial networks. In: Proceedings of the IEEE International Conference on Computer Vision, pp. 2223–2232 (2017)

Author Index

A

Abramova, Valeriia 255
Akbar, Agus Subhan 69
Aljuboory, Mariam 264
Alves, Victor 79
Amod, Alyssa R. 241
Anazodo, Udunna C. 200, 241
Anwar, Syed Muhammad 221
Arbel, Tal 300

B

Baid, Ujjwal 278
Baltruschat, Ivo M. 58
Barakat, Mohannad 200
Bouget, David 11
Brilian, Ahmad Hayam 69
Buchner, Josef A. 177

C

Capellán-Martín, Daniel 221
Cattin, Philippe C. 35
Chen, Cancan 355
Chen, Jianpin 140
Chen, Jieneng 190
Chen, Ke 233
Chen, Ziru 291
Cheng, Junlong 140
Cheng, Xi 291
Chopra, Agamdeep 165
Clèrigues, Albert 255
Combs, Stephanie E. 177
Confidence, Raymond 200

D

Dammann, Philipp 79
Dawant, Benoit M. 372
Deng, Zhongying 140
Durrer, Alicia 35

E

Egger, Jan 79
Ekenel, Hazım Kemal 94
Elsharkawi, Sarah 221
Erdur, Ayhan Can 177

F

Fan, Yubo 372
Fang, Zhirui 128
Farzana, W. 312, 322, 332
Fatichah, Chastine 69
Ferreira, André 79
Fortson, Lucy 152

G

Glandon, A. 312, 322
Gosai, Advait 211
Granados, Alejandro 3
Guan, Cuntai 386
Guirao, Marc 255
Guntuku, Sharath Chandra 278
Guo, Sizheng 140
Guo, Yanqing 128
Gupta, Aashray 278
Gupta, Aayush 278

H

Hamadache, Rachika E. 255
Han, Luyi 364
Hashmi, Anees Ur Rehman 264
He, Junjun 140
Hernández, José Armando 341
Honey, Ethan 165
Huang, Liqin 106
Huang, Ziyan 140
Huo, Jiayu 3

I

Iftekharuddin, K. M. 312, 322, 332

J

Jakhetiya, Vinit 278
Janbakhshi, Parvaneh 58
Javaji, Shashidhar Reddy 211
Jiang, Zhifan 221
Joubert, Pearly 241

K

Kleesiek, Jens 79
Kriz, Anita 300
Kurt, Mehmet 165

L

Lal-Trehan Estrada, Uma M. 255
Lam, Van 221
Ledesma-Carbayo, María J. 221
Lenga, Matthias 58
Li, Di 128
Li, Jianning 79
Li, Tianbin 140
Li, Xianhang 190
Li, Yi 128
Lin, Hui 291
Lin, Ruikai 386
Linguraru, Marius George 221
Liu, Han 372
Liu, Xinyang 221
Liu, Yang 3
Lladó, Xavier 255

M

Maani, Fadillah 264
Magdy, Noha 200
Mann, Ritse 364
Mantha, Kameswara Bharadwaj 152
Mathis-Ullrich, Franziska 24
Mehta, Raghav 300
Mei, Jieru 190
Mistry, Sahaj K. 278
Mohapatra, Sovesh 211
Motchon, Dodzi 241
Mutsvangwa, Tinashe E. M. 241

N

Nichyporuk, Brennan 300
Nisar, Hareem 221

O

Öksüz, İlkay 94
Oguz, Ipek 372
Oliver, Arnau 255
Ourselin, Sébastien 3

P

Parida, Abhijeet 221
Pedersen, André 11
Peeken, Jan C. 177
Phiri, Ethel 200

Q

Quetin, Sébastien 241

R

Rahman, M. M. 312, 322, 332
Rai, Sunny 278
Raymond, Confidence 241
Rebala, Harshitha 165
Reinertsen, Ingerid 11
Ren, Tianyi 165
Rueckert, Daniel 177

S

Sadique, M. S. 312, 322, 332
Saeed, Numan 264
Saini, Sourav 278
Salvi, Joaquim 255
Sankar, Ramanakumar 152
Schlaug, Gottfried 211
Scholz, Daniel 177
Sharma, Abhishek 165
Shen, Yiqing 140
Smith, Alexandra 241
Sobirov, Ikboljon 264
Solak, Naida 79
Solheim, Ole 11
Sparks, Rachel 3
Su, Yanzhou 140
Suciati, Nanik 69

T

Tan, Tao 364
Tapp, Austin 221
Temtam, A. 312, 322, 332
Tovar Sáez, Francisco Aarón 255

Author Index

W
Wang, Dawei 355
Wang, Guotai 46
Wang, Haoyu 140
Weng, Ying 233
William, Jjuuko George 200
Wolleb, Julia 35

X
Xie, Cihang 190
Xie, Xin 128
Xu, Kaixin 386
Xu, Zhoubing 372

Y
Yalçın, Cansu 255
Yang, Siwei 190
Yang, Xiao 117
Yang, Xulei 386
Yaqub, Mohammad 264
Yazıcı, Ziya Ata 94
Ye, Jin 140

Z
Zeineldin, Ramy A. 24
Zhang, Dong 200, 241
Zhang, Juexin 233
Zhang, Rongguo 355
Zhao, Ziyuan 386
Zheng, Jiahao 106
Zheng, Shaohua 117
Zhong, Lanfeng 46
Zhou, Yubo 46
Zhou, Yuyin 190

www.ingramcontent.com/pod-product-compliance
Lightning Source LLC
Chambersburg PA
CBHW072016120125
20267CB00006B/82